Your Guide To
COPING WITH
BACK PAIN

Judylaine Fine

McClelland and Stewart

McClelland and Stewart Limited
The Canadian Publishers
25 Hollinger Road
Toronto, Ontario
M4B 3G2

Canadian Cataloguing in Publication Data

Fine, Judylaine.
    Your guide to coping with back pain

Includes index.
ISBN 0-7710-3139-4

1. Backache – Treatment. 2. Backache.   I. Title.

RD768.F56 1985   617'.56   C85-098883-7

The information in this book is not intended to replace the services of a
physician. While most back pain is of a chronic nature, any pain can be the
result of a disease that should be diagnosed and treated only by a physician. I
strongly recommend that you consult a doctor about your back pain, if only to
rule out the possibility of disease as opposed to chronic degenerative
processes. Any application of the treatments set forth in this book is at the
reader's discretion and sole risk.

For more information about the Back Association of Canada and its quarterly
journal, *BACK TO BACK*, contact the Back Association of Canada,
111 Avenue Road, Concourse Level, Toronto, Ontario, M5R 3J8, telephone
(416) 967-4670.

Printed and bound in Canada

Contents

Introduction: There Is a Light at the End of the Tunnel / 9

PART I — THE BASICS OF BACK PAIN

Chapter 1. Anatomy of a Back / 17
Chapter 2. What Goes Wrong with Human Backs? / 31

PART II — GEARING UP TO COPE WITH BACK PAIN

Chapter 3. Pain: To Say It Is Complex Is Too Simple / 59
Chapter 4. Some Practical Advice for Dealing with Health Care
               Professionals / 73
Chapter 5. Drug Addiction: Facing the Possibility / 79

PART III — THE MEDICAL MODEL

Chapter 6. The M.D.'s Diagnosis: If You Know a Few Things, You
               Can Learn a Great Deal / 89
Chapter 7. The CT Scanner: Revolutionary Radiology / 99
Chapter 8. Myelograms and Discograms / 104
Chapter 9. Surgery: Only the Chosen Few Need Apply / 111
Chapter 10. Discotomy by Microsurgery: A Morsel to Ponder / 119
Chapter 11. Chymopapain: Myth or Miracle? / 124
Chapter 12. Orthopaedic Physicians: Manipulative Medicine / 131
Chapter 13. Acupuncture: Pinning It Down / 138
Chapter 14. Physiotherapy: Treatment to End All Treatment / 145
Chapter 15. Psychiatry: If Your Back Hurts, Try Using
               Your Head / 152

Chapter 16. Traditional Exercises: Margaret Duffy's Twenty-Minute Workout for the Back / 157
Chapter 17. Posture: The Best for Your Back / 175

PART IV – THE HOLISTIC ALTERNATIVES

Chapter 18. Chiropractic: All That It's Cracked Up To Be? / 191
Chapter 19. Hypnosis: The Power of Suggestion / 205
Chapter 20. Massage: There's the Rub! / 212
Chapter 21. The Alexander Technique: Heads Up! / 217
Chapter 22. Yoga: Tying It All Together / 224
Chapter 23. Feldenkrais Method: The Israeli Connection / 230

PART V – ADVICE FOR SPECIAL SITUATIONS

Chapter 24. Sports: Good or Bad for Your Back? / 241
Chapter 25. Scoliosis: Don't Let It Throw Your Kid a Curve / 259
Chapter 26. The Cervical Spine: That Pain in the Neck / 264
Chapter 27. Osteoporosis: Prevention Is the Key / 271
Chapter 28. Pregnancy: Is Back Pain Inevitable? / 281

Acknowledgements / 289
Bibliography / 293
Index / 300

For Jo

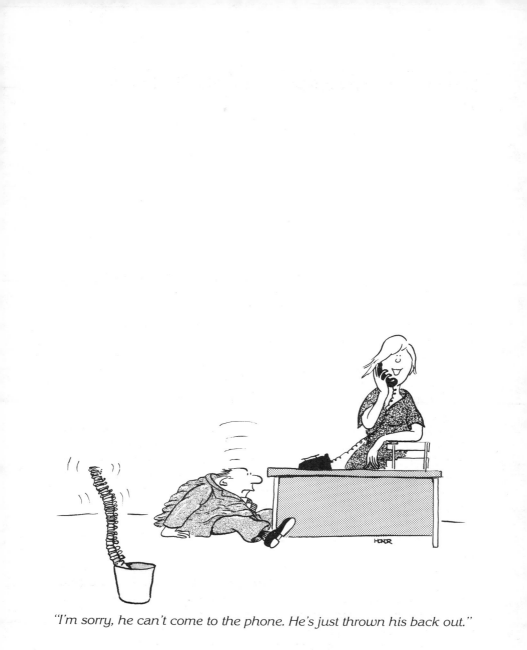

"I'm sorry, he can't come to the phone. He's just thrown his back out."

Introduction: There Is a Light at the End of the Tunnel

The trouble I have with most of the existing books on back pain is that they are written by people with one point of view, in most cases that of a medical doctor. There is nothing inherently wrong with subscribing to one point of view, if that's what you believe. But after talking to more than 3,000 people who suffer from back pain and several hundred of the professionals who treat them, it has become clear to me that nearly all of the methods used to treat this epidemic-sized ailment do work – at least for some of the people, some of the time. The $64,000 question that has never been asked, let alone answered, is which treatment works for whom and when?

Few studies comparing the various treatments have been initiated. "Observations" have been made by various physicians around the world. Swedish orthopaedic surgeon Dr. Alf Nachemson (who is famous for his research on disc stress caused by various body positions) has reported that he has not noticed any significant difference in the length of time it takes patients to return to their former pain-free state whether the treatment has been physiotherapy, manipulation or – amazingly enough in some cases – nothing at all. Unfortunately, only these three treatments were observed.

A few comparison studies have been done. One which compared microsurgery for disc removal to the standard discotomy procedure (see page 123) indicated that with microsurgery, the less radical method, there were fewer adverse side effects and a shorter recovery time for patients than with the standard procedure.

However, no independent, non-partisan group has come up with either the resources (which would be formidable) or a method to evaluate all the different treatments for back pain, one against the other.

In truth, the task may be impossible. Even if the financial resources could be found, the stickler would be diagnosis since diagnosing back pain is fraught with difficulties; the issue conjures up an image of a huge n with the myriad of diagnosticians making educated guesses, most patients.

.ct is that no foolproof method exists to divide the majority of
 ain sufferers into like groups so that the members of each group
 . be subjected to the different treatments and the success of each treatment measured and evaluated.

One of the most frequently used tools for diagnosing back pain is the conventional X-ray. Dr. Carl Sutton, director of orthopaedic surgery at St. Mary's Hospital in Montreal, explains the problems associated with this method: "If you were to put 300 randomly chosen spinal X-rays up on a screen, you'd find that in about half of them, there would be definite signs of degenerative changes – general wear and tear, narrowing of disc spaces, arthritic changes. You'd also likely find that 150 of those 300 patients had back pain to varying degrees. But the crazy thing is that there would likely be very little, if any, relationship between those who are in pain and those who have signs of degenerative changes.... I've seen X-rays of backs that look as if they should belong to veritable cripples, and yet the person has no pain at all. By the same token, I've seen patients whose X-rays look perfectly normal but who suffer from severe back pain."

Making a clinical diagnosis is frequently just as difficult. What a diagnostician looks for depends, for one thing, on his or her training bias. An orthopaedic surgeon, for example, will tend to look for gross abnormalities which are correctable by surgery; performing surgery is the orthopaedic surgeon's job. A physiotherapist, on the other hand, is more apt to gravitate toward soft tissue problems, ligaments and muscles. Many of the holistic-type practitioners, having no access to testing facilities (and no training in their interpretation in any case) gravitate toward conditions with general names – such as *structural imbalances* – when prodded by patients to tell them exactly what is wrong. I, myself, have had at least a dozen different diagnoses, and if the 3,000 other back pain sufferers I have spoken to are any indication, I am certainly not alone.

The statistics on back pain are astounding. Although Canada does not collect statistics on back pain on a nation-wide basis, the American numbers, divided by ten to account for the difference in population, are considered to be more or less accurate:

• Seventy-five million Americans (approximately 7.5 million Canadians) currently suffer from back pain.

• Some 16 million Americans (1.5 million Canadians) visit their doctors each year because of back pain. This figure doesn't include the number of visits to chiropractors, massage therapists, physiotherapists, etc.

• The number of workdays lost per year due to back pain in the United States has been estimated at 93 million (almost 9.5 million in Canada). Backaches are second only to respiratory infections as the cause of absenteeism from work.

10

• On any single day, the number of Americans in bed due to back pain has been estimated at 6 million (600,000 Canadians).

• The annual bill for back pain (not including lost productivity, lowered morale, costs for retraining, lost skills and absenteeism) has been set at $14 billion by the U.S. federal government (almost $1.5 billion in Canada), but to many professionals this figure seems low.

After five years as executive vice-president of the Back Association of Canada and editor of BAC's journal *BACK TO BACK*, I have made several observations of my own. One of them is that it is unlikely that the proponents of the different methods of treatment for back pain will ever be interested in sorting through the maze, assuming a reliable diagnostic method could be found.

Closer to the truth of the matter, I'm afraid, is that back pain is no Camptown Racetrack. It is big business and many of the people who own a big share of the pie have no intentions of losing it. Those who have traditionally wielded little power have been finding lately that their scant territory is expanding as the incidence of back pain increases. Alternative methods of treatment for back pain have also been getting better press as more consumers take health matters into their own hands; it is also unlikely that the members of these alternative professions would be interested in initiating studies to compare treatments.

But in researching and writing this book, a light has emerged. I remember the first flicker when it dawned on me that I was hearing the same sorts of things from professionals of different disciplines who considered themselves to be worlds apart.

At the time, I had been interviewing people about posture and its contribution to back pain.

Physiotherapist Margaret Duffy was the first person I saw. She talked about the fact that so many people's knowledge of biomechanics – how, for example, to stand without strain – was lacking. Massage therapist Kristi Magraw saw an additional component: slouching – which *is* poor biomechanics – is frequently connected to one's self-image and the need to hide feelings such as anger or sadness. In her view, you can't correct one without the other. Alexander Technique teacher Robert Rickover used the word *disorganized* to describe poor posture, pointing out that slouching actually requires an enormous amount of unnecessary muscle strain. Yoga teacher Esther Myers talked about poor posture in terms of lost "unity," the fact that in our modern sedentary society, people have become almost totally unaware of how they use their bodies. Moshe Feldenkrais, the Israeli who developed the Feldenkrais Method of Movement, talked about biomechanics in the efficient terms of the physicist which, among other things, he was. (Feldenkrais died in the fall of 1984.) Psychologist Dr. Rickey Miller, who frequently uses hypnotherapy, talked about "pain behaviour" – hunching up the shoulders, for example – and its relationship to back pain. Psychiatrist Dr. Stanley Greben talked about the effects back pain caused by poor posture can have on a person's confidence and self-esteem, sounding a lot like Kristi Magraw if you ask me. Chiropractor Dr. Adrian Grice, whom I had interviewed for *BACK TO BACK*, talked about posture in terms of "realigning" the spine. The same day, general prac-titioner Dr. Ahmed Sakoor said that a lot of people's backs would probably hurt less if they would learn to sit up straight!

The language, as you can see, is different but the essence is much the same.

Similarities became evident in other areas. The theme of body aware-ness and mind awareness and their relationship to each other and to back pain came up time and time again. Some of the advocates of the western-type disciplines spoke of "endorphins" – powerful pain-killers that can be produced by the brain. Some of the proponents of the more eastern-type philosophies talked about restoring "natural energy flows." The means to the end were different; the end in each case was the same.

A question began to interest me: Could it be that most of the methods that are used to treat back pain work for some of the people some of the time *because of their similarities* rather than their differences? With some exceptions – obviously surgery and other invasive procedures as well as manipulation in certain circumstances – I think that the answer is yes. As important as the choice of therapy is the therapist (the gunner not the gun!). As important as the choice of therapist is whether you, the patient, feel *comfortable* with a particular technique.

Comfort is an interesting word in this context. In many instances, it boils down to personality. I have a penchant for working on my own at my own pace, so swimming is more appealing to me than an exercise class whose pace is controlled by someone else. I have a spiritual leaning toward things western and scientific, so the explanations of physiotherapy, hypnosis and Feldenkrais "touch me" in a way that the more transcen-dental philosophies of the Alexander Technique and yoga do not. It's more a matter of predilection than the quality of the therapy and yours, on the other hand, may be totally opposite from mine.

Nevertheless, I firmly believe that when it comes to choosing a treatment for your back pain, there is one universal wisdom and that is *caveat emptor*/"let the buyer beware." For better or worse – and probably for better since you've lived with it longer than any therapist – it is up to you to figure out your own answer for your own back.

I can, however, offer you some ground rules and some practical advice to ensure that this task is not only within your grasp but also enjoyable:

• Don't allow yourself to be intimidated by professionals. While the best of just about any discipline can give you invaluable advice and the worst can send you packing with a backache that is worse than when you came, you should regard everyone who treats back pain as a consultant whose opinion you may, or may not, decide to accept. Chapter 4, "Some Practical Advice for Dealing with Health Care Professionals," will provide you with some specific ideas on how to accomplish this feat.

• If you are interested in pursuing a conservative, or non-invasive, therapy for your back pain, first consult a physician who can *eliminate* from the list of possible ills the rare, but potentially fatal, ailments that can cause back pain, such as a tumour or kidney disease. If a physician feels that you may be suffering from a severe localized problem that can be corrected by surgery (for example, a herniated disc), you will likely be sent to an orthopaedic surgeon or neurosurgeon for a consultation. From that examination, you should expect to find out if you are a good candidate for surgery (less than one chance in ten!) or if you are not.

• Once you have determined that you are one of the approximately 75 million North Americans who is suffering from nothing more than ordinary, albeit excruciating, backache, it is time to make some decisions for yourself with the help of a professional.

First of all, you should not be embarking on any new exercise or body awareness program while you are in an acute phase of back pain. Pain is a warning sign that should not be ignored. Bed rest is recommended until the acute phase subsides. Second of all, nobody can guarantee that any treatment will work for you. If one of the conservative methods for controlling back pain *sounds* like it will fit your physical and mental/emotional needs, you will have to try it to find out if it is really the right discipline for you.

There are, however, a couple of ways to explore a treatment. One is as a supplicant who jumps nervously at the practitioner's every phrase. The other is from a position of knowledge as an informed customer. I suggest the latter very strongly.

Bone up on the principles of a discipline before you try it. Ask the professional you choose some pointed questions about why he or she thinks it may work for you. Some therapists tend to sweep aside philosophical questions posed by patients saying that the "whys" and "hows" are less important than results. I disagree; if you are interested, then it's important. I don't see how a therapist can inspire confidence in a patient if he or she doesn't respect the philosophy of "informed consent," used in the broadest sense of the phrase.

With the therapist set some goals:

• It is often unrealistic to expect to be totally pain-free. Most back pain can be controlled but not cured.

• Ask your therapist how many weeks, or months, should pass before you will re-evaluate the treatment together. When that time comes, don't let the blame be placed on you if the treatment is not working – unless you are clearly not following the advice.

• If the treatment is not working, you must decide together if it can be modified to suit *your* needs or if it is simply not the answer for you. (Don't buy a suggestion – either direct or implied – that you are "the only person who has ever expressed dissatisfaction.")

• Be patient. Most episodes of back pain subside within two or three months, but an episode that goes on for six or even eight months is not uncommon.

• There does come a time, after conservative therapy shows no results, to again explore the possibility that a more radical type of treatment – surgery or a chymopapain injection, for example – may be indicated after all. At that point, you will probably have to undergo some additional diagnostic tests. These, like the various treatments, are more likely to provide you and your physician with the information you both need if you approach them calmly and knowledgeably—that is, if you know what to expect. This is the objective of the chapters on diagnostic techniques.

This book will help you gain the confidence to do all of these things. Chapter 1, "Anatomy of a Back," explains in plain English how a back ought to work. The next chapter, "What Goes Wrong with Human Backs?", explains most of the reasons why backs so often don't function as they ought to. Chapter 6, "The M.D.'s Diagnosis," will help you decide just where you fit in. I suggest that you read them thoroughly. Afterward, choose the chapters that interest you. They are organized in such a way that you can read them in any order you like. Whether it's acupuncture or yoga, physiotherapy, the Alexander Technique – whatever – somewhere in these pages is an answer that has worked for thousands of back pain sufferers and will work for you.

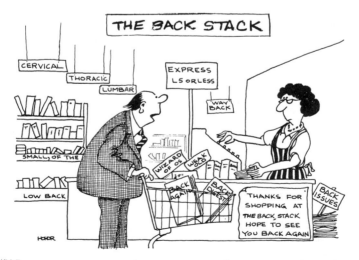

"When are you expecting your next shipment on facets?"

I
The Basics of Back Pain

1

Anatomy of a Back

When it is functioning the way it was intended to work, the back is an engineering feat. The spinal column itself is so flexible that it can be bent to form two-thirds of a circle. At the same time, it is able to support a 12- to 16-pound head at the top and an approximately 90- to 120-pound torso. It has a lifting capacity of up to 300 pounds per square inch. As if that were not enough, the spine is also able to manage the body's communication system – the spinal cord and its huge complex of nerves which branch out on either side, running to and from every organ and bit of tissue that make up the body.

From the side, the normal spine has three gentle curves. The two that curve forward – one at the top, the other near the base – are each called a lordosis. The third curve – a kyphosis – arches the opposite way.

All of these curves develop shortly after birth. When they are in balance, they help absorb shock – both when the body is erect, but stationary, and when it is in motion. When they are either excessive or inadequate, however, the muscles and ligaments of the back and abdomen must work harder to keep the body erect and in balance.

Altogether, the spine consists of 24 mobile vertebrae (which are separated from one another by a disc) plus the sacrum and the coccyx. The sacrum is attached by strong ligaments, several on either side, to the two large bones of the pelvis, called the ilia. Hence the name *sacroiliac* for each of these two joints.

The top seven vertebrae, which form the first of the two lordotic curves, are called the cervical vertebrae. The next 12, which form the kyphosis, are called the thoracic vertebrae and each is attached to one of the 12 ribs. The lowest five vertebrae, which form the lower of the two lordotic curves, are called the lumbar vertebrae.

The cervical vertebrae are labelled C1 to C7, starting at the top. The 12 thoracic vertebrae are labelled T1 to T12. The five lumbar vertebrae are labelled L1 to L5.

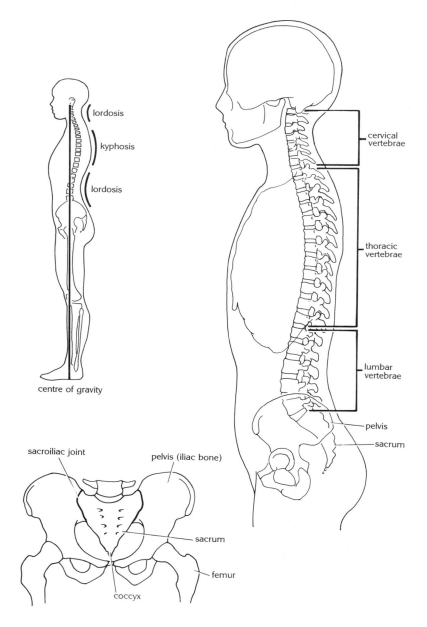

Diagram 1   The Spine

Below these 24 vertebrae lies the sacrum. At birth it is made up of five separate vertebrae, but during the first few years of life, they fuse together into one arrowhead-shaped bone. Even when they are fused, however, it is easy to see where each section of the sacrum begins and ends, so these are labelled S1 to S5.

Below the sacrum is the coccyx (pronounced cock-six) which, in humans, is all that's left of the bone that was once a tail. It consists of four, or on occasion three, small vertebrae, which usually fuse together by the age of 20.

Some health care professionals describe the spine as having 33 or 34 vertebrae; they add the five bones of the sacrum and the three, or four, bones of the coccyx to the 24 mobile vertebrae of the cervical, thoracic and lumbar regions to reach that total. Others prefer to total the number of vertebrae at 26, counting the mobile vertebrae as 24 and adding two more – one for the sacrum and one for the coccyx.

The Mobile Vertebrae

Although they differ in size (and the top two, called the atlas and axis, are somewhat unique in shape), the 24 mobile vertebrae are fairly similar in

POSTERIOR   ANTERIOR

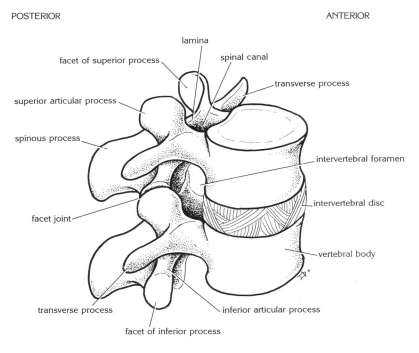

Diagram 2   Normal Vertebrae, Lateral Oblique View

design. A close look at one will give you a pretty good idea of what all the mobile segments look like and how they function.

Each vertebra is made up of two parts. The anterior section is the part which is closest to the front of the body; the posterior section is the part closest to the back. The only part of the spine you can actually feel when you run your fingertips up and down your back is the very tip of the posterior section.

The anterior section of each vertebra is shaped like a drum. The bottom of one drum is solidly attached to the top of a disc; and the top of the drum below is attached to the bottom of the same disc. You could say that the two vertebrae are like the two slices of bread in a sandwich separated by a disc filling (see Diagrams 2 and 3).

The function of the drumlike section of each vertebra is to bear weight and, in fact, the largest ones of the lumbar spine can support up to several hundred pounds per square inch.

The vertebra's posterior section is more complex. It is made up of the spinal canal, the back section of which is called the lamina.

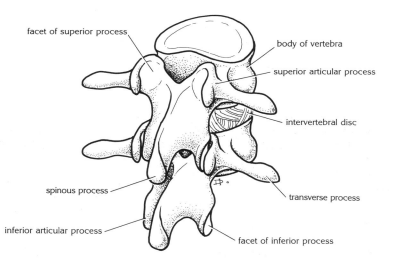

facet of superior process

body of vertebra

superior articular process

intervertebral disc

spinous process

transverse process

inferior articular process

facet of inferior process

Diagram 3   Normal Vertebrae, Posterior Oblique View

Facet Joints and Processes

From the lamina emerge seven projections. Four of these projections are called articular processes. The two at the top are called superior articular processes. The two at the bottom are called inferior articular processes. At the end of each process is a facet.

20

The two superior articular processes of one vertebra join with the two inferior articular processes of the vertebra above. The resulting structure, or joint, is called a facet joint, or occasionally, an apophyseal joint. Each facet is capped with smooth cartilage to help it move frictionlessly against its partner and each facet joint is encased in a strong, fibrous capsule that prevents the two facets from separating. This capsule, however, is roomy enough to allow movement of the facets inside of it.

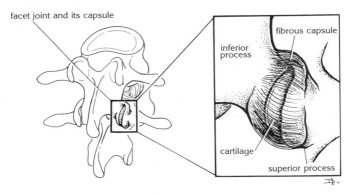

Diagram 4   A Facet Joint with Its Capsule

The three other projections are also called processes. The two that stick out sideways, like wings, are called the transverse processes. The other one, called the spinous process, points back, with a downward slant. This is the bit of spine you are feeling when you run your fingers down your back.

The Discs

Between the 24 mobile vertebrae are the 23 discs. The discs of the lumbar spine are slightly thicker than the ones at the top, but added together they measure approximately six inches. Each disc separates the vertebrae above and below, creating a space called the intervertebral foramen, which you can see clearly in Diagrams 2 and 3. Discs also act as shock absorbers. They are labelled according to the two vertebrae between which they are located. For example, the disc between the first and second lumbar vertebrae is called L1-L2. (Sometimes this is shortened to L1-2.) The disc between the lowest lumbar vertebra and the first one of the sacrum is called L5-S1.

Like the vertebrae, each disc is made up of two sections. The outer section, called the annulus fibrosus, is composed of tough, criss-crossed, fibrous layers, much like the layers of a radial belted tire. Gradually, moving toward the centre of the disc, these layers become less fibrous. Finally, they turn into the nucleus pulposus, a compartment filled with a pulpy mass which looks like jelly in an infant and crabmeat in an adult. Because this mass is mostly water, it is highly elastic; it can change its shape and then return to its original form.

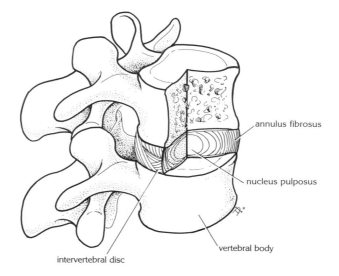

annulus fibrosus

nucleus pulposus

vertebral body

intervertebral disc

Diagram 5   The Intervertebral Disc

At birth, this nucleus is 90 per cent water. Gradually, with age, the percentage of water decreases, although not by much; at age 70, a nucleus' water content is still approximately 70 per cent.

The 23 discs also lose and absorb water on a daily basis, much like a sponge soaking up water and then being wrung out. During the day, while gravity is exerting its force on the body, water leaves the discs' centres and they lose a bit of height. At night, without the pressure of gravity, water – along with nutrients – soaks into the discs from the blood. The average person is approximately two inches taller in the morning than at night. After 84 days in space at zero gravity, Skylab Mission astronaut William Pogue had "grown" almost four inches. By the time he came down to earth, however, he had returned to his normal size.

The Ligaments of the Spine

Ligaments are tough bands of connective tissue that bind bone to bone. They support the spine and also help prevent us from making excessive movements that may be damaging, such as moving a facet joint beyond its normal range. The ligamentum flavum (sometimes called the yellow ligament), the interspinous ligament and the supraspinous ligament provide support for the facet joints. The longitudinal ligaments provide support for the discs and the vertebral bodies.

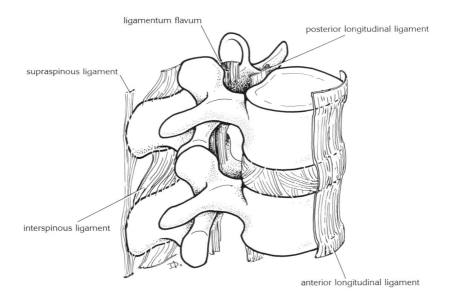

Diagram 6   The Ligaments of the Spine

The anterior longitudinal ligament runs the length of the spinal column. It is attached to the front section of the vertebral bodies and discs. The posterior longitudinal ligament also runs the length of the spinal column but is attached to the back of the vertebral bodies and discs. No one will disagree with the fact that both these ligaments are essential for spinal stability; however, just how much of a role they play in the matter of back pain – and what that role is – depends upon whom you ask. This controversy is explained in further detail in Chapter 2.

The Muscles of the Spine

The muscles of the spine come in different sizes. The shorter muscles, whose main function is to expand and contract enabling us to make delicate movements, also support the spine. As the ones attached to the processes expand and contract, the processes are pulled and released like levers, and the body can bend and twist within the limitations set by the ligaments.

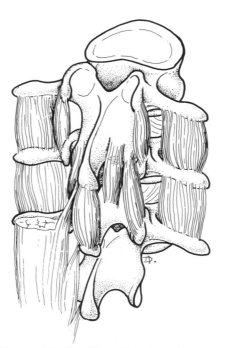

Diagram 7   The Short Muscles of the Back

When the short muscles attached to the facet joints expand and contract, the facet joints are also pulled and released like levers. But in this case, the plane of each facet joint determines its ability to move in certain directions – forward, backward and sideways. Those at the top of the spine, for example, are more horizontally oriented than those of the lumbar region. Because of this orientation, they are better suited for rotational movements than are the facet joints of the vertebrae lower down.

Over the short muscles are many layers of longer back muscles. Some are medium-length muscles which stretch from one vertebra to another several inches away. Covering these medium-length muscles is the group of muscles that runs the entire length of the spine – the erector spinae. When it is contracted, the erector spinae arches the spine backward. When only one side of it is tightened, the spine bends sideways. The erector spinae also braces the spine from the rear and prevents it from falling forward – much like the guy wires that keep a flagpole from toppling forward.

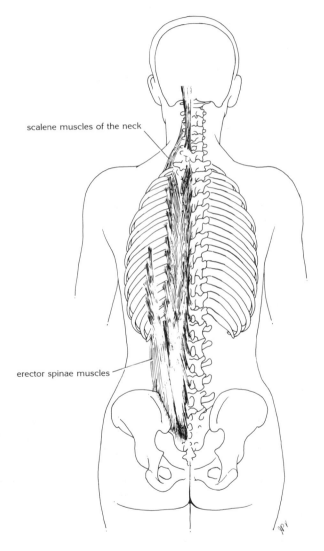

scalene muscles of the neck

erector spinae muscles

Diagram 8   The Erector Spinae Muscles

25

The Muscles of the Abdomen

If you look at Diagram 9, you'll notice that there are very few muscles attached to the front of the vertebrae to help the spine bend forward. The psoas muscle is one exception, but its main function is to move the legs rather than the spine. That leaves the job of bending forward to the muscles of the abdominal wall, of which there are several layers running in different directions. The innermost layers (called the obliquus internis and the obliquus externis) are not visible in Diagram 9. They run diagonally from the hip bones to the ribs. The middle layer (called the transversus ab-

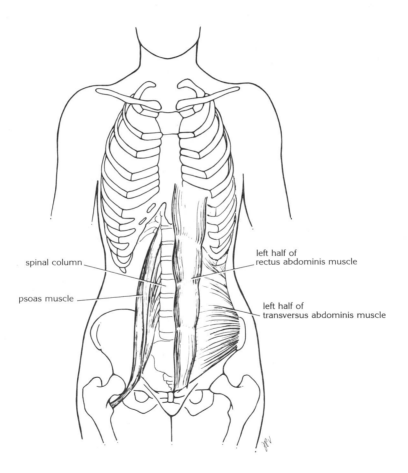

spinal column

psoas muscle

left half of
rectus abdominis muscle

left half of
transversus abdominis muscle

Diagram 9   The Abdominal Muscles

dominis) crosses the innermost layer. The outermost layer (called the rectus abdominis) runs vertically. When they are all contracted, the spine bends forward.

But the abdominal muscles have other jobs as well. For example, when those on one side of the spine are contracted, the spine is pulled sideways. More importantly, however, they provide the other side of the "guy wire" system, keeping the spine from toppling backward. When the erector spinae and the abdominal muscles are more or less equal in strength, they work in tandem and maintaining an erect posture is a relatively easy job for the body to perform. When the abdominal muscles are considerably weaker than the muscles of the back, the spine is more vulnerable to both wear and tear and injury.

The Spinal Cord and the Nerves

The most complex part of the back is the spinal cord and its many branches, called nerves. The cord itself runs from the base of the brain down through the spinal canal, the tubelike structure attached to the "drum" of each vertebra. Several layers of fibrous tissue cover and protect

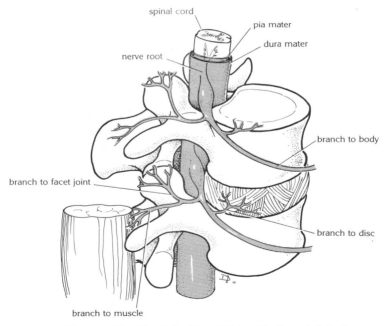

Diagram 10   The Spinal Cord, Nerve Roots and Spinal Nerve Branches

the spinal cord. The innermost layer is called the pia mater and the outermost layer is the thick, fibrous dura mater.

Before birth, while the embryo is at an early stage of development, the spinal cord extends from the brain all the way to the sacrum. The vertebrae, however, grow faster than the spinal cord and by birth, the cord only reaches from the brain to the level of the third lumbar vertebra. This uneven growth continues during the developing years and by age 12, the end of the cord is at the first lumbar vertebra. The point at which the cord ends is called the conus medullaris.

The spinal cord has many small branches which deliver messages to and from the organs and tissues of the body. These small branches develop from 62 main branches – 31 on each side of the cord – called nerve roots. Each nerve root emerges from the spinal column through an intervertebral foramen, the space that exists between two vertebrae due to the thickness of the disc. Just past the point where it emerges, each nerve root splits into smaller branches. One of these nerve branches delivers messages to and from the nearest facet joint. Another delivers messages to the disc nearby. And another services the closest muscle. But another, much longer branch, winds away from the spine where it branches, rebranches, and combines with other nerves. Some of these nerves supply power to the body's muscles. Others supply sensation to the skin, both normal and painful. Still others supply information to the organs. This network, like the telephone system of a large city, is bewildering in its complexity.

The branches of the cervical nerve roots send and receive messages to and from the upper regions of the body, and the branches of the lumbar nerve roots send and receive messages to and from the lower regions of the body. For example, branches of the nerve roots that exit from between the third and fourth cervical vertebrae (as well as the ones that emerge from between C4-C5, C5-C6, C6-C7 and C7-T1) wind all the way to the arms passing, en route, between the muscles that move the shoulders.

The pair of nerve roots that emerge from between the fourth and fifth vertebrae of the lumbar region (called the L4 nerve roots) and the four nerve roots below it (the L5, S1, S2 and S3 nerve roots) merge at hip level, beneath the gluteus maximus muscle. The combination of these five nerves forms the thickest nerve of the body – the sciatic nerve. The sciatic nerve runs down the back of the thigh and divides into two just above the knee. One of these branches runs down the front of the shin into the big toe; the other branch divides again, running down the back of the leg to the heel and winding again toward the front of the leg to the smaller toes. And these are only the *main* branches of the sciatic nerve! Each has so many tiny offshoots that they would be impossible to show in a drawing.

If you look at Diagram 11, you'll see an interesting difference between the nerve roots that exit above the first lumbar vertebra and those that exit below it. Because the spinal cord ends at L1, the nerves that eventually exit from between the lower lumbar and sacral vertebrae must run down the length of the spinal canal for longer and longer distances as they make their way to the lower lumbar and sacral regions. The strands of

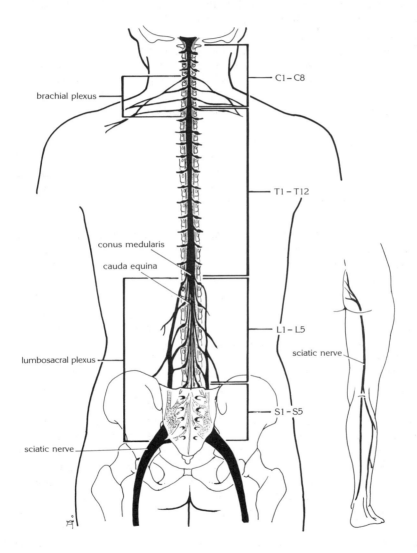

brachial plexus

conus medularis

cauda equina

lumbosacral plexus

sciatic nerve

C1 – C8

T1 – T12

L1 – L5

sciatic nerve

S1 – S5

Diagram 11   The Nerve Roots

nerves that run through the spinal canal look like the strands of hair in a horse's tail; they are appropriately called the cauda equina, which means "horse's tail" in Latin.

Many of the nerve endings are sensitive to pain, but some are not. It is only recently that researchers have begun to study the various tissues of the body in general and the spinal column in particular to see which contain "pain receptors" and which do not. For example, there are pain receptors in the nerve endings that branch to the facet joints, the dura mater, the blood vessels which supply the muscles of the back, and the ligaments of the spine. There are, however, no pain receptors in the nerves that supply the nuclei of the discs and none in the annuli, except at the spot where each annulus is attached to the posterior longitudinal ligament. As well, there are more pain receptors in some of these structures than in others. The significance of pain receptors is explained in more detail in Chapter 3, but it is interesting to keep this new evidence in mind when reading Chapter 2.

2

What Goes Wrong with Human Backs?

By the time we are in our mid-twenties, the bones of the spinal column will have reached their mature size. Ironically, it is precisely at this moment that the spine "begins to degenerate," as the process is commonly described by medical professionals.

If you think about it for a moment, the word *degenerate* is not particularly ominous; it simply means the opposite of *generate*, which means growth. While cells in our bodies are constantly wearing out and being replaced, during the growth years, bone and other tissue is created faster than it is destroyed and the net result is generation. After maturity, however, slightly less bone and other tissue is produced than destroyed and the net result is degeneration. In this sense, the spine is no different from any other organ of the body. Each goes through a slow process of degeneration with age.

When you think of it in this way, the term *degenerate* is accurate. But it is also unfortunate. Conjuring up the image of vertebrae turning to dust or discs disintegrating into nothingness, the concept of the "degenerating spine" has left thousands of people in fear for their long-term well-being and, in some cases, their lives. The fact of the matter is, that while it can be the cause of severe back pain, this degenerative process is, in itself, perfectly normal. It is also usually minor and, except in extremely rare instances when the spinal cord itself is damaged, certainly no more life-threatening than, for example, the common cold. The truth is that more than 90 per cent of us are suffering from either temporary, or chronic but quite manageable, back pain.

The Natural Aging Process of the Spine

In many respects, the process that the human spine goes through as it ages can be compared to the natural process that the skin begins to go through at about the same time. The spine's degenerative process, however, is actually ultimately advantageous in the majority of cases: by the time most people have reached the sixth or seventh decade of life, the degenerative changes of the spine render it less flexible, more stable and less susceptible to both injury and pain. According to the statistics, the majority of back pain sufferers are in their late twenties, thirties, forties and early fifties. Back pain, say the authorities, tends to get better with age, rather than worse.

But let's take a closer look at the aging skin analogy. When we are in our mid-twenties, our skin begins to both dry out and sag. Tiny lines – they are actually minuscule cracks – appear, for example, around the eyes. The tautness of the skin, which is a characteristic of youth, begins to diminish.

By the same token and around the same time, the water content of the intervertebral discs' nuclei begins to decrease. The fibres of the annulus, which encapsules the nucleus, begin to wear out. Like the plies of a slightly worn radial belted tire, they sometimes fray. Often, they develop concentric tears, which start near the nucleus and work their way toward the shell's outer edge.

When a disc's annulus tears, it tends to tear toward the back rather than toward the front, simply because the back sections of intervertebral discs are congenitally weaker than the front sections. But the fibres at the front of a disc's annulus also tend to weaken, if not tear, and this can also contribute to back pain.

As well, the body's ability to lubricate the facet joints – and, in fact, many of the body's other joints – diminishes. As a result of this, the facet joints frequently begin to suffer from general wear and tear.

At the same time, the ligaments of the spine frequently begin to lose some of their strength becoming lax. Lax ligaments also contribute to wear and tear of the facet joints. This happens because the facet joints, which were not intended to bear weight, rely on the spinal ligaments for support. If these ligaments begin to sag – and usually this is due to chronic strain caused by poor posture – the facet joints can become wobbly, or unstable, and misaligned. Most professionals believe that once a spinal ligament has lost its tautness, this process cannot be reversed completely, even if a person corrects his or her posture. When the ligaments have lost some of their ability to support the spine, it is more important than ever to have strong muscles to compensate.

The muscles that help support the spine and enable us to move can also lose their strength. This problem is more prevalent among people who lead sedentary lives, getting little or no exercise. Sometimes these muscles respond to the degenerative changes of the spine's discs, ligaments and joints by going into spasm. The purpose of muscle spasm in

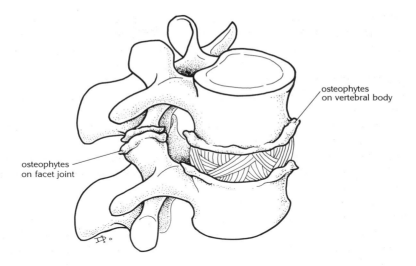

osteophytes
on vertebral body

osteophytes
on facet joint

Diagram 12   Osteophytes

this instance is to protect the area around a worn disc, or joint, by limiting movement. But muscle spasm can also be very painful. Unlike ligaments, however, muscles have great recuperative powers. By correcting the posture and exercising, a person can regain muscle strength.

In response to changes such as the ones just described, other characteristics that ultimately stabilize the spine begin to appear. For example, where a disc is attached to the vertebra above and below it, osteophytes — arthritic growths of bone which are also sometimes called lipping, or bone spurs, because of their shape — begin to form. Eventually, these osteophytes render the spine less flexible, but more stable and generally less susceptible to the problems caused by the degeneration of the discs.

Similarly, bone growths frequently appear around the facet joints and, over the years, they achieve the same end: diminished flexibility with the positive side effect that these joints become less susceptible to the problems caused by less lubrication or general wear and tear.

In the same way that the term *degenerate* is unfortunate when used in reference to the natural aging process of the spine's discs and joints, the terms *arthritis*, *osteoarthritis* and *arthritic changes* are also unfortunate. Nevertheless, all of them are used interchangeably by doctors and other health care professionals to describe these osteophytes or bony growths.

The first syllable of *arthritis* is a derivative of the Greek word *arthron*.

It simply means "joint." *Itis* means nothing more than "an inflammation of." And *osteo* simply means "bone." Hence *osteoarthritis* – an inflammation of a bony joint.

Arthritic changes such as these are as normal, and common, as the degenerative changes of the discs. And yet the mere mention of the word *arthritis* often conjures up the image of other, totally unrelated, extremely serious types of arthritis (such as rheumatoid arthritis). Because of this, thousands of back pain sufferers who are told that osteoarthritis is at the root of their problem react as if they were being handed a death sentence rather than a description of a very natural occurrence.

The Common Causes of Back Pain

It is while, rather than before or after, these changes are taking place that most people experience bouts with back pain. In fact, it is the rare and truly fortunate individual who escapes back pain completely. It is also true, however, that a significant amount of back pain could be avoided, or at least diminished, if people understood more about the details of these processes and the various ways to mitigate their effects.

At the root then of more than 90 per cent of all back pain are:
1. the changes in the spinal ligaments which are meant to support the spine;
2. the normal degenerative changes of the intervertebral discs;
3. the changes of the facet joints due to normal wear and tear, diminished lubrication, loss of disc height or strain from sagging ligaments and weak muscles;
4. the bony growths, or osteophytes, that develop on the vertebral bodies above and below the discs and around the facet joints in response to normal wear and tear;
5. the muscles that become weakened from chronic strain and lack of exercise and cannot perform their job. As well, weak muscles have a greater tendency to go into protective spasm, usually in response to the degenerative changes of the joints, discs and ligaments.

(The rarer, and sometimes more serious, causes of back pain such as Spina Bifida, Spondylitis, and Spondylolisthesis are discussed at the end of this chapter. Scoliosis and Osteoporosis are discussed separately in Chapters 25 and 27.)

Often, more than one of these five problem areas is involved simultaneously because the functioning of discs, facet joints, muscles and ligaments, and the formation of osteophytes are all interdependent. In fact, the complexity of this interdependence is one of the factors that makes the diagnosis of back pain so difficult. Nevertheless, the simplest way to get a grasp of what sorts of things generally cause backs to hurt is to look at each problem area separately.

How Ligaments Become Strained

The function of the spinal ligaments is to support the spine. Unlike muscles, however, which are built to expand and contract, ligaments are only slightly elastic. They can stretch, on the average, about 25 per cent of their length. Any more and they will tear. A partially torn ligament is called a sprain.

But sprained ligaments are not usually the thorn in the back pain sufferer's side. Ligaments will only stretch beyond their 25 per cent limit under *extreme* stress, and usually it is ligaments other than those of the spine which are torn. For example, when a skier takes a bad fall, he or she will sometimes tear ligaments in the knee. When a runner stumbles on an unexpected bump, he or she will sometimes sprain an ankle.

Chronic *strain* is a far better term to use when describing what usually happens to the ligaments of the spine over years of misuse. A person who sits in a chair that offers poor support, hunched forward over a desk eight hours a day, year after year, will strain a number of the spinal ligaments. Have another look at Diagram 6 on page 23. It's easy to see that bending forward will put strain on the back sections of the intervertebral discs; we hear about this all the time. But this posture also strains the posterior longitudinal ligament, the supraspinous ligament, the ligamentum flavum and the interspinous ligament. If you strain these ligaments for years on end, they will lose some of their ability to support the various structures of the spine.

Orthopaedic surgeons tend not to talk about ligaments very much, but chronically strained ligaments can certainly cause pain. For one thing, like muscles and nerves, ligaments contain pain receptors called nociceptors (see page 65). When they are under chronic strain, the firing rate of these receptors will increase, meaning that messages will arrive at the brain telling it that there is trouble afoot.

Strained ligaments can also lead to other problems which cause pain. For example, while the four ligaments mentioned above will stretch with prolonged sitting in a hunched forward position, the anterior longitudinal ligament will contract. The joint capsules at the back of the facet joints will also be chronically stretched, but the front part of the joint capsules will contract. *Adaptive shortening* is the term professionals use to describe what happens to tissue that is chronically contracted. As the term suggests, the tissue tightens up, or shortens. A facet joint whose capsule is stretched at the back and shortened at the front will simply not function properly. The term *misaligned* is sometimes used to explain this phenomenon.

Another posture that tends to strain the ligaments of the spine is standing for long periods of time, especially when a person extends, or arches, the lower back, a posture which increases the lumbar lordotic curve. In the case of chronic hyperextension, another set of adaptive shortening changes takes place. The anterior longitudinal ligament becomes stretched while the others become shortened. The front part of the facet joint capsule also becomes stretched while the back part shortens. This too affects the alignment of the joints resulting in pain. (It's almost impossible, by the way, to avoid hyperextension if you wear high heels.)

As I have already mentioned, when ligaments under chronic strain become lax, they lose some of their ability to support the spinal structures. Eventually, without the assistance of the appropriate ligaments, the facet joints will be forced to bear weight, which they are not designed to do. If the front part of a disc's annulus also becomes weakened, still more weight will be placed on the facet joints behind it. It is believed that when the facet joints are forced to bear weight, the normal degenerative process that these joints undergo as a result of age is speeded up. Once a facet joint has suffered some wear and tear, its status cannot be reversed. Strong muscles, however, can reduce a worn facet joint's burden. This is why exercise will frequently eliminate back pain, if not completely, then at least to a degree that does not encumber your life.

How Sacroiliac Joint Strain Occurs

In the 1920s, before it had been linked to disc degeneration, back pain was frequently attributed to sprains and strains of the ligaments of the sacroiliac joints — the joints that attach the sacrum to the hipbone, one on each side. Then, in the 1930s, disc trouble was "discovered" by two American surgeons and sacroiliac strain went out, almost like last year's fashion. Fashions, however, almost always return if one waits long enough, and over the past few years strains of the ligaments of the sacroiliac joints have been receiving more press.

The fact is that a host of ligaments attach the ilium to the sacrum on each side (see Diagram 36 on page 283). This is not the issue. The bone of contention is that some health care professionals believe that (other than during pregnancy) the "SI" joints move scarcely at all and that only a severe trauma, such as a car accident, could exert enough force on these ligaments to cause them to be strained. Others disagree, insisting that the SI joints do move and that strains of these joints are a significant cause of low back pain. Chiropractors, for example, do believe in SI joint strain and frequently manipulate these joints. Orthopaedic physicians (see Chapter 12) go one step further, sometimes using sclerosing injections to tighten up lax ligaments of the SI joints.

How Disc Degeneration Causes Back Pain

Around the third decade of life, the balanced process whereby discs absorb and lose both water and nutrients from the bloodstream on a daily basis

36

(see page 22) begins, very gradually, to fail. Over a period of time, slightly more water is lost than absorbed.

As each of the 23 discs dry out, it loses a bit of thickness, or height, and its annulus weakens. On the average, a disc will lose about an eighth of an inch in thickness over the years, although strictly speaking, the lower discs, which are larger and must bear more of the body's weight, tend to lose more than an eighth of an inch, and the upper discs lose a little less. An eighth of an inch seems like a meagre amount, but if you multiply an eighth of an inch by 23, it begins to make sense why people are usually a few inches shorter at age 70 than at age 17.

Losing a couple of inches in height is as normal and inconsequential – except perhaps from vanity's point of view – as having your hair turn grey. Other consequences which stem from those 23 plumped-up shock absorbers ending up looking more like raisins than grapes can, however, cause back trouble. Loss of disc height, for example, stimulates the growth of osteophytes, which can sometimes come into contact with pain-sensitive tissue. The loss of disc height and the weakening of the annulus can also affect the alignment of the facet joints.

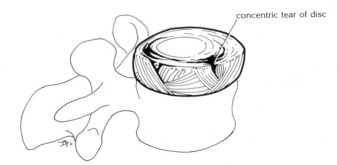

concentric tear of disc

Diagram 13   Concentric Tears of Intervertebral Disc

But the truth of the matter is that the drying out process that the discs' nuclei undergo probably eliminates more back problems than it causes.

If you think of the two aging processes in the disc going on simultaneously – the nucleus drying out and the fibrous annulus, or outer shell, beginning to fray – it will make sense that as its liquid content diminishes, the nucleus will exert less force against the fibres of its annulus. Think of a balloon; the more air you pump into it, the more important it is that the rubber sides be firm in all places so that it can withstand the pressure of the air. But if you leave a blown up balloon for a few days, a bit of the air will usually leak out. The pressure on the sides of the balloon will diminish, and they will not give way as easily even if there is a weakness in one or two spots.

THE HERNIATED DISC • In the best of circumstances, the aging process of the disc's nucleus and annulus will take place in harmony: the annulus will lose some of its strength and, as if to compensate, the nucleus will lose a percentage of its water, therefore exerting less stress.

Sometimes, however – and it is really not that common – nature's balancing act fails completely. In less than 10 per cent of people with a back problem, the cause is a disc – and almost always a lower lumbar disc – that has "herniated." In this situation, the annulus weakens *before* its nucleus has had a chance to dry out. Then, one day – sometimes after what can seem like a totally inconsequential act – the annulus ruptures. Like a tire that blows out, the nucleus, or at least part of it, oozes out and presses against a nerve root, causing severe pain. It is interesting to note, however, that since discs contain no pain receptors (except where they attach to the posterior spinal ligament), a herniation can be completely painless if the bit that oozes out does not come into contact with a nerve root. When it does meet up with a nerve root, however, the pain that a true disc herniation can cause – called sciatic pain – can be excruciating and is most often felt in the leg. When the functioning of the nerve is actually disrupted by the bit of disc pressing against it, numbness and muscle atrophy will occur. This is the condition that is so often referred to as a "slipped disc," a misnomer really, since nothing is slipping at all.

Sometimes a disc will herniate because its annulus is congenitally weak; the results of some recent studies have suggested that a disc's propensity to herniate may be an inherited condition related to genetics. In other instances a herniation just happens; some studies suggest that a life of hard labour increases a person's risk of a disc herniation. Other studies suggest, however, that people who lead sedentary lives, hunching over desks for hours each day, year after year, are at higher risk.

Whatever the cause, disc herniations are uncommon. Most physicians estimate that fewer than ten per cent of back pain patients are suffering from a herniated disc that is pressing against a nerve. And yet, almost everyone who has a back problem *thinks* that a herniated disc is the cause. Ask ten people to explain the source of their back pain and nine will say that "a disc has slipped and is pinching a nerve." These people also tend to hold the erroneous conviction that whenever their back has "gone out" it is because they have "slipped a disc," and that discs frequently move into and out of place, sometimes in a matter of seconds. Nothing could be further from the truth. While a frayed annulus can repair itself, in the sense that like other tissue of the body it forms scar tissue, this process is slow, sometimes taking many months.

In some instances, the bit of nucleus that has oozed through the annulus will break away completely from the rest of the disc and lodge against a nerve root in the spinal canal. In this situation, that bit of nucleus material will remain in the spinal canal even if the annulus has completely healed.

This rare type of herniation is called a sequestrated disc, *sequestrated* simply meaning "alone" or "isolated," as when a jury is sequestered to render a verdict. More frequently, however, the bit of nucleus that has herniated through the annulus remains attached to the rest of the nucleus as shown in Diagram 14.

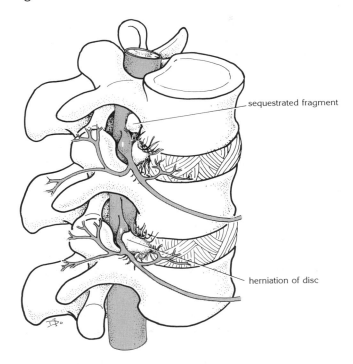

sequestrated fragment

herniation of disc

Diagram 14   A Herniated Disc and a Sequestrated Disc

In one respect, the small percentage of people with a herniated disc can be considered lucky. They are the ones whose back pain is due to a specific, localized problem. In many instances, with time, rest and conservative treatment, a herniated disc will heal. When it does not, it can be pinpointed by a myelogram, discogram or CT Scan, and then removed — either surgically or by a chymopapain injection. The invasive procedure usually eliminates the localized problem and, with it, the pain.

Sometimes, however, surgery or a chymopapain injection fails to relieve the pain caused by a herniated disc. No doubt, at least in some cases, the technical skill of the surgeon is at fault. But other times, the finger is pointed at "adhesions," which were not spotted and therefore not removed at surgery. (In fact, when a chymopapain injection is used to treat a disc herniation, removing adhesions is not even an option.) The theory is that at the time of the original injury – that is, when the disc herniation occurred – there was an amount of swelling at the site of the injury. Due to poor circulation, or muscle tension, the fluid that built up – and built-up fluid is what swelling is all about – was not able to dissipate. Over a period of several months, this fluid dried out and became a sticky, viscous mass that "adhered" to pain-sensitive tissue; hence the term *adhesion*.

The two lowest discs of the lumbar spine – the L4-L5 disc and the L5-S1 disc – tend to herniate more frequently than the other discs of the spine. The reason is simple: these two discs bear more of the body's weight than the others. Studies have also shown that the rear portion of the disc's annulus tends to be weaker than the front portion. Therefore, if a disc does herniate, it tends to do so at the back, near the intervertebral foramen. The bad luck of the matter is twofold: the rear portion of the annulus is the one area of a disc that contains pain receptors. As well, it is through the intervertebral foramen that the nerve roots which branch off from the spinal cord exit from the spinal canal. Thus the nerve roots are susceptible to compression when a disc herniates.

If you think back to Chapter 1, and have a second look at Diagram 11 on page 29, you'll recall that branches of the nerves which exit from between L4-L5 and L5-S1 join together in the hip area with other nerve branches to form the two sciatic nerves. The sciatic nerves, one on each side, run down the leg all the way to the foot. For this reason, the pain or numbness that accompanies a herniation of one of the lower lumbar discs is usually more severe in the buttock and leg than in the back. Depending upon the extent of the pressure against the nerve from the offending bit of disc, the pain or numbness may extend down the leg to the knee or even as far as the big toe or the heel.

In a lot of cases, however, patients with herniated discs do experience at least some back pain as well as buttock and leg pain. Some physicians feel that the back pain is caused by the fact that the many branches of our nerves are interconnected, and sometimes the brain gets confused about the source of a pain, referring it from one location to another. (See page 46.) Other physicians believe that the back pain is caused by the ligaments or muscles in the damaged area. Both contain pain receptors. As well, the muscles in the damaged area frequently go into spasm to limit movement.

Some patients with a herniated disc, however, experience no back pain at all; they arrive at their doctor's office complaining of excruciating leg pain only to find out that the source of the pain is a herniated disc in the lumbar spine.

THE BULGING DISC • In the majority of cases – in my case and probably in yours – a problematic disc doesn't actually herniate. If the annulus of a disc weakens before its nucleus dries out, the pressure of the nucleus will cause it to bulge – sometimes minimally, other times severely – rather than to blow out.

Like a herniated disc, a bulging disc can also come into contact with a ligament or nerve root. Most often, however, a disc that is bulging doesn't exactly *press* against, or pinch, a nerve root sufficiently to interfere with its functioning; a better way of describing the situation is to say that a bulging disc *irritates* a nerve root.

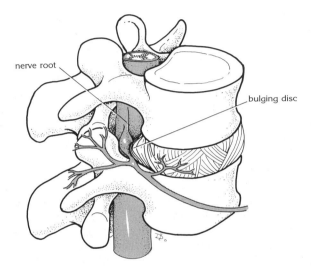

nerve root

bulging disc

Diagram 15   A Bulging Disc

Nevertheless, when a nerve root is irritated, it can cause pain, a tingling sensation or numbness in a buttock or leg, and sometimes these symptoms can be extremely severe. It is unusual, however, for the sensation – whether severe or mild – to extend below the knee. If a ligament is irritated by a disc, the firing rate of the nociceptors in it will increase, causing pain. Either of these two situations can also cause painful, protective muscle spasm, called secondary muscle spasm.

If your back problem is caused by a weak annulus that has a propensity to bulge, you will most likely suffer from the type of annoying backache and/or leg pain that comes and goes several times a year. And, as I just mentioned, because the back of the annulus tends to be its weakest section, bending forward – which puts additional stress on the rear wall – will cause it to bulge.

Dr. Alf Nachemson, a Swedish orthopaedic surgeon who is renowned for his work on discs, designed a study to demonstrate the amount of strain that various postures place on the discs of the lumbar spine.

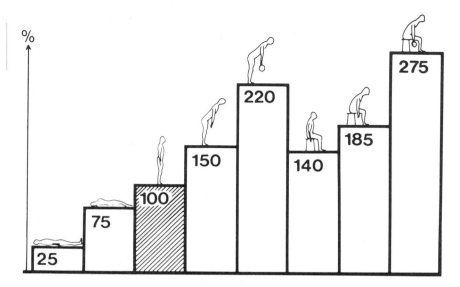

Diagram 16   Dr. Alf Nachemson's Postural Study

Most people are surprised to learn that sitting puts more strain on the lumbar discs than standing. Sitting hunched over a desk, or standing bent over a table, a shovel or a vacuum cleaner, puts more strain on the discs of the lumbar spine than any other posture. When you realize this, it makes more sense why a long day in the garden bent over a hoe, a few hours of vacuuming or an afternoon hunched over a typewriter will put extra pressure on a weak annulus, causing it to bulge.

Usually, a minor bulge, along with the pain, will subside after a good night's rest. Other times, however, a bout with a bulging disc can be so severe that the pain will take months to subside completely. In some cases the pain drags on for much longer than what seems logical; studies have shown that even a badly herniated disc will generally heal within nine months. When the pain continues after this length of time, some physicians blame adhesions. Their feeling is that while the disc herniation may have healed, the adhesions it has caused have not dissipated. Some doctors believe that adhesions can take up to several years to dissipate completely.

It is also important for chronic back pain sufferers to understand how difficult it is to diagnose a bulging disc with total certainty, and that it is even tougher to pinpoint it as *the source* of a back ailment.

A regular X-ray, for example, reveals only bone — not the soft tissue of which discs are composed. For this reason, while a regular X-ray is able to show that the space between two vertebrae looks narrower than normal, it cannot show the outline of the disc's actual bulge. (See page 10.)

Even the films provided by a myelogram test, during which radiopaque dye is injected into the spinal canal (see Chapter 8), reveal only the outline of the canal, not the discs themselves. If a disc is actually impinging into the spinal canal sufficiently to distort the canal's shape, the indentation in the canal will be revealed on the X-ray screen. A disc that has a small bulge, however, will not cause a definite indentation and the diagnosis will be negative or at least suspect. Likewise, the results of a discogram will be negative unless there is a herniation, or a large bulge.

Clinical examinations can also be misleading. A true herniation at the rear portion of a disc's annulus will likely result in nerve root compression, but the signs and symptoms of a mere bulging disc are frequently tough to pin down. Another consideration is that there are studies which show that disc displacement cannot always be correlated with pain. Sometimes, for example, a myelogram will be performed to pinpoint a herniated disc of the cervical spine on a patient with a *neck* problem and the test will reveal an additional herniation in the lumbar spine which is causing no low back pain whatsoever. Autopsies have been performed for various reasons on people who have no history of back pain and these too have revealed severe herniations.

Most of us who have suffered from severe chronic back pain have wished that a disc problem could be diagnosed and cured surgically – the magic bullet solution which requires no effort on our part! It would, however, be unethical for a doctor to prescribe radical treatment whenever there is *some* evidence of a bulging disc. Before a back pain patient is considered a candidate for disc surgery, there must be conclusive evidence of a true herniation. This evidence must be corroborated by both clinical and radiological evidence. This condition is relatively rare.

Sometimes, a patient will suffer off and on for many years from a bulging disc and then, suddenly, the disc will actually herniate. In most cases, however, a bulging disc will stabilize over the years rather than herniate. As the nucleus dries out and loses a bit of height, osteophytes will develop, limiting mobility. As well, when there is less water in the nucleus, correspondingly less pressure will be exerted against the annulus.

The trick is to find the conservative treatment that works for you while your discs are going through this process.

The Worn Facet Joint

While the drying out of a disc's nucleus results in *less* pressure being exerted on its annulus, it can also result in *more* pressure being exerted on the facet joints – the small joints at the back of each vertebra which link it to the vertebra above and the one below.

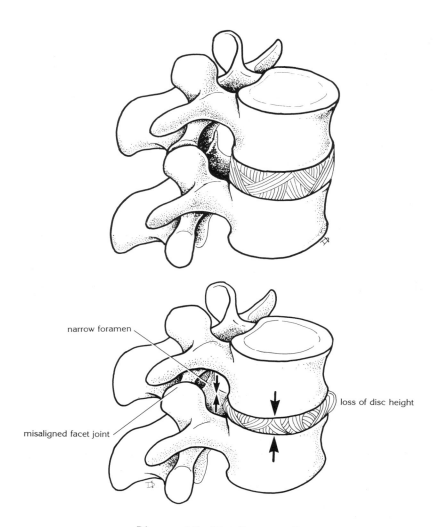

Diagram 17   Disc Degeneration

Compare the two discs in Diagram 17. The first illustration shows the disc of a 20-year-old. Because the disc's nucleus is still plump, the disc has not lost any height. In the second illustration, the disc has aged about 30 years and is about a quarter of an inch thinner. The disc, of course, separates two vertebrae, and it's obvious that when it loses a bit of height, those two vertebrae will settle closer together. The result is that the facet joints at the back of the vertebrae move closer together as well.

Other degenerative changes can cause facet joints to "settle" closer together. As discussed earlier, ligaments that have stretched from years of poor posture cannot provide the facet joints with the support that they need. Without support, facet joints must bear weight and since they were not intended to be weight-bearing joints, this extra strain can also cause them to settle closer together. A third cause is the stretching of the annulus at the front of a disc. This degenerative change can also result in the settling of a facet joint.

The results of this settling? Very simply put, if the two parts of a joint become too close, their alignment will change and they will rub against each other when they move. Eventually, if this rubbing goes on for long enough, the smooth cartilage which lines each joint will become worn and rough.

The thought of having a couple of your facet joints rub together every time you move is as frightening to think about as the degeneration of a disc, or osteophytes growing where the disc attaches to a vertebra – that is, until you stop a moment and think calmly about what really occurs.

For one thing, we're talking about a process that can take decades to develop; facet joints don't settle and start rubbing together overnight. For another thing, just as small, stabilizing osteophytes form where a disc attaches to its vertebra, stabilizing osteophytes frequently form around worn facet joints, ultimately limiting their mobility.

The image of worn facet joints that most people conjure up in their minds – that of two joints grinding together like two gears that don't mesh – is as uncommon as, or perhaps even more uncommon than, the truly herniated disc.

Again, a more appropriate word to use is *irritation*. As a pair of facet joints start settling a tiny bit closer together, they don't start grinding, they merely cease to function as well as they once did. Just as a disc bulges slightly because its annulus is weak, a pair of worn facet joints lose a bit of their youthful ability to operate frictionlessly and in most cases nothing much more.

However, although the pathology is usually minor, there are nociceptors in the facet joints and this friction can result in pain. While bending forward will aggravate a disc that has a tendency to bulge, the opposite motion – arching the back into a posture of hyperlordosis – can aggravate worn facet joints. Why? Have another look at Diagram 1 on page 18. When you arch, or extend your back, you bring the facet joints closer together. If they're already a bit worn, it makes sense that this posture will accentuate the problem. On the other hand, reducing the spine's lower lordotic curve – for example, doing the proverbial pelvic tilt which is described on page 167 – will ease the back pain that is caused by a pair of worn facet joints.

Just as a bulging disc can cause leg pain as well as back pain, most physicians maintain that a worn facet joint can cause leg pain too. In fact, several studies during which a saline solution was injected into a facet joint have confirmed that sensations from a worn facet joint can actually refer pain all the way to the foot! The pain, however, is far less severe and less specific than the neurological pain caused by a disc pressing against a nerve. Patients generally describe leg pain that originates from a facet joint as vague. Sometimes they can't even pinpoint exactly where the pain is, whereas the leg pain caused by a herniated disc literally shoots down the leg and is often described as electric, or burning.

To understand more about how facet joint pain can "radiate" into the leg, take a look at Diagram 10. While one branch of the nerve runs down the leg, another branch moves off toward the facet joint, another supplies the muscles nearby, and still another serves the outer layers of the adjacent disc.

Let's take, as an example, a woman who has a slightly worn pair of lumbar facet joints and who spends an evening at a party standing in high heels. You'll recall that this posture accentuates the normal lordosis of the lumbar spine.

After several hours, her anterior longitudinal ligament will be feeling the strain, and this could be the source of her pain. But more likely, the source is the facet joints. While her back is arched, her already worn joints jam together and are therefore taxed more than usual, with the result that they become irritated.

Very basically, this irritation produces signals which travel to the spinal cord via the particular branch of the nerve that serves the facet joints. At the spinal cord this "information" is processed and then relayed to the brain where the pain is identified. How this all happens is discussed in more detail in Chapter 3.

While the body's communication system is brilliant in many respects, it does, like most systems, tend to have the odd flaw. One of them is that it sometimes gets confused about the precise source of a signal. The nervous system sometimes thinks that signals emanating from one source are coming from another. In other words, the system can become confused about which branch of a nerve is transmitting the information. When this happens, we say that the signal – the pain in this case – is being "referred." A good analogy is a passenger at the main depot of a train station who is looking out of the station's tunnel as a train is pulling in. Although he knows that trains from many places arrive at the main depot, it is difficult for him, as he stands at the terminus, to determine where the train originated. The brain sometimes has the same problem.

Our woman at the party is another good example. The initial signal that there is irritation originates at the end of the nerve branch that serves the facet joint. This information is sent via the nerve root to the spinal cord, and then up the cord to the brain. Keep in mind that the nerve root also has other branches, one of which runs down the leg. Sometimes the brain gets confused and thinks that the pain is coming from the sciatic branch of the nerve as well as the facet joint branch; after all, these branches both emerge from the same nerve root. When pain whose source is a facet joint is felt in the leg, or more commonly the thigh, it is called referred pain. The more severe the irritation of the facet joint, the farther down the leg the referred pain will be felt.

Sometimes a situation like this can become even more complex. At the same time as the signal is getting its wires crossed, an impulse — which travels via the nerve branch that serves the muscles in the area — will alert those muscles that there is trouble afoot. They will respond by going into spasm in an attempt to limit movement and thus ease the irritation, nature's version of a protective splint. When these muscles go into spasm, others frequently tighten up to compensate, and the area of pain becomes even more widespread.

To the brain, a situation like this can be very confusing. Sometimes, it can't answer the question, where did the problem begin? All it knows is that a branch of a branch of another branch of a nerve has delivered a message that says "pain." Although it may know that the pain is coming from the left side of the body rather than the right, below the waist rather than above, much more than that may be difficult to compute. By the time you arrive at the doctor's office with pain that originates from a worn facet joint, which is referring pain to the leg and is causing muscle spasm as well, it is frequently as difficult to pinpoint the worn facet joint as the source of that pain as it is, in other circumstances, to identify a bulging disc.

Another type of facet joint problem can also cause pain. Sometimes, if you twist very suddenly or move beyond your normal range, the capsule surrounding the joint can get nipped by the joint itself. Try to visualize the capsule as a balloon that has lost its air after having been blown up for several days. It is loose and a bit saggy. It has to be in order for the facet joints contained within it to have room enough to move. But because it is loose, the capsule can get nipped between the two ends of bone, in the way that the inside of your cheek can get nipped between your teeth. When this happens, the capsule can become bruised. Inflammation may follow, leading to protective muscle spasm in the area. This is frequently what has happened when you twist suddenly and feel a twinge of pain.

A third type of facet joint problem is probably more common, but is very poorly understood. It has to do with the synovial fluid (see page 193) contained within the capsules of all facet joints. Prior to a storm, barometric pressure frequently drops suddenly causing this synovial fluid to expand. You would think that discovering exactly how this mechanism works and why it so frequently causes back pain would be a topic researchers would be keen to address. But over the past five years, despite inquiries and many searches through many journals, I have yet to come across a single documented research study dealing with this well-known phenomenon.

In any case, the irritation, muscle spasm and pain caused by over-straining a worn facet joint or bruising its capsule will usually subside after the cause of the irritation is removed. Most doctors agree that if the source of back or leg pain is a facet joint, the acute stage does not generally last as long as a bout of back pain caused by a bulging disc. If our woman at the party goes home, gets a good night's rest, wears sensible shoes and avoids arching her back for several days, chances are good that the irritation in her facet joints will subside. If you twist badly in your sleep or while playing a sport, nipping a joint capsule in the process, the pain will likely be gone after two or three days. Likewise, as the storm clouds disappear, back pain caused by a drop in barometric pressure usually fades away.

The trick is to incorporate the needs of your slightly worn joints, or discs, into your life-style so that you can avoid beginning a new bout of pain almost as soon as you have gotten over the last one. While you are learning to do this, nature too is at work to diminish your vulnerability to back pain. It is busy stabilizing your spine, a process which will ultimately limit your susceptibility to the pain caused by degenerative changes such as these.

Osteoarthritis (Osteophytes, Bone Spurs or Lipping)

A number of years ago, the spines of 195 Swedish men and women were X-rayed and compared. Several interesting things showed up on the films.

Of those who were in their forties, 72 per cent had evidence of osteo-phytes growing either on the rims of the vertebral bodies, or near the facet joints, or both. Of those who were in their sixties, 97 per cent had evidence of osteophytes. And yet, curiously enough, there was little correlation between the degree of degeneration and whether or not a person had back pain.

As I have already mentioned, osteophytes (also referred to as bone spurs, lipping, and arthritic changes) are generally an aid to back pain, not the cause of it. When their shape has become established, and they have actually accomplished their purpose of stabilizing the discs or joints on which they are growing, osteophytes will usually eliminate back pain. As they limit mobility, they may be the cause of stiffness in the back, particularly in people over the age of 65. But as far as actual pain is concerned, many physicians feel that osteophytes are the villain in relatively few cases.

When osteophytes do cause trouble, the ailment is called spinal stenosis.

Spinal stenosis is another potentially scary term which has a rather benign meaning. *Steno* is from the Greek word *stenos*, which means "narrow." And *osis* means "a condition of" or "a process." Basically, this highfalutin term means nothing more than "a condition where there is narrowing."

There are two types of spinal stenosis: central spinal stenosis (sometimes called midline stenosis) and lateral spinal stenosis.

If you are told that your back problem is caused by central spinal stenosis, it means that your spinal canal, through which your spinal cord runs, is narrower than normal in a particular area. Sometimes the condition is congenital, and at other times it develops as the bony spinal canal, which is normally heart-shaped, thickens, leaving less room for the nerves running through the canal. Very simply, when they have less room, the nerves can become irritated. Sometimes this condition is so mild that it remains undetected. At other times it can cause severe back pain. Central spinal stenosis can most easily be diagnosed by a CT Scan. The procedure is described in Chapter 7.

There are different opinions about whether or not a congenitally narrow canal will actually cause pain or simply *predispose* a person to back pain, meaning that a narrowish spinal canal is, if you will, less forgiving than one that is normal in diameter.

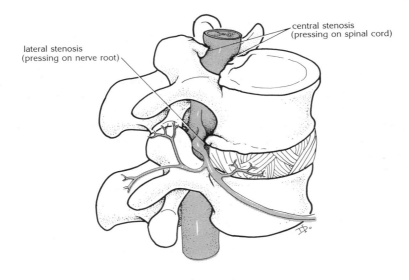

central stenosis
(pressing on spinal cord)

lateral stenosis
(pressing on nerve root)

Diagram 18   Central and Lateral Spinal Stenosis

An interesting study by two British physicians, Richard Porter and David Ottewell, seems to indicate the latter. While studying the spines of pain-free patients as well as those who suffer from back pain, these physicians discovered that about ten per cent of the population have lumbar spinal canals less than half an inch wide. At the opposite extreme, about ten per cent of the population have lumbar spinal canals that are nearly three-quarters of an inch wide. The most interesting aspect of the study, however, was that a large proportion of people who did suffer from back pain fell into the small group of people with very narrow canals. Out of 154 patients who suffered from sciatic pain, 56 per cent had spinal canals less than half an inch wide!

Lateral spinal stenosis is a narrowing of an intervertebral foramen, the space at the back of a vertebra out of which the nerve roots exit. Many things can cause lateral spinal stenosis – an injury, severe settling of facet joints due to a disc which has lost an abnormally large amount of height, spondylolisthesis (see page 55), or an abnormal variation in the shape of a vertebra.

Osteophytes, however, are the most common cause of lateral spinal stenosis. When they form around the edges of a vertebra, they sometimes encroach into the spinal canal. These bony growths may then irritate a nerve root as it makes its exit through the foramen.

When the encroachment is minimal, the back pain caused by lateral spinal stenosis is usually minor – perhaps the occasional ache after strenuous activity. In the rare instances when it is severe – that is, when a nerve root is actually being pinched by bone – lateral spinal stenosis can be corrected by surgery. A laminectomy is performed (see page 113) and the excess bone is removed.

How Much Do Strained Muscles Contribute to Back Pain?

Muscles, unlike ligaments, are extremely elastic, routinely expanding and contracting to enable our bodies to move. For this reason, they tend to overstretch rather than tear. While you often hear of sprained ligaments, you rarely hear of a sprained muscle. A muscle that has been *strained*, however, can cause severe pain.

How frequently strained muscles are the cause of back pain is a controversy that has been debated for decades.

The issue is a difficult one to resolve. For one thing, ligaments and muscles – like discs – are made of soft tissue, and soft tissue does not show up on X-rays. For this reason, it is very difficult to either counter, or confirm, a diagnosis of muscle strain, particularly if a deep, rather than superficial, muscle of the back is in question.

There is, as well, another area of confusion when the subject of muscle strain as a cause of back pain comes up. As I've already mentioned, the small muscle groups may go into painful spasm with the purpose of immobilizing an area when there is trouble in a nearby facet joint or disc. Certain questions, however, remain unanswered. Is the majority of the actual pain caused by the muscle spasm, the joint or the disc? The answer depends upon whom you ask. And is it appropriate to say that the *source* of the pain is the muscle spasm? Or the irritated joint? Or the bulging disc? Do muscle spasms sometimes remain long after an irritated joint or disc has healed? And do muscles sometimes go into spasm even when there is nothing wrong with the facet joints or discs? In other words, can stress or over-exertion without significant degeneration cause muscle tension?

Most of the people I have spoken to believe that when muscles are involved in back pain, they are a secondary cause; they believe that in almost all cases, the primary cause is the degenerative process of ligaments, discs or facet joints. But it also seems to me that physiotherapists and massage therapists, for example, believe that the contribution of muscle spasm to back pain is significant. This attitude is logical since their training concentrates as much on soft tissue (muscles and ligaments) as hard tissue (bones). On the other hand, orthopaedic surgeons, whose training bias is toward bones, tend to talk less about the contribution of muscle spasm to back pain.

Whether physiotherapist or surgeon, however, most health care professionals agree that in most cases, when muscle strain is involved, it tends to subside on its own after a few days or weeks. A muscle strain usually does not become the source of chronic pain.

Nevertheless, it often helps to be reminded that, although muscle pain is not generally long-lived, it can be extremely severe. Recent studies have shown that the complex system of blood vessels that run throughout the muscles of the spine are dense with pain receptors. At times, when I have a backache so painful that I have been convinced that something terrible must be wrong, I try to remind myself of this as well as an experiment so simple that it makes me laugh. A physiotherapist showed it to me years ago and thinking about it has often put my frazzled mind to rest.

Hold a copy of a formidable book in your hand — a concise version of *Webster's Dictionary* will do nicely — and then extend your arm in front of you so that it is parallel to the ground. Now count to 60, extremely slowly.

By the time a minute has passed, the pain caused by the strain of the muscles in your hand and arm should make it apparent that the severity of pain does not necessarily correspond to the severity of its pathology. Severe pain doesn't necessarily mean that something terrible is wrong, although it does usually mean that the pain will subside when the source of the irritation is removed.

And how do you remove that irritation? Sometimes, I have come to learn, with a very subtle approach. For some people, simple changes in posture, or a few exercises done consistently, will do. For others, practising one of the other disciplines described in this book has worked miracles.

I have also come to learn that half of the battle of beating back pain is conquering your fear of it. Once you have accomplished that feat, you'll have an excellent chance of taking control.

Other Specific Causes of Back Pain

ANKYLOSING SPONDYLITIS (Marie-Strumpell Disease) • *Ankylosing* means stiffening. *Spondy* means "spine" and *itis*, as in arthritis, means "inflammation." Put them all together and you've got the rare condition that affects men twice as often as women and usually begins in the late twenties.

The symptoms are severe inflammation of the spinal joints, which stiffen and cause severe pain. The hip and knee joints are also frequently affected. Eventually some, or all, of the vertebrae fuse together. Typically, the disease begins at the base of the spine, affecting the sacroiliac joints first, and then the lumbar vertebrae. Over a period of years the disease progresses up the spinal column. When more than a few of the vertebrae fuse, the disease will actually hunch a person over until he or she can

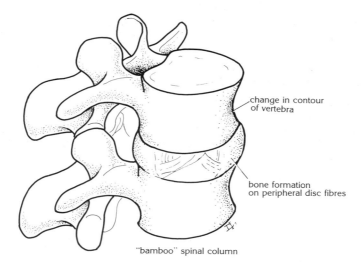

change in contour of vertebra

bone formation on peripheral disc fibres

"bamboo" spinal column

Diagram 19   Ankylosing Spondylitis

barely see ahead. At this point, the fused joints resemble a bamboo rod — for this reason, the disease is sometimes referred to as "bamboo spine." The cause is unknown — although recent research points to genetic factors. It is also unknown why this disease may go into remission spontaneously.

The treatment for ankylosing spondylitis is usually pain-relieving and anti-inflammatory drugs, exercise and attention to posture. In extremely severe cases, surgery will sometimes be performed to fuse the spine. If the disease is not severe, a person with ankylosing spondylitis can live a nearly normal, albeit painful, existence.

RHEUMATOID ARTHRITIS • Unlike osteoarthritis, which is a local problem, rheumatoid arthritis is a body-wide illness. It attacks the joints — specifically a joint's synovial membrane — of the hands, wrists, elbows, knees, ankles, feet, hips and sometimes the facet joints of the spine. The result is severe inflammation, swelling and painful stiffness. Rheumatoid arthritis, unlike osteoarthritis, will usually destroy a joint as it progresses, as well as the tissue nearby.

Rheumatoid arthritis can be crippling. For reasons that are not known, it strikes three times as many women as men. In fact, the cause of the disease is largely unknown, although recent research points to a genetic disorder that may be triggered by a virus but only when a person is particularly susceptible because of a deficiency in his or her immune system. Stress may also play a role in the onset, or exacerbation, of the disease or its symptoms.

Rheumatoid arthritis can begin at any age. Even young children can develop it. It is sometimes difficult to diagnose. An antibody called the rheumatoid factor may be present in the blood, and this will alert a physician that the patient has the disease. At other times, however, the rheumatoid factor is not present, and the presence of rheumatoid arthritis can only be "confirmed" when all other diseases that produce similar symptoms have been ruled out.

At present there is no cure, only treatments that can reduce, or slow down, the onset of symptoms. Once damage has been done to a joint, it is largely irreversible. However, for reasons that are not understood, a rheumatoid arthritis patient will sometimes go into remission for years at a time.

Until a cure is found, the treatment will continue to focus on controlling the disease. Specialists, called rheumatologists, supervise the treatment, which consists of drug therapy to relieve the pain and inflammation, exercise to prevent the affected joints from stiffening further, and resting splints to prevent or reduce deformities. Aspirin, gold salts, cortisone and other anti-inflammatory drugs are all used, the choice depending upon the individual's tolerance and reactions. In severe cases of rheumatoid arthritis, a destroyed joint can be replaced surgically.

53

SPONDYLOLYSIS • *Spondyl*, once again, is from the Greek word which means "vertebra." *Olisis* is from the Greek word which literally means "loosen." Put them together and you have a condition called spondylolysis, in which a defective vertebra becomes loose because it has cracked.

Spondylolysis occurs across the back of a vertebra. Usually, the crack, or fracture, is hairline — so minor that it remains undetected unless an X-ray is taken for another reason. It is surprisingly common; in North America, it is estimated that one in twenty people have a mild spondylolysis. In some populations, notably the Eskimo population of northern Alaska, nearly 30 per cent of the people have a spondylolysis.

Although the cause of spondylolysis is unknown, some researchers speculate that it is related to a hereditary weakness combined with prolonged stress. This theory would explain why so many Eskimos, who probably fall frequently on ice as children, are susceptible to the condition. The crack often occurs in early childhood and fails to heal.

Generally speaking, mild spondylolysis causes neither back pain nor mechanical problems. In rare instances, however, the hairline crack will widen. When this happens the condition is called spondylolisthesis, which can cause back trouble.

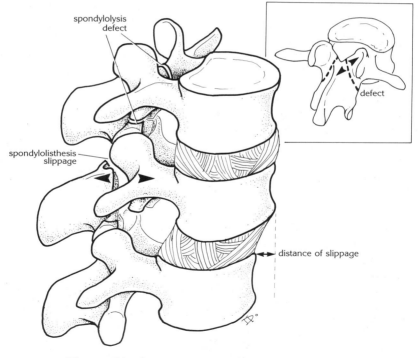

spondylolysis
defect

defect

spondylolisthesis
slippage

distance of slippage

Diagram 20   Spondylolysis and Spondylolisthesis

SPONDYLOLISTHESIS • It sounds unpronounceable, but if you break it down the condition becomes straightforward. *Spondyl* means "spine" and *olisthesis* is from the Greek word which means "slip." Ironically, the misnomer "slipped disc" is better known than the condition where actual slippage does take place.

For a person to develop spondylolisthesis, spondylolysis (see above) must first exist. if the spondylolysis, or crack, at the back of a vertebra widens sufficiently, the front portion of the vertebra, which is detached from the rear, can gradually slip forward in relation to the vertebra below.

In its very mild form, spondylolisthesis may remain undetected. More severe cases usually respond to conservative treatment, which consists of rest during a flare-up and some form of exercise to strengthen the area when the acute pain subsides. A flare-up may be caused by physical overexertion. In extremely severe cases, surgery may be performed to fuse the slipping area. (See page 115.)

SPONDYLITIS • *Itis* means "inflammation" and *spondyl* means "spine." But this type of inflammation does not affect a joint. Instead, spondylitis refers to the inflammation caused by an infection or a reaction to a chemical.

Bacteria can sometimes cause a spinal infection. When bacteria invade the spine, the term *osteomyelitis* is generally used. This condition can be caused by an infection elsewhere in the body spreading to the spine; or sometimes as a result of surgery when the unfortunate event of incisional infection occurs post-operatively. Treatment generally consists of antibiotics and rest. In rare circumstances, spondylitis can take several years to subside completely.

In other rare cases, the cause is a chemical that irritates the spine; for example, when diagnostic tests are conducted on the spine (such as a discogram or a myelogram) and the patient develops an infection. These types of infections are also treated with antibiotics and rest.

SPINA BIFIDA • Like spondylolysis, spina bifida is a condition that rarely causes back pain and often remains undetected. It is at least as old as the mummies of Egypt in whose vertebral remains "holes" have been found.

The condition sounds much worse than it is. Basically, in the process of developing, the bony ring which forms the back of each vertebra fails to close completely, leaving a tiny gap at the rear. Generally this gap is filled with scar tissue and is so minimal – one or two millimetres – that it is totally insignificant. Only on very rare occasions is the gap wide enough to be a serious birth defect.

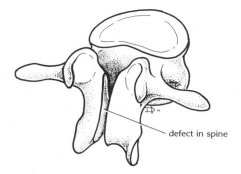

defect in spine

Diagram 21 Spina Bifida

SPONDYLOSIS • Take the term apart (*spondyl* meaning "spine"; *osis* meaning "condition of") and you get to the bottom of the meaning of this term – which is no meaning at all. Unfortunately, it is sometimes used by health care professionals who forget that to most lay people medical jargon can produce fear and anxiety. If you hear it, ask the person who has used it what he or she means!

LUMBAGO • Of all the terms used to describe back ailments this takes the cake. It's even less meaningful than spondylosis! Basically it means "pain in the lumbar region," which means pain in the lower back.

PRIMARY CANCER OF THE SPINE • Primary cancer of the spine, which is a type of cancer that develops in a vertebra, the bone marrow or the muscles of the spine, is extremely rare. When it does occur, however, the symptom is usually pain that does not respond to conservative treatment or rest. If a patient complains of unrelenting back pain throughout the night, a physician may suspect a tumour. Because the cells in a malignant tumour divide more quickly than normal cells, they can be detected by means of a bone scan. However, this test is not always conclusive and other tests – usually blood tests and X-rays – will be done. Surgery, if the tumour is accessible, radiation therapy and chemotherapy are all used in the treatment of primary cancer of the spine.

SECONDARY CANCERS OF THE SPINE • Although secondary cancers of the spine are also rare, it is more common for a cancer that has developed in another organ of the body to spread, or metastasize, to the spine than to originate in the spine. Breast cancer, for example, sometimes spreads to the bones of the spine as does cancer of the prostate and the lung. The diagnosis and treatment of secondary cancer of the spine is similar to that for primary cancer of the spine.

II
Gearing Up to Cope With Back Pain

3

Pain: To Say It Is Complex Is Too Simple

Pain is universal. We have all felt its clutch at one time or another, for this reason or that. Describing how pain *feels*, however, is another matter completely. You can say that pain throbs, burns, aches, pounds, stabs, sears – to name just some of the words that have been used to describe it. Yet none of them grasp the enormity of pain's impact, or the anguish which is part and parcel of the experience.

In her essay, *On Being Ill*, author Virginia Woolf poignantly explains the inadequacy of language when it comes to describing pain: "English, which can express the thoughts of Hamlet and the tragedy of Lear, has no words for [pain].... The merest schoolgirl, when she falls in love, has Shakespeare and Keats to speak for her; but let a sufferer try to explain a pain . . . to a doctor and language at once runs dry."

When she made the comment, Virginia Woolf was talking about headache, rather than backache. But Montreal graphic artist Judith Franklin's recollection of her first bout with back pain, six years ago, expresses the same frustration with the limitation of words.

"I reached down to pick up a newspaper and I couldn't get back up," she recalls. "Each time I tried, I felt as if something in my back was about to rip. It was like a vice grip, or a clamp, had attached itself to my lower spine, although nothing I say could adequately describe the fear, the sick feeling that welled up in my gut when I realized that a sensation of this intensity could be coming from within me."

A hot pack, a few muscle relaxants and two days in bed "cured" Judith Franklin of her episode with back pain and, mercifully, it has never returned with the same magnitude.

Acute Pain

Like the pain that all of us have felt – from toothache, childbirth, surgery, a cut or a bruise – Judith Franklin's experience falls into the category of "acute" pain. Acute pain can be terrible, like hers. Or it can be mild and merely irksome, a discomfort that you realize is over only after it has faded away.

The most obvious characteristic of acute pain is that it is short-lived. As well, acute pain usually serves a purpose, alerting the body to the fact that something is wrong. In some instances, that something is an infection; the pain alerts us to the fact that medication may be required. At other times, the pain from an injury, such as a strained back muscle, serves to protect us from making further movements which could exacerbate the injury. Acute pain can sometimes prevent injury by producing the lightning type of reflex action that causes us to remove a thumb from a hot stove *before* damage can take place. In all of these instances, the pain has a physical source that you can point a finger to, and physicians therefore say that it is "organic," in the sense that it emanates from an organ. Sometimes, however, acute pain occurs for reasons which cannot be explained; this phenomenon underscores the complexity of pain.

Chronic Pain

There is, of course, another type of pain. It is called "chronic pain" and it is very different in nature from acute pain. Chronic pain persists, lasting for many months and sometimes for years. Chronic pain serves no useful purpose; unlike most episodes of acute pain, it is not a warning sign at all.

In some cases, chronic pain is organic; its origins are obvious but, given the state of the art of medicine, nothing can be done to alleviate the misery it causes. In other cases, chronic pain continues long after the acute injury that caused it in the first place has healed. In still other cases, there never was an acute precursor; the origins of the pain are mysterious. In these situations, as in some cases of low back pain, the source of chronic pain may be tension, anxiety or stress, and the pain will be labelled "functional" or "psychogenic," its origin being the psyche. But pain whose origin is the psyche is as real as pain that has an organic source. The tension that tightens the muscles of the lower back can be just as painful as a tumour that is pressing against a nerve.

More important is the impact chronic pain can have on one's life. While acute pain can be debilitating, it is not *depressing* in the way that chronic pain can be. Acute pain can be severe enough to make you cry out for relief. But it does not change your personality or your perception of the world. People who are suffering from acute pain look forward to the moment when it will end. On the other hand, people who face chronic pain day after day, year after year, often come to feel as if they have donned a pair of "grey coloured glasses." They frequently lose their motivation to carry on. In many instances, fear, tension and anxiety are triggered by the pain, causing it to increase even more.

But sometimes, it is a person's emotional state that profoundly influences their chronic pain rather than the other way around. For example, a man with a relatively minor injury that nonetheless prevents him from working, may begin to feel useless, or "unmanly," and, as if to justify his state of inactivity, the subconscious intensifies the pain to a point that is far out of proportion to the injury. A woman with an inattentive husband may discover that when she is suffering from back pain, he comes home directly after work; ironically, it is in her best interest – or at least her subconscious' best interest – to have her back pain magnified. Or, a person who has been in a car accident and is awaiting a trial may find that the pain has increased in proportion to the possibility of financial gain. In all of these cases, however, the pain is *real*, not imagined. These people are not malingerers; they are not faking what they feel. Nevertheless, if there is a change in the situation or emotional state that has caused the pain to become magnified, it will often decrease.

The Statistics on Pain

The statistics on the number of people who face pain on a daily basis are shocking. According to Seattle anaesthesiologist Dr. John Bonica, the eminent researcher who founded the International Association for the Study of Pain, approximately a third of North Americans suffer from recurrent or persistent chronic pain. Other researchers have estimated that some 80 million North Americans suffer from chronic back pain. Said Dr. Bonica in a 1984 interview for *Time* magazine, "Chronic pain disables more people than cancer or heart disease and it costs the American people more money than both." By his calculations, chronic pain costs Americans $70 billion each year in medical costs, lost working days and compensation.

Pain – both acute and chronic – is the most common reason why people consult their physicians and take medication. In Canada, in 1980, almost $13 million worth of prescriptions for pain-killers were handed out. And yet, ironically, physicians have not been able to come up with a definition of pain which satisfies themselves, let alone their patients. Dr. Angela Mailis, a Toronto Western Hospital staff physician who is director of the hospital's Pain Investigation Unit, says that no one definition of pain means the same thing to everybody. "Pain," she says, "means one thing to the philosopher, another to the clinician, and yet another to the individual who is experiencing it."

Trying to Define Pain

The imperfect definition which most researchers believe works best is the one which London, Ontario, psychiatrist Dr. Harold Merskey has proposed. Dr. Merskey defines pain as "an unpleasant sensory and emotional experience associated with actual or potential tissue damage, or described in terms of such damage." While "unpleasant" is rather an understatement, the definition's strengths are two-fold. The first plus of Dr. Merskey's definition is that it allows for a *loose* association between the degree of injury and the amount of pain. In certain circumstances, a small injury will produce a lot of pain. In other circumstances, a severe injury will produce little pain. And sometimes, the mere memory of pain with no new injury at all will produce excruciating pain.

Second of all, Dr. Merskey's definition recognizes the *emotional* dimension of pain along with its sensory aspects. Pain hurts, but it also conjures up memories, fears, desperation and a whole host of other emotions that can make it seem even worse.

The Gate Control Theory of Pain

While Dr. Merskey can be credited for defining pain, another Canadian, McGill University professor of psychology Dr. Ronald Melzack, helped to change science's entire concept of pain. In 1965, he and British professor of anatomy Dr. Patrick Wall proposed the Gate Control Theory of Pain. Before that, scientists had believed that a person's perception of pain was on a one-to-one ratio with its source. In other words x amount of injury produced x amount of pain.

The Gate Control Theory introduced, for the first time, the concept of inequity where pain is concerned. Melzack and Wall proposed that the amount of pain "input" at the site of an injury need not be equal to the amount of pain that is felt when the message finally arrives, and is registered, in the brain.

For example, just because x amount of painful sensation is received by your big toe at the point where it has made contact with a big rock, does not necessarily mean that you will perceive x amount of pain. The perception of pain, said Melzack and Wall, can be *modified* on its way from the big toe to the brain. On one occasion, your brain might perceive more pain than would ordinarily be expected by such an impact. On another occasion, less pain might be perceived.

Basically, what Melzack and Wall were proposing was this: that by the time a pain message runs along a nerve fibre to the spinal cord, then up the cord to a centre in the brain called the thalamus, then farther along to the cerebral cortex (where pain becomes defined and emotional components are added), the original message may have become altered. What was doing the alteration, they proposed, was a "pain gate," hence the name Gate Control Theory of Pain. When the pain gate is completely open, they theorized, pain messages would breeze through to the brain with the speed of Mercury. When the pain gate was *partly* open, pain sensations of a diminished quality would get through. If the pain gate was completely closed, however, no pain messages at all would find their way up to the brain.

Even before the Gate Control Theory was proposed, researchers knew that soldiers in battle, or players in the middle of a crucial game, could be suffering from tremendous injuries without feeling any pain. They also knew, as I have mentioned earlier, that people with minor injuries could be suffering great amounts of pain. What they lacked was a theory to explain how this could be so. Melzack and Wall's theory did just that: the soldier felt no pain because his pain gate was shut. At the same time, the theory accounted for those back pain patients who had very minor amounts of discernible pathology but tremendous amounts of pain. If a closed gate could prohibit pain messages from getting through to the brain, a wide open gate would facilitate their arrival. No physiological "gate" has ever been found, however, and now, 20 years later, researchers know that the mechanisms of pain are far more complex than Melzack and Wall first proposed.

The Anatomy of a Pain Message

The basics of the physiological mechanisms that transfer a pain message from the big toe to the brain are not difficult to understand. Nor are the basic principles behind the mechanisms that might alter these messages en route. Many physicians who work with chronic pain patients take the time to explain these mechanisms to their patients. It is now known that, in some cases at least, understanding these mechanisms can help chronic pain sufferers to gain control of their pain.

Take, as the example, the big toe which has made contact with a big rock. At the turn of the century, researchers had the notion that pain messages from the big toe were transmitted *uninterrupted* from the toe to the brain. You stubbed the toe and "presto" — the message zoomed along a nerve fibre to the spine and up the spine to the cerebral cortex where it was perceived as mild, or severe, depending upon the quality of the altercation with the rock.

Today, scientists know that this concept is faulty. Pain messages from the big toe do not run non-stop all the way to the brain. They travel from the toe only as far as the dorsal horn, an area which runs the entire length of the spinal cord (see Diagram 22). At this point, there is a gap in each nerve fibre called a synapse.

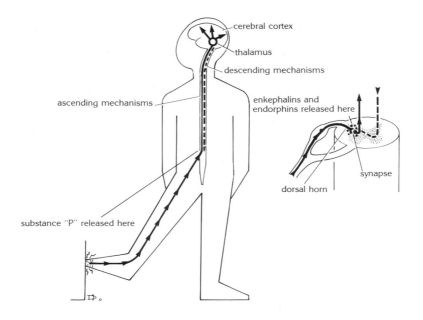

Diagram 22   Transmission of Pain

If a message from the big toe is going to travel to the brain, it must bridge this synapse. It can do this only when a chemical, called a neurotransmitter, is produced within the nerve fibre and excreted at the synapse. There it acts like a biochemical ferry, transmitting the message to the next nerve fibre. The message can then travel up the spinal cord to the thalamus where a second synapse is found.

The thalamus is where we first become conscious of a sensation and respond with what is called a reflex reaction, a sort of black and white, all or nothing response that causes such behaviour as the rapid withdrawal of the toe from the rock. This, however, is not the end of the message's journey. From here, it must bridge a third synapse in order to travel to the cerebral cortex where the location of the sensation and its intensity is perceived. The cortex is also the place that adds the "colour" to the picture, making decisions about the appropriate cognitive response. Taking into account emotional states and past experiences with pain, it consults its roster of possible replies and picks one, or more.

Frequently, the cortex decides that the appropriate reaction is to scream, or cry out, or wring the hands in woe. Sometimes, however, it may decide that it is more important to get on with the war, or winning the game, in which case no response to the pain message will occur because no pain will be felt.

When Melzack and Wall first proposed their Gate Control Theory, the first synapse at the dorsal horn was where they thought the pain gate was located. In fact, there are several places along the route where a pain message can be altered on its way to the cerebral cortex.

To understand how a pain message can be altered, it is necessary to learn about the journey in chemical terms. If you cut the nerve to the big toe cross-sectionally and look at it under a microscope, you'll see some interesting things. First of all, you'll see many bundles, each of which contains huge numbers of nerve fibres. There are many different types and sizes of fibres. Some carry sensory messages such as touch, heat and cold. Others carry pain messages. At the toe end of all fibres are receptors, which receive the messages that are constantly coming in.

Specific receptors called nociceptors at the end of certain small fibres *receive* pain messages; these small fibres conduct these pain messages. At the end of larger fibres are mechanoreceptors which receive sensations such as touch and pressure, and thermoreceptors which receive sensations such as warmth; these larger fibres conduct these messages.

During a normal walk down a normal path, minutes before the inevitable collision of the toe with the big rock, both types of receptors are busy picking up sensations from the world. They are also "firing," meaning that the messages they are picking up are travelling along the fibres at a normal rate.

What is perceived by the brain — soft earth, a warm breeze — is based on the premise that only a certain amount of sensory information can be processed by the nervous system at any one time. In normal circumstances, the large fibres fire at a higher rate than the small fibres, and the incoming sensations from them dominate. In other words, the sensations of soft earth and a warm breeze prevail. The relatively few sensations travelling along the small pain fibres are ignored.

Things change very rapidly, however, when the big toe meets up with the big rock. Very quickly, at the point of contact, a number of potent chemicals are produced. One is called brandykinin. It sensitizes the pain fibres, and their firing rate increases dramatically. Other chemicals are called prostaglandins. They, too, sensitize the pain fibres in order to increase their firing rate, but prostaglandins have another job as well. They increase circulation to the big toe, causing swelling, or inflammation. Infection-fighting white blood cells are attracted to the area. They reduce inflammation and fight any bacteria that have entered the system. As well, inside the fibres, a powerful neurotransmitter is being produced. It is called Substance "P", the *P* standing for Pain.

By now, the situation in the dorsal horn will have changed. Far more messages will be coursing along the small pain fibres than along the large sensory fibres, and this is where the Gate Control Theory comes into play. Since only a certain amount of information can be perceived at any one time, a choice must be made. Will it be the messages from the large fibres, or the ones from the small? Before the big toe's close encounter with the big rock, there was no contest. Now, however, the picture has changed. As a result of brandykinin and prostaglandins, the small fibres are firing at a far greater rate than the large fibres.

Now, far more messages from the small fibres than the large fibres are arriving at the dorsal horn. In Melzack and Wall's terms, the pain gate is open. Perceptions of soft earth and a warm breeze fall by the wayside. The small fibres have a monopoly on the situation and the predominant message – the one that is perceived – is PAIN.

Up the dorsal horn they go, and if they are strong enough, they bridge the second synapse at the thalamus. Here pain is first perceived, although at this point, it is as colourless as a dull November sky. Reflex reactions such as the instant withdrawal of the big toe occur. But it is not until the pain messages bridge the next synapse to the cerebral cortex that cognitive sensations like "severe" and responses like "ouch," or rubbing the sore toe, occur. And sometimes these responses are very different from what one would expect.

For example, if someone is afraid of pain, perhaps because of a memory of pain in the past, the cerebral cortex may intensify the sensation. Anxiety, or stress, about the impact the pain may have on one's life can do the same thing. People also learn responses to pain from their parents as youngsters; in some cultures, people learn to tolerate quite high amounts of pain with little response, and the cortex is "aware" of this propensity. In other cultures, people are vociferous about their aches and pains. Studies have shown that Jews, for example, tend to be concerned about the meaning of pain; if they can discover the cause, or understand its mechanisms, its functional aspects will often subside to some degree. Italians seem to be more interested in immediate relief, the underlying cause being of less consequence than this goal.

On the other hand, positive thoughts or emotions can reduce the amount of pain that is perceived. The anticipation of a meeting with an old friend, or a large cheque waiting in the mailbox at the end of the path, are reasons why the cerebral cortex may not perceive the pain as severe. In parts of India, hooks embedded in the flesh of the back during ceremonial rituals cause no pain at all! These decisions, however, are not made consciously. They are within the realm of the subconscious, that vast, largely unexplored recess which is more complex than any human-built computer.

The physiology of pain modification is far from completely understood. But basically, scientists believe that there are two ways that pain can be reduced once it has begun. Either the impulses that are coursing along the small pain fibres can be inhibited, or decreased. Or, the input into the large fibres can be facilitated, or increased. The latter, if great enough, can over-ride the input into the small fibres, preventing its transmission.

Rubbing the sore toe, for example, will result in increased firing of the large fibres which conduct the sensations of touch and warmth. A hotpack can accomplish the same thing. According to the Gate Control Theory, if you rub the toe hard enough, the messages in the large fibres will over-ride the messages in the small fibres, thus opening the large fibre gate and closing the small. The electrical stimulation of a TENS machine (see page 148) is thought to work on this principle. A recent study of manipulation (see page 194) suggests that it, too, may accomplish this feat.

Decreasing the firing rate of the small fibres can accomplish the same end. When you take an aspirin tablet, for example, the production of prostaglandins is inhibited, thereby reducing the firing rate of the small fibres. Other analgesic drugs, such as morphine and related opiates, also reduce the firing rate of the small fibres but work in a different way.

Endorphins and Enkephalins

Research into the anatomy and physiology of pain blossomed during the late 1960s and 1970s, and as more and more information emerged, many researchers abandoned some of Melzack and Wall's conclusions. No one failed to stress, however, that it was the Gate Control Theory of Pain which was responsible for this new research. Because of it, new concepts, which illustrate that pain is a much more complex phenomenon than Ronald Melzack and Patrick Wall originally thought, have emerged. Most researchers have ceased to think of the "gate" as a physical entity to continue searching for; rather, it has become more of a metaphor, a symbol of the fact that the body can modify pain messages.

One of the major breakthroughs occurred in 1975. In that year, it was established how morphine, and other opiates, work. The research was done by a group of Americans who had been convinced for some time that morphine worked as a pain-killer because of the existence of special "opiate receptors" throughout the nervous system. The molecular structure of these opiate receptors was thought to be the biochemical *opposite* of the structure of opiates; in other words, a morphine molecule could fit into an opiate receptor molecule like a key fits into a lock. In 1975, these receptors were found.

Because of this research, a question was begged: Why would the body have developed these opiate receptors when humans don't go around ingesting morphine day after day? The answer to this question – which was the third major breakthrough in the area of pain research – was discovered by University of Aberdeen pharmacologists John Hughes and Hans Kosterlitz.

Hughes and Kosterlitz postulated that the purpose of the opiate receptors was to receive powerful, pain-killing, opiate-like chemicals that the human body itself produced, and that's what they decided to look for. When they found them, they called them endorphins and enkephalins. Enkephalins were found in the pituitary gland of the brain, endorphins in the brain and the spinal cord itself.

Finding these chemicals changed the way scientists thought about pain yet again. Not only was it possible for messages on the way up to the brain to be altered (by stimulation of the large fibres, for example), but, if analgesic chemicals were being produced up top, there must be *descending* mechanisms that could alter pain messages as well.

Some researchers talked about the endorphin discovery in terms of a sequel to Melzack and Wall's Gate Control Theory. They postulated that the stimulation of large nerve fibres was causing endorphins to be produced. Once produced, they would inhibit the production of brandykinin and prostaglandins, thus decreasing the firing rate of the small fibres.

Other researchers, however, explained the mechanisms of endorphins as an alternative, rather than a sequel, to the Gate Control Theory of Pain. They were also beginning to see that the mechanisms which control pain are so complex that, with the discovery of these opiates, more questions were arising than were being answered. When, a few years later, several other opiates and some non-opiate pain-altering chemicals were discovered, the mechanism of pain blurred again, rendering the field more complex than anyone had ever dreamed.

The research continues. Some scientists are searching for analgesics that can be received by the body's opiate receptors but are not addictive like morphine. Other researchers are looking for drugs that may activate the body's non-opiate descending systems.

Still others are responding by searching for a drugless answer. In the same *Time* magazine article, Dr. Bonica talks about his vision of a day when people will look to their own innate mental powers to relieve themselves of pain. "I don't think it takes too much scientific license to say that we will discover mental activities that can produce specific analgesia," he says. "In 10 or 15 years, perhaps we can begin to teach people to control their own pain."

Already, the results of a number of studies have shed at least some light on the issue of chronic pain.

For example, research suggests that people with healed back injuries who continue to suffer pain could perhaps be deficient in their ability to produce endorphins and other pain-decreasing chemicals. Those who advocate acupuncture, for example, theorize that in some instances, the treatment may "kick a faulty endorphin system back into gear." Indeed, experiments conducted at the University of Toronto on the brain cells of cats have shown that acupuncture causes endorphins to be produced.

In many people whose lives have been dominated by pain for a long time, depression sets in. Some studies indicate that depression can cause endorphin production to decrease.

Other studies have shown that chronic pain can cause the small nerve fibres to become "sensitized." Whereas, in normal circumstances, a certain amount of painful stimuli are necessary to provoke the perception of pain, much less is required by a sensitized fibre. When the firing rate of fibres is abnormally high for an extended period of time, just a small amount of additional input will be enough to tip it over the edge.

Other studies have associated the efficacy of placebo pills with endorphins. *Placebo* is Latin for "I will please." Doctors have found that when patients are given placebo pills – usually they contain nothing but sugar which, of course, is meaningless as a drug – their pain is decreased about a third of the time. Researchers at the University of California in San Francisco have shown that placebo pills can stimulate the body's endorphin system. Some studies show that jogging, and other activities which the participant finds relaxing, can also stimulate the production of endorphins. Other studies have shown that laughter, too, can stimulate the body to produce endorphins.

Pain Clinics

In medical school, doctors are taught precious little about pain other than which diseases typically cause pain and what sort of pain they cause. When he conducted a survey of 17 standard medical textbooks in 1983, Dr. Bonica found only 54 pages out of a total of 22,000 that even discussed pain.

As a result of the paucity of their knowledge, many doctors feel uncomfortable with chronic pain patients for whom they can find no, or little, organic cause for pain. Some doctors dismiss such patients as neurotic. Many chronic pain patients have found themselves wandering from specialist to specialist, in search of a non-existent magical cure.

Fortunately, at least some of these people find help at one of the world's approximately 150 multidisciplinary pain clinics, the majority of whose patients suffer from chronic back pain. The sole criterion for entry is chronic pain. Generally speaking, the duration of that pain must be six months at least, although the average pain clinic patient has been suffering much longer than that.

Many pain clinics focus on teaching patients how to *manage* their pain. They are staffed by a variety of health care practitioners from a variety of disciplines. For instance, Dr. Carl von Baeyer, who is a clinical psychologist, consults to the Pain Management Service at University Hospital in Saskatoon.

"Our efforts are spent on controlling pain, minimizing its disruptive effects on patients' lives without necessarily expecting it to be cured," he says. "Patients must learn to accept responsibility for much of their own progress." The physicians and other health care workers at a pain clinic act as teachers and consultants, the patients being active as opposed to passive, which is what the word *patient* means. "The goal," says Dr. von Baeyer, "is self-reliance."

The concept of the multidisciplinary pain clinic was pioneered in the early 1960s by Dr. Bonica. From his experiences in dealing with wounded World War II combat soldiers, he realized that if the management of chronic pain was going to be successful, the knowledge and perspectives of professionals from many disciplines would need to be used. He honed his theories at the University of Washington Medical Center's Clinical Pain Service in Seattle. Today, most major North American cities have at least one pain clinic, usually at a teaching hospital. To become a patient, a chronic pain sufferer must have a referral from a general practitioner. Often there is a waiting time of several months.

Some pain clinics are literally "clinics," the members of the team having offices under the same roof. In other cases, physicians, psychologists, nurses, physiotherapists, social workers, occupational therapists, dance and movement therapists, chiropractors, dieticians and dentists get together to collaborate but, usually due to financial constraints, do not have a building to call their own.

If you were to visit a pain clinic, your first appointment would be co-ordinated by one of the team members, often a psychologist or a nurse. The first visit would not seem all that different from any other visit to a doctor: a physician takes a medical history and conducts a clinical diagnosis, ordering X-rays and other tests if necessary. Medications are reviewed. But here is where the similarity ends. At a multidisciplinary pain clinic, patients see a psychologist, psychiatrist, or social worker. Says Dr. von Baeyer, "The emotional aspects of chronic pain must be assessed." In most cases, family members are interviewed as well.

When the information has been collected, the pain team will meet to form a plan. At many centres, patients are encouraged to attend this conference so that they can begin to take control right from the start.

In some centres, four groups are used to "type" patients. The first group, into which only 10 to 20 per cent of chronic pain patients seem to fit, is the "organic" group. For these people, the source of the pain is obvious – although not always curable – and while there may be emotional and psychological overtones to the pain, they are minimal. In the fourth group are the one to two per cent of individuals who are "malingering." They feel no pain. They, themselves, don't even think they feel pain. A much rarer phenomenon than it was thought to be in the past, malingerers are simply lying for one reason or another.

The great majority of chronic pain sufferers fall into the other two groups. Their pain has both an organic and a functional, or psychological, source. In some cases, the ratio is about half and half. In other cases, the organic source is minimal while the functional source has become very large. The results of a recent study conducted at a Boston pain clinic showed that about two-thirds of its patients had significant pain relief as a result of their experience. (A year later, 75 per cent had maintained their gains.) Says Dr. Mailis, "The ones with the large organic source and the minimal functional source make the most gains. When social, financial and emotional factors are involved in the generation or magnification of the pain syndrome, it is very hard to find a treatment."

Part and parcel of the treatment plan at a typical pain clinic is the contract that the patient, the patient's spouse if there is one, and the treatment co-ordinator all sign. Several specific goals are sought: working toward managing the pain without drugs; recognizing and adjusting to the limitations of the pain; decreasing the importance of the pain relative to the rest of the person's life; and being able to accept an occasional increase in pain without becoming frightened and without seeing the increase as a sign that the pain is once again taking control.

Some programs last for a couple of weeks, others for several months. Some are conducted on an in-patient basis, but most people are able to continue living at home.

Patients attend educational sessions, relaxation training sessions and physiotherapy sessions in which better posture and exercises are learned. Many of these sessions are held in groups so that people with chronic pain can share their experiences with others in similar circumstances. It is essential to learn which activities provoke pain, how long it usually lasts, and what techniques work to diminish it.

Where back pain is concerned, techniques such as hypnosis, or relaxation exercises, are almost always used to help people cope with tension and stress. TENS machines and acupuncture are often used to reduce pain. But far more important is changing people's attitudes toward pain, teaching them how to make it less intimidating. Just as stress and tension can exacerbate pain, decreasing tension can work the opposite way.

Above all, patients who have been sitting around focusing on their pain are kept busy. Each day has a purpose and at the end of it they usually can sleep. Says Dr. Mailis, "People who are busy and diverted don't feel their pain quite as much." The principle is the same as the soldier busy with his battle or the athlete who is concentrating on winning the game.

Gary Birk, a 50-year-old chemical engineer sought help at a Toronto pain clinic after four years of constant low back pain. He had injured his back when he fell off a ladder while painting his eaves. When it failed to improve, his back pain ultimately cost him his job.

"When it seemed like my marriage was about to go the same route, I was ready to try anything," he says.

When Gary Birk was assessed, it was felt that while there was definitely an organic component to his back pain, it was also being magnified by functional factors. At first he was more than a bit intimidated by the idea that even a part of his pain was psychological. "I didn't understand that 'functional' pain is as real as 'organic' pain," he says. "I thought that the psychological part was unacceptable, that any mature person should be able to beat it on their own. Learning that functional pain produces pain messages in the cortex of the brain that are as real as the messages produced by an organic source validated it for me. I think it also helped my wife to understand my pain better. And it helped us both to see the kinds of behaviour patterns we had fallen into." Two years had passed since Gary Birk had lifted a bag of groceries, mowed the lawn or washed a dish.

Within four months, Gary Birk was back to work part time. Now, a year later, he is employed full time. He is faithful to the daily exercise program he was taught during his three months at the pain clinic. He is careful about his posture, particularly while sitting at his desk, and when he feels tension building, he can usually reduce it with self-hypnosis. "I wouldn't say that I don't have any back pain," he says by way of evaluating his pain clinic experience. "What I would say is that the back pain I do have no longer dominates my life. I hurt to some extent, but I'm not afraid of hurting. I know that the slightest twinge is not going to mean that my life is once again ruined. I even do a couple of things like gardening and bicycling that increase my pain for about a day. I do them because I like them; it's worth it to me. You could say, I guess, that because of my experience I recognize the patterns of my back pain. I know what will cause it to increase and how long it will take to subside. I know that for me, the drop in barometric pressure before a storm is difficult to cope with because it's something I can't control. But I also know that it will pass. I know the difference between hurt and harm. I guess you could say that it is I, rather than it, who is in control."

4

Some Practical Advice for Dealing with Health Care Professionals

"After ten years and probably as many doctors," says Mary Gardstein, a 45-year-old librarian, "it has finally dawned on me that in many respects, I know as much about what is happening to my back as they do. I know when my back pain is worse because of stress. I know when I need more exercise, less exercise, more rest, or less rest. I know when I've done something really stupid – like shifting a piece of heavy furniture on my own because I was too impatient to wait for help. I know when taking pain-killers for a few days is the only thing that will work . . . . What I am saying, basically, is that I no longer seek out doctors with the preconceived notion that they know everything and I know nothing. Instead, when I do go, it's with my bit of knowledge that I hope to combine with their bit of knowledge. You might say that I think of doctors as 'consultants.' Hopefully, what we come up with together will be greater than the sum of each of the two parts."

Dr. Ahmed Sakoor has a family practice in Toronto which includes many back pain sufferers. While some members of his profession might have a tendency to feel intimidated by comments such as Mary Gardstein's, Dr. Sakoor is thrilled to hear someone express such a responsible attitude toward her own health.

"Patients have to remember that when it comes to back pain, we're operating in a very grey area," he says. "Nothing is more frustrating to me as a professional than a person with a back problem who walks into my office with the attitude 'You're the doc – *you* tell me what's wrong and what to do' without giving me the slightest clue about what is going on."

Clearly, the relationship between doctors and their patients has been undergoing some changes in recent years, mostly because patients have been honing their skills as consumers.

In the United States, for instance, some medical schools have responded to this new patient attitude by *requiring* students to enroll in courses that teach them how to develop, and maintain, good rapport with their patients.

In Canada, such undergraduate "communications courses" are, for the most part, voluntary. It is not until they reach the post-graduate level that most doctors receive in-depth education in the area of doctor-patient rapport.

Most two-year residency training programs in family medicine stress the importance of the doctor-patient relationship. Many of these programs aid students by videotaping examining sessions so that young doctors can actually see how they are coming across and where they could improve. The emphasis is on dealing with patients as human beings rather than as "units" to be moved through a system. "The new philosophy," says Dr. Sakoor, "is that patients are entitled to as much information about tests and procedures as they feel they need."

Your Relationship with Your GP

While the attitudes of doctors are certainly less paternalistic than they have been in the past, it seems that in some cases at least, their evolution has not been as rapid as ours. When it comes to their relationship with their general practitioners, chronic back pain sufferers seem to have two major grievances.

The first is that while doctors' *intentions* may have improved, communication skills (especially in the case of specialists) are still not their strong suit. The second most common complaint of patients is that general practitioners are sometimes poor treatment co-ordinators. Most patients feel that their GP should be taking the responsibility of co-ordinating their treatment: making sure that records and test results are sent, in advance, to any specialist who may be consulted; and taking the final responsibility for ensuring that anything a specialist discovers is explained to them in plain English.

When it comes to the issue of communication, it's often difficult to lay blame. In many cases, patients' descriptions of visits to the doctor are so jumbled, that it is impossible to sift through the rubble to determine exactly how and when communication broke down. The scenario that was typical of a visit to the doctor by Mary Gardstein, before her metamorphosis ten years ago, illustrates the point.

" . . . I would leave my doctor's office with all sorts of new information about what was causing my back pain," she recalls. "I'd have in my mind what he was going to do about it, how long it was going to take until I could see some results, and what we were going to try next if that didn't work. . . . I would start to tell my husband about it over dinner and suddenly, you know, my mind would go blank. What was that term he had used to describe my problem? [The term was *spinal stenosis* but, at the time, all Mary Gardstein could remember was that it sounded like *stenographer*!]

What had he said about the medication he was going to prescribe? Something about possible side effects and taking the drug with meals, but I honestly couldn't remember what. What side effects had he said I should call him about immediately?"

"First ask yourself some questions," says Dr. Sakoor. "Did your doctor express himself, or herself, well? Did he speak plainly or use a lot of medical jargon? Did he seem open to questions? Did he try to clarify concepts you found difficult? Did he seem happy to give you all the time you needed?"

If your answer to most of these questions is no, the only reasonable choice might be to find a new doctor. But if most of the answers are yes, and you are still finding yourself in situations like the one Mary Gardstein describes, then some more questions should be asked.

"Have you ever considered bringing along a small notepad when you visit your doctor?" Dr. Sakoor suggests. At the time you might believe that the four-syllable word used to describe your condition – spondylolisthesis at six syllables is a wonderful example – will remain imprinted in your brain for life, but it's a better idea to write these things down. In the case of chronic back pain sufferers, this ritual is especially important since so many of the terms used to describe back conditions (spondylitis, spondylolysis and spondylosis, for example) sound similar.

"In fact, it's not a bad idea to write down a number of things," says Dr. Sakoor. He lists as examples: side effects of medication; length of hospital stay if there is to be a trip to the hospital for either tests or treatment; and when you can expect to go back to work.

Sarah Miles, a back pain sufferer who works as a waitress, is a good example of someone who would have benefited from taking notes. She went into hospital for some "minor surgery" on her foot, which was contributing to her back pain. It *was* minor. But it also required her to wear a foot cast for several weeks. Her doctor, perhaps not realizing that her job required her to be on her feet, had not told Sarah exactly when she could go back to work. Focusing on the word *minor*, Sarah hadn't thought to ask!

Another good idea is to write down some questions *before* your visit when you're more relaxed and clear-headed. Some people make a checklist and cross questions off as they come to them. "It's up to you to tell us if you can't understand what's being explained," says Dr. Sakoor. "It's also up to you to ask again if it's not registering. Confirm that you understand what is being said by repeating the answer in your own words: 'Are you saying that my chances for recovery are excellent, around 90 per cent, and that if you were in my position you'd go for it?' is not as silly as it might seem."

It is also not silly to give your doctor the information necessary for a proper diagnosis. Most patients obviously think they are doing just that. But many doctors feel that patients frequently edit information – perhaps, in some cases, because they feel pressured not to take up too much of their physician's time.

But there are other reasons, too, why some patients withhold information. Says Dr. Sakoor, "Patients often don't want to tell me that they've already had a certain test, because it came back normal the first time. Their hope is that if the test is repeated, it will come back positive the second time, and there will be something concrete to substantiate the very real pain they've been experiencing.

"What they don't realize is that with back pain, almost 80 per cent of the diagnostic tests I order come back normal. X-rays and blood tests for back pain don't mean all that much, except to rule out the rare possibilities such as infection. High technology is not always the answer for diagnosing a back problem . . . . If nothing shows up on a test, we're not saying that you're making this up or that there isn't really any reason for your pain. We're just saying, okay, now we know that a CT Scan doesn't show us anything, so let's go on to something else. Or let's stop worrying about exactly *what* is wrong and start treating the symptoms. I don't mean pain-killers when I say this. I just mean that many treatments for back pain are general. If, for example, physiotherapy is going to work, it probably doesn't matter all that much if we determine whether your facet joint problem is at the L5-S1 or at the L4-L5 level. The same exercise program, mobilization, or heat treatments will work in either case.

"In the end," Dr. Sakoor stresses, "What I need to go along with the signs I find is a good subjective description from the patient."

If you're wondering whether or not you have been providing such a description, consider these aspects of a back problem:

• Does exercise help you, or make you worse?

• Are some days better than other days, or is your pain constantly the same?

• If some days are worse than other days, what is happening on the bad days? Bad weather? A bad night's sleep? Too much sleep? (Some conditions are actually exacerbated by lying too long in one position.) Or did your boss come back from his three-week trip out of town?

"This is all valuable information," says Dr. Sakoor. "Sometimes I find out months after the fact that my patient's marriage was on the verge of collapse or that he was in terrible financial shape. I think patients worry that we'll dismiss their back trouble as 'just stress' if they tell us about their emotional problems. In fact, that's not it at all. It's just that with a back problem, stress is bound to affect what is going on and it helps us to know."

The issue of the general practitioner's role as treatment co-ordinator is also complex. Ensuring that any specialist who is called in gets briefed in advance and that the specialist's report is explained clearly to the patient is not always as easy as it seems.

Says Dr. Sakoor, "Having your family practitioner act as treatment co-ordinator is ideal. And yes, time constraints notwithstanding, it is the general practitioner's responsibility to ensure that a specialist has all the necessary background information about your case when you arrive.

"But, difficult as it may be to believe, it is sometimes impossible for me to get reports back right away from a specialist. I've had cases where the patient has actually been recovering from back surgery before *anything* from the surgeon has reached my hands. I can telephone. And the communication will generally be better if we both have privileges in the same hospital and work together frequently. But the ability of a family practitioner to influence a specialist to send reports or test results quickly, or return phone calls right away, is sometimes more limited than many patients realize."

Don't Be Intimidated by a Specialist

Where the patient is concerned, Dr. Sakoor suggests the same technique for dealing with a specialist as a family practitioner. Go in with written questions. Take your time. Be polite but firm. If you don't understand something that is being explained to you, ask for it to be repeated. Says Mary Gardstein, "It may be difficult to get used to the idea of being firm with a doctor, especially a specialist who can be pretty intimidating. But once you've tried it, you'll get to like it. And you'll kick yourself for not having done it years ago."

Mary Gardstein's account of her first brave venture in the role of confident consumer is amusing, as well as edifying.

"It happened one day when I went to see a new orthopaedic surgeon. It was one of those delightful conversations that we have all had in our heads but that never come true. I was feeling particularly good that day, fairly pain-free, and I guess, because of that, I was less vulnerable than usual. Perhaps, I've since thought, no one should go to see a doctor for the first time when they're ill!"

Mary Gardstein walked in, gave the nurse her insurance number and filled in a few forms. Then she was led into a small examining room and asked if she would like to undress. "Much to my surprise I found myself saying 'No thank you, I wouldn't!' The nurse looked at me a little quizzically and I added for emphasis, 'I don't generally take my clothes off for someone I haven't yet met!'"

A few moments later, the surgeon walked in. He looked even more surprised than the nurse. "I offered my hand for him to shake, saying

'How do you do?' in that tone of voice that really means, 'Won't you have a seat?' Since I was sitting in the only chair in the room, he ended up on the examining table while *I* asked the first half dozen questions. We've had an excellent relationship ever since!"

What are those half dozen questions? Most of them have to do with the issues Dr. Sakoor has already touched on. Some apply to specialists in particular, others to any doctor you might see:

• Ask all doctors which hospital, or hospitals, they have privileges in. (One of the advantages of a teaching hospital is that it is likely to have the latest equipment. One disadvantage – if it bothers you – is that you will likely be asked to submit to examinations by interns and residents as well as your own doctors.)

• Ask about house calls. As a rule, specialists do not make them, and only a few general practitioners still consider house calls to be part of what they bargained for when they took the Hippocratic oath. Some general practitioners restrict house calls to their elderly patients. Others avoid house calls completely, believing that true emergencies should be dealt with by hospitals.

• If you're seeing a general practitioner for the first time, ask which specialists he or she uses. Your best bet is to choose a family physician who has a group of specialists (orthopaedic surgeon, neurosurgeon, general surgeon, urologist, internist, gynaecologist), all of whom work out of the same hospital.

• You may also be interested to know which types of "Continuing Medical Education" courses your doctor opts to take? For Mary Gardstein, it was important that her doctor be the type of person who was interested in at least some of the less orthodox alternatives, such as acupuncture and hypnosis. "It wasn't important to me that he be a *specialist* in all of these procedures," she says. "But had he been unable, or unwilling, to discuss these approaches, or had he dismissed them as bunk, I hope that I would have had the guts to leave."

• You may also want to know if your doctor takes phone calls during the day. Some doctors prefer to save up their messages and return everyone's phone calls at the end of the day. A bit of advice is to keep a piece of paper with your questions near the phone so that when your doctor finally does return your call, you are prepared to be concise. "Having the ability to keep it to the point," says Dr. Sakoor, "can be to your advantage when your doctor has a list of calls to return that's half a mile long."

Says Mary Gardstein, "The key is to think of yourself as an equal. My doctor has six years of medical training, which I don't have. But I have the same amount of training as a librarian, which he doesn't have. If he came to me wanting a computer search on disc disease, I would treat him with respect. He'd be a customer. I expect to be treated the same way and perhaps because I expect it, I get it."

5

Drug Addiction: Facing the Possibility

At a July 1981 meeting of the Canadian Medical Association at Halifax, Nova Scotia, drug abuse among patients was cited as one of the greatest problems facing the medical profession today. It is particularly a problem for doctors whose practices include a large number of patients with chronic back pain.

"There isn't a prescription medication that's really good for chronic pain," says Dr. Marion McIntosh, head of family and community medicine at the Addiction Research Foundation in Toronto. "Life becomes one big sleep for people when they're on all those strong prescription pills."

How Addiction Begins

The chronic back pain patient's scenario is so typical that you can practically predict what someone will say about drugs. The story told by Howard Lang, a forty-three-year-old accountant, nicely sums up the drug experience of the long-term back pain sufferer: "My back has troubled me off and on for several years, mostly on for the last two. In the beginning, I'd take a couple of aspirins every few hours when the pain was really bad. During one particularly difficult episode that lasted several months, I began to take between four and six 222's a day. Looking back, I guess I'd have been better off taking a few days off work. But you know how it is with deadlines and pressure. I went to my doctor. I think he felt a little sorry for me and perhaps a bit frustrated. He prescribed 292's and I promised to take it easy."

That time, Howard Lang was lucky. His back pain settled down within a few weeks and he stopped popping the pills. But six months later, he found himself back up the chronic creek, so to speak.

"It was tax time. I had a lot of stress at work. I couldn't shake that pain and I didn't have time to go to bed. I convinced my doctor to give me Percodan, a really strong pain-killer similar to morphine. I was on Percodan for three days when I had my wisdom teeth out and they'd worked great then. A couple of weeks later, my doctor went on holidays. My orthopaedic surgeon, who didn't know about the first prescription, gave me a second prescription for Percodan. He also suggested that Robaxisal, a muscle relaxant that also contains aspirin, might work better and wrote out a prescription for that. When my GP returned, I managed to get a third prescription for Percodan. He didn't know about the second one. For a couple of months there I was taking Percodan, 222's and Robaxisal every day."

How does this happen? Howard Lang is neither stupid, nor unaware of the potential for addiction where these drugs are concerned. And what about his doctors?

Dr. McIntosh has seen many drug-addicted back pain patients who have been taking 292's, Tylenol 2 or Percodan over a long period of time. "The physicians who did the original prescribing are not bad doctors," she stresses. "Often, they only want to save their patients from what they know can be excruciating discomfort." They prescribe these drugs, intending them to be used for short-term relief, and they are unaware that another doctor is prescribing the same thing.

Says Howard Lang, "My orthopaedic surgeon didn't ask me what my GP had prescribed, and I didn't offer the information. If he had asked, I can't say for sure, but I just possibly might have lied. When my back pain is at its worst, I care far more about masking it than the possibility of addiction."

"Patients can sometimes be very suave about their pain and multiple other things," says Dr. McIntosh. "And once patients are on the pill-popping road, it's difficult to get them off."

"It's a bit like smoking," says Howard Lang. "Even though you have a lot of motivation to stop — I mean, you can read; you know the possible consequences — there's still the desire to take just one more. I guess it's somewhat of a compulsion. You're controlled by the drug a little bit. But just a little bit. You don't want to admit more than that even to yourself."

Dependence on drugs prescribed for pain can be either physical or psychological. You may not be aware that you are physically in need of a drug like Percodan until you are taken off it. At that point, you *may* experience some or all of the classic narcotic withdrawal symptoms (sweating at first, followed by tremulousness, stomach cramps, diarrhea, runny nose and nasal congestion), or you may not. Some people can use high doses of drugs like Percodan and *not* become physically dependent, even over periods of time that would normally be expected to produce that response.

How can this be? "That's a question I think a lot of people would like to be able to answer," says Dr. McIntosh.

Those people who do not have a tendency to fall victim to physiological dependence do usually succumb to what doctors call a psychological dependence. This is generally described as a yearning for the drug without any of the physical components. People often feel a desire to take another pill, even though the level of pain on a particular day doesn't warrant it.

Howard Lang can testify to that. "Something in your *rational* brain clicks off. I have friends who describe the same sort of feeling when they're on a diet and the hostess walks in with the chocolate cake. You're sorry afterward and you make all sorts of promises to yourself about never doing it again. But while it's happening, it's as if you're not really all there. With a pain-killer, it's even easier to 'fall off the wagon.' It takes five minutes to eat a piece of chocolate cake, but only a second to pop a pill."

How can you recognize if you are developing a dependence — at least a psychological one — on a drug prescribed for pain? The hallmark of psychological dependence is generally described by clinical pharmacologists as a "striving for some effect of the drug itself, either euphoria or sedation, as well as relief from pain." In other words, if you take a drug and then wait for the buzz, you should seriously consider the possibility that you have a psychological addiction. And, if you get to the point where you are taking twice as much of a drug as the prescribed dose — two tablets every two hours instead of every four — you'd be crazy not to do some serious thinking.

A Family Member Can Sometimes Help

Often, as was the case with Howard Lang, a family member is the first one to become aware that "something fishy is going on."

"My wife began to notice that I was drowsy awfully early in the evening," he says. "I'd dismiss her remarks, saying that I'd had a few beers after work. But she knew I'd never been much of a social drinker."

If you do suspect that a family member or a friend is using too much of a drug, you might call your pharmacist for help. Most doctors stress that there is a fine line between violating confidentiality and just seeking advice. They suggest that you start the conversation by saying, "My spouse may be increasing his medication without the doctor's knowledge, but I'm not sure." This advice will only work if the person about whom you are concerned is not at the point of using multiple pharmacies to throw people off guard.

How to Prevent Drug Addiction

In order to prevent drug dependence from developing in the first place, Dr. McIntosh stresses the importance of sticking to one pharmacist. And people who are taking multiple drugs should always carry a drug history card in their wallets. For obvious reasons, a drug history card is invaluable if you are involved in an accident of any sort.

Your doctor should automatically be asking you what medication you are taking – or were taking in the past – and should also be reminding you that non-prescription drugs are an essential part of a drug history. If your doctor doesn't ask, you should volunteer this information. And that goes for information about side effects, dosages and the effects that alcohol and other drugs have on your prescribed drugs as well. In a perfect world, the doctor would always be diligent about this sort of thing. In this world, it is up to the consumer to protect his or her best interests.

Naprosyn is a good example to use as far as the issue of side effects is concerned. It is one of the non-steroid, anti-inflammatory types of drugs that are sometimes used to treat backache when it is suspected that facet joint inflammation is involved. It has the reputation of being an "all or nothing" drug; either it works wonders or not at all. Most doctors will tell you that Naprosyn can cause stomach upset and should be taken with food or milk, but very few doctors advise their patients that Naprosyn sometimes causes depression as well.

Here is a list of questions that you should know the answers to before taking any prescription drug:

• Can your medication be taken on an empty stomach?

• Should it be taken with water, fruit juice, or milk?

• Some drugs – several types of antibiotics, for example – shouldn't be taken with dairy products; is your prescription one of them?

• Is your medication likely to cause drowsiness?

• Can you stop taking it suddenly, or is it the type of drug you should be weaned from?

• Stopping some medications "cold turkey" can sometimes cause depression and other side effects; will yours?

Apart from asking these questions of your doctor, it is a good idea to own one of the books on drugs written for the layman. *The People's Pharmacy* by Joe Graedon, Avon, 1976; *The Pill Book* by Harold Silverman and Gilbert Simon, Bantam Books, 1979; and *The Essential Guide to Prescription Drugs* by James Long, Harper & Row, 1982, are all excellent choices.

Over the long term, either good old-fashioned aspirin or acetaminophen is generally the safest and best type of drug for those days when you feel you absolutely have to take something for your back pain. As well as being a pain-killer, aspirin can reduce mild inflammation in back muscles, joints and ligaments. Acetaminophen works in a similar way to aspirin as a pain-killer but has no anti-inflammatory properties. Its advantage over aspirin is that it does not irritate stomach tissue; it is often recommended for people who suffer from ulcers or other stomach conditions.

But the main plus of both these drugs is that they contain no opiates; they are not addictive, which is particularly significant for those of us who suffer from chronic back pain.

Drug	Indications and Contraindications
Aspirin Excedrin A.S.A. 217 Anacin Bufferin Acetophen	Non-prescription anti-inflammatory analgesics. Do not take regularly for more than 10 days without consulting your doctor; pain is a warning sign and you may have something that needs further investigation. If you have a stomach ulcer, tell your doctor before taking. Also inform your doctor if you are breast-feeding, pregnant or trying to become pregnant. Best not to drink alcohol since the combination of these drugs and alcohol can cause stomach problems.
Coated A.S.A. Entrophen Novasen Ecotrin	Non-prescription anti-inflammatory, analgesic, coated A.S.A. Effects not immediate – peak reached six to eight hours after dose. Best for chronic pain. Eliminates, or diminishes, gastric distress during long-term treatment. Call doctor if you develop nausea, vomiting, diarrhea, sweating, flushing, fever, dizziness, drowsiness, thirst, skin eruptions. Do not use if you have ulcers.
Tylenol Campain 500 Atasol	Non-prescription analgesics made with acetaminophen rather than aspirin. No anti-inflammatory properties. Generally recommended for people who cannot tolerate aspirin because of stomach disorders. Do not take regularly for more than 10 days without consulting your doctor. Call doctor if you develop stomach pain, diarrhea, fever, unusual weakness, easy bruising or bleeding. Call doctor if medication does not relieve symptoms.
Tylenol 1 222's Atasol 8	Non-prescription analgesics with codeine. Tylenol 1 and Atasol 8 contain 8 mg of codeine as well as acetaminophen. 222's contain 8 mg of codeine as well as aspirin. Do not take more of this medicine than your doctor has prescribed. Could become habit-forming. The medicine works best if you take it when the pain first begins. Do not drink alcoholic beverages while taking these drugs without the approval of your doctor. Call doctor if you develop fever, unusual weakness, easy bruising or bleeding, unusual nervousness, stomach pain.
Tylenol 2 Tylenol 3 Tylenol 4 Empracet 30 Empracet 60 Atasol 15 Atasol 30	Prescription analgesics: acetaminophen with codeine. Tylenol 2 and Atasol 15 contain 15 mg of codeine. Tylenol 3 and Atasol 30 contain 30 mg, Tylenol 4 contains 60 mg. Empracet 30 contains 30 mg of codeine. Empracet 60 contains 60 mg of codeine. Do not take more than what your doctor prescribes. Can become habit-forming or you could overdose. Follow your prescription rather than waiting until the pain becomes unbearable. Call your doctor if you feel like taking the drug more often than it is prescribed. Do not drink alcohol without doctor's approval. Be sure that your doctor knows about all other medications you are taking. May cause dizziness, drowsiness, constipation. Inform doctor if you develop fever, yellow skin or eyes, bruising, bleeding, shortness of breath, stomach pain or difficult urination.

Drug	Indications and Contraindications
292 282 294	Prescription analgesics: aspirin with codeine. 282's contain 15 mg of codeine, 292's contain 30 mg of codeine, 294's contain 60 mg of codeine. Do not take more than what your doctor prescribes. Can become habit-forming. (See information on prescription Tylenol.) Must be swallowed whole. Same information re alcohol and other medications as prescription Tylenol. Inform your doctor if you are pregnant, trying to become pregnant or breast-feeding. Side effects may include ringing in your ears, stomach pain, dizziness, fever, severe constipation, difficulty in urinating, easy bruising or bleeding. Inform your doctor if you notice any of these symptoms.
Darvon 642	Prescription analgesics: contains propoxyphene. Related chemically to the "narcotics" drugs but not as potent and therefore not as habit-forming as drugs such as Percodan or 292's. Do not take more than what your doctor prescribes – has the potential to become habit-forming. Usually works best taken when pain first becomes uncomfortable rather than waiting until pain is unbearable. Same precautions apply re pregnancy, breast-feeding, and alcohol as prescription Tylenol and 292's. Call doctor immediately if you develop skin rash, facial swelling, difficulty in breathing, hives or itching. Carry identification card indicating that you are taking this medication.
Percodan Percodan-Demi	Prescription analgesics: aspirin and oxycodone, which is a codeine derivative. Do not take for more than ten days without doctor's permission. Can become habit-forming. Do not wait until pain becomes unbearable before taking. Inform doctor if you have a stomach ulcer. Same information as 292's re pregnancy, breast-feeding, alcohol. Call doctor immediately if you develop skin rash, facial swelling, difficulty in breathing, itching. This drug is extremely potent.
Valium E-Pam Robaxisal Robaxisal with Codeine Flexeril Vivol	Prescription sedatives used to relieve tension, help relax muscles. Robaxisal also comes with codeine as Robaxisal C. Robaxisal plain contains aspirin. Vivol, Valium and E-Pam are not codeine-based. Check with your doctor if you do not know why you have had this medication prescribed. Flexeril is not recommended for periods longer than two to three weeks. Same information as for 292's re pregnancy, breast-feeding, alcohol. Obtain medical advice before taking *any* other medicines including analgesics, sleeping pills, allergy medications, or weight reduction medication. Valium, Vivol and E-Pam cause dizziness or drowsiness. Possible side effects include skin rash, itching, nasal stuffiness, blurred vision, fever, ringing in the ears, stomach pain, confusion and blood-shot eyes. *Do not stop taking these medications suddenly without consulting your doctor.*

Anti-Inflammatories—Non-Steroidal	Generally not very effective for mechanical disorders, which are 90 per cent of back problems, unless drug has analgesic properties such as Motrin. These drugs are best for osteoarthritis or spondylitis of the spine, also rheumatoid arthritis. Do not use during pregnancy or when nursing. May cause nausea, heartburn, diarrhea, dizziness, headache, depression, skin rash, itching, blurred vision, decreased appetite, fluid retention.
Motrin Novonaprox Clinoril Novomethacin Indocid Tandearil Orudis Butone Tolectin Butazolidin Voltaren Sterazolidin Naprosyn	
Anti-Inflammatories — Steroidal	Same indications as for Anti-Inflammatories — Non-Steroidal.
Prednisone	

III
The Medical Model

6

The M.D.'s Diagnosis: If You Know a Few Things, You Can Learn a Great Deal

To understand how back problems are diagnosed by medical doctors, it is first necessary to know the difference between two terms: *signs* and *symptoms*.

A *sign* is something unusual, or abnormal, that a doctor who is examining you can observe and measure. In this sense, signs are both objective and quantitative. A scoliosis (a sideways curvature of the spine); the loss of muscle power in a foot; or evidence of reduced mobility when you attempt to bend forward, are all signs.

Symptoms, on the other hand, are not visible. They are what you — the patient — report, and in this sense they are both subjective and qualitative. The most common example of a symptom is pain. But when you describe how much your back pain depresses you, or causes you anxiety, you are also reporting symptoms rather than signs. It has long been known that different people tolerate pain differently. But recent studies have also shown that the variability of pain thresholds from patient to patient is more marked for back pain than for almost any other condition.

For this reason, it is important to realize that while your symptoms may seem infinitely clear to you, and certainly can provide a physician with excellent clues about the nature of a back problem, they are very difficult to measure. Even more essential to understand is that the most detailed description of a back problem's symptoms will rarely shed light on the precise source of that problem. For example, a surgeon cannot base a decision about surgery on a patient's subjective symptoms; it is essential to find a precise sign. Therefore, when it comes to making a medical diagnosis of your back problem, correlation between symptoms and signs is crucial.

The complexities of the matter of diagnosing back pain take on yet another dimension when you realize that the precise cause of a sign can also be ambiguous. Furthermore, some signs are more ambiguous than others. Broadly speaking, there are two types of signs: specific and non-specific.

A scoliosis, for example, is a specific sign. So is a neurological deficit – the loss of muscle power, for example – which indicates that a particular nerve which ought to be conducting messages to a particular muscle is not functioning properly. Say you have lost the ability to raise the big toe of one foot upward against the downward pressure applied by the examiner. The diagnosis will probably be a compression of the L5 nerve root, the nerve root which emerges from between the fifth lumbar vertebra and the sacrum; the L5 nerve conducts abnormal sensations (pain, numbness or tingling) down the leg and into the big toe. But precisely *what* is causing this problem is far more difficult to determine. An osteophyte pressing against the nerve could be preventing the nerve from functioning properly. Or, the problem could be a herniated disc that is pressing against the nerve root just as it emerges from the spine. Say it is a disc. Which disc is it? Most likely, it will be the L4-L5 disc simply because the law of averages has shown that when the L5 nerve root is being pinched by a disc, the L4-L5 disc is almost always the culprit. However, in certain instances the disc below, the L5-S1 disc, can also impinge upon the L5 nerve root when the disc has herniated more laterally.

Frequently, the physician who is conducting the clinical diagnosis must order a specific test, usually a CT Scan or a myelogram, to pin down the cause of such a specific sign; even then we're talking about a judgement call, not a 100 per cent sure thing.

Most of the signs that a back problem will exhibit, however, are not specific. Pinpointing the cause of non-specific signs is even harder than pinpointing the cause of specific signs. The most common non-specific signs of back pain are: a reduction in mobility in one or more directions; evidence of general degeneration on an X-ray; or a stiffness in a particular area of the spine, for example the lumbar spine.

Frequently, it is virtually impossible for a physician to figure out the precise cause of a non-specific sign.

Look at it this way. Say you have signs of reduced mobility when you try to bend sideways. The problem could be caused by an irritated facet joint, which might or might not have been initiated by a bit of disc degeneration, which might or might not have been caused by ligaments that are lax due to chronic poor posture – any of which may or may not be causing muscle spasm, if you happen to have muscle spasm, which may or may not be the actual cause of your pain! Furthermore, exactly *which* joint and/or *which* disc is the culprit is almost always impossible to say. Trying to get this kind of information across to a patient who is in the mood for a cut and dried explanation of why he or she looks and feels like a pretzel has left many physicians at a loss for words.

As if all this weren't complex enough, making a diagnosis is sometimes more difficult still. Many times, an examination of a back will reveal no signs at all. Many people have severe back pain – that is, severe *symptoms* – without any signs, or just vague signs. And ironically, plenty of people have X-ray evidence of degeneration and signs of limited mobility with no pain. With those sorts of complexities in mind, we can now proceed to the matter of the medical doctor's diagnosis.

The Clinical Examination

Most of us become extremely interested in back pain when we exert ourselves either consciously, or unconsciously, and discover that what we had always thought was a figment of the imaginations of the lily-livered, can be one of the most excruciating types of pain known to mankind. First, there is the struggle to find a comfortable position and a telephone to call the physician. Then, for most people, there is the slow realization that while their backs have "bothered" them from time to time over the years, the difference between that sort of pain and this is like the difference between Dr. Jekyll and Mr. Hyde. Only a minority of people experience one of these excruciating attacks without previously having suffered from mild backache.

For most people, the telephone call to the family physician will supply a suggestion to stay in bed for a couple of days and then call back. In many cases, the pain will subside completely and life will return to normal, at least for a while. For many people, this "pain-rest-in-bed-for-two-days" scenario occurs once or twice a year, and that's all there is to it.

For others, however, the pain will not subside substantially, and there will be a visit to the general practitioner for an examination. Generally speaking, this will entail a number of tests – blood tests, a urine sample, and perhaps some plain X-rays – which are all designed to rule out the possibility that the pain is being caused by an infection or other serious ailment. A clinical examination – meaning an exam that takes place in a clinic or office – generally follows. If there is nothing obviously wrong, a mild pain-killer or perhaps an anti-inflammatory drug may be prescribed along with more rest. If, however, several weeks go by without much improvement, a thorough clinical examination will be performed.

Sometimes a general practitioner will feel competent to do the clinical exam. Frequently, however, he or she will prefer to refer you to an ortho-paedic surgeon (or sometimes a neurosurgeon) for an assessment.

It is at this point that a lot of back pain sufferers experience frustration. The source of it, in my opinion, stems from the fact that most back pain sufferers fail to comprehend the orthopaedic or neurosurgeon's training bias. The main job of the surgeon is to determine if the patient he or she is examining is a candidate for surgery and, if so, to perform that surgery. (It is a very different bias, for example, from that of the physiotherapist to whom many surgeons refer their non-surgical patients for what is commonly called conservative treatment. In Chapter 14, you'll get a pretty good idea of the differences between the philosophy of the physiotherapist and that of the orthopaedic surgeon when it comes to assessing a back pain patient.)

During the clinical examination, an orthopaedic surgeon will look for all sorts of signs. He will listen to an account of your back pain and a description of your symptoms. A *good* clinical diagnostician who communicates well with patients will also try to give you an idea of what is wrong with your back even if you are not a surgical candidate. But because of their orientation, orthopaedic surgeons tend to concentrate on specific signs rather than non-specific signs. In particular, they look for gross neurological signs — muscles that have lost a substantial degree of their power, or areas that have lost their sense of touch due to the inability of a compressed, or pinched, nerve to ferry messages to them. Those are the types of back problems that can be corrected by surgery.

Most of the time, however, severe specific signs will not be found. Says Dr. Marvin Tile, deputy surgeon-in-chief of the Sunnybrook Medical Centre in Toronto, "It is unfortunate that some orthopaedic surgeons will then say, 'I can find nothing wrong with your back.' What they really mean, and what they should be saying, is that they can find nothing wrong with you *that makes you a good candidate for surgery.*" If you have no serious neurological signs, Dr. Tile emphasizes, it does not necessarily mean that there is nothing wrong with your back. It should not imply that you are making too much out of nothing. It does mean that what is wrong with your back need not be corrected surgically at that time, and that is true for more than 90 per cent of people with back pain.

A physician's clinical diagnosis will generally begin with a history of your back pain. The doctor will want to know: when the pain began; what it feels like; where it hurts; what activities cause it to hurt more; and whether or not resting your back relieves the pain, at least to some degree. Says Dr. Tile, "Say a patient in his mid-thirties comes in saying that he never had back pain in his life, has not had a major injury, but woke up six weeks ago with severe back pain that began radiating into his heel a couple of days later and now the heel is numb. From this description, I'd get a pretty good idea that he has a herniated disc. I'd also figure that the S1 nerve root (which emerges from a foramen of the sacrum) is involved, and when I performed the actual examination, I'd be on the look-out for signs to confirm this suspicion." An osteophyte can also be the cause of a pinched nerve, Dr. Tile reminds us, but patients with severe osteoarthritic changes are generally more elderly than those with herniated discs, and the onset of their pain is not generally so sudden.

"On the other hand, if I'm taking a history and someone says that his back has been bothering him for years and that a recent golf game has made the pain unbearable, I'd be more inclined to suspect a flare-up of a chronic facet joint problem," says Dr. Tile. However, the information he gets from a patient's history can be ambiguous. "You can get leg pain from a facet joint problem, for example, and so I need to know more about the nature of that leg pain." Generally speaking, leg pain that is being "referred" to the leg from a worn facet joint will be a different kind of leg pain than what you'd get from a pinched nerve. Neurological pain (which is what a disc, or an osteophyte, impinging on a nerve root will provoke) is often described as "electric." It's associated with a burning sensation, numbness or sometimes tingling. It usually hurts more with flexion (bending forward), coughing or sneezing. The referred leg pain that occurs from a worn facet joint doesn't often go below the buttocks. It rarely goes below the knee and is usually worse with extension, or arching, rather than with flexion. Nor is it associated with that burning quality. As well, patients who have referred leg pain from a facet joint problem often find it difficult to pinpoint exactly where in the leg it hurts. Referred pain is often described as "very vague."

Most of the time, back and/or leg pain will subside, at least to some extent, when a patient is resting. "If I hear a patient who has been in bed for six weeks still saying that the pain is constant or worse at night, that it frequently keeps him up or awakens him, then I might begin to worry about a tumour," says Dr. Tile. In such a situation, a bone scan X-ray, which can locate tumours, would be ordered. Bone scans work on the premise that when a tumour invades bone, both blood supply to the area and bone growth in the area increase. A harmless, radioactive substance called technetium polyphosphate (which is absorbed by bone cells) is injected into the bloodstream. A few hours later, a special X-ray is taken, and if there is a tumour in one of the bones of the spine, it will usually show up as a "hot spot." Not all bone tumours are malignant, however. If a tumour is discovered by a bone scan, it must then be biopsied. A sample of the tumour's cells must be studied in a lab to determine whether they are benign or cancerous.

After listening to the patient's history, the doctor will begin the clinical examination. While some of his colleagues may vary the order in which they conduct their exam, the procedure that Dr. Tile uses is more or less standard.

To begin with, the patient stands. "The first thing I want to do is inspect the whole back and look for deformities, red spots and muscle spasm," says Dr. Tile. By deformities, he means a scoliosis, an abnormal kyphosis or an abnormally prominent lordosis, any of which may, or may not, be contributing to the patient's back pain.

Next, he will flex the patient's neck forward, an action which puts stress on the spinal cord. "If there is a herniated disc, this type of neck flexion may provoke a sharp pain down a leg," he explains. With the neck still flexed, he will next ask the patient to cough, which puts even more strain on the spinal nerves. "If a cough provokes leg pain," he says, "then I'll be on the look-out for a disc herniation. If it doesn't, I may be more inclined to begin thinking about a facet joint problem, or perhaps spinal stenosis."

Pressing the carotid arteries in the neck puts pressure on the jugular veins which are behind them. This action will change the pressure within the spinal fluid, and that is what Dr. Tile does next. "This may also produce leg pain," he says, explaining that for every problem there are at least several tests. "You're looking for a correlation between many different tests for the same thing."

The next part of the procedure involves putting the spine through its range of motions. The first is bending forward. "This can be ambiguous since even a person with a totally fused spine (ankylosing spondylitis) can almost touch their toes because the hip joints will still rotate," says Dr. Tile. The trick, he explains, is to watch the spine carefully to see if each of its levels move. Some physicians use a tape measure and watch to see how much the tape stretches. A mobile spine will stretch a tape about four inches. A totally fused spine will bend forward, but because it is the hip joints that are doing the actual rotating, the tape measure won't stretch out at all.

Forward bending is also a test for a herniated disc. Dr. Tile explains: "If a person bends forward a little bit, gets severe pain down the leg, and the back goes into spasm and can't move much more, then you can be almost certain that you're looking at a disc problem."

The next movement is extension, or bending backward. Anyone who is suffering from an abnormally narrow spinal canal (spinal stenosis) is likely to feel pain with extension. This is because the space in the spinal canal tends to be reduced even more in the extension posture. "You might also feel numbness, or tingling, in the legs or toes," says Dr. Tile, "and many people who are suffering from spinal stenosis also find that walking any distance exacerbates their symptoms." What makes the diagnosis of spinal stenosis so difficult, however, is that pain which originates from a worn facet joint, or as a result of osteoarthritic growths on a facet joint, will also increase with extension. This is because facet joints are jammed together in the extension posture, and if they are worn, pain will result. The simplest way to verify a clinical picture of spinal stenosis is with a CT Scan (see Chapter 7). The clinical diagnosis of a severely degenerated facet joint can be confirmed by a regular X-ray, although many radiologists feel that a CT Scan can provide a much clearer view.

The third movement in the range of motion test is lateral bending. When you bend to the side, your hand should be able to reach slightly beyond the knee level without causing you pain. "Again, if this causes severe pain down a leg, it could be the sign of a disc problem, although this test is less conclusive than some of the others," says Dr. Tile.

The last range of motion test is rotation. With your feet flat on the floor, you should be able to turn a full 90 degrees to both the right and the left. If the range is restricted, a facet joint problem is likely the cause.

Says Dr. Tile, "If any of these movements produce a neurogenic type of pain, then it's likely that you're looking at a disc problem. If they produce backache, or vague leg pain above the knee, then it's more likely that a facet joint, spinal stenosis or muscle spasm is the cause." In some cases, more than one problem exists.

By this time, the physician will have a sense of what is going on and can begin the specific neurological examination to determine if any nerves have been affected. During this part of the examination, the physician will try to find specific neurological signs.

To start with, the patient remains standing. First the functioning of the S1 nerve is tested; this is the nerve that runs down the back of the calf into the heel, supplying power to the muscles of the calf along the way. To do this, you raise one foot several inches off the floor and then move up and down on the toes of the opposite foot ten times. You then switch feet and repeat the test. Dr. Tile explains; "If you can only do this once instead of ten times – that is, if you get up on your toes once and are simply too weak to continue – I'll get a pretty good idea that the S1 nerve root is involved in the problem." But even if it can be determined that your S1 nerve is not supplying enough power to the muscles of your calf to allow you to perform this test, the cause cannot always be conclusively determined. The culprit could be a disc. Or an osteophyte could be pinching the nerve. An experienced diagnostician can get a pretty good idea of which it is, but in the end, if surgery is contemplated, there will have to be a correlation between the clinical diagnosis and the one that is made as a result of a myelogram, discogram or CT Scan test.

Next, the patient kneels on the seat of a chair with his or her back toward the examiner, feet pointing toward the floor. This is the best position for testing the ankle reflex by hitting the ankle with a reflex hammer. If the S1 nerve is conducting messages properly, the foot will respond by involuntarily jerking backward. If the nerve is not conducting properly, there will be no response. "I also look for subtle differences between the left and right reflexes," says Dr. Tile.

Next, the patient sits on the chair. The knee reflex is tested with the same hammer. If it is absent, this indicates that there is a problem with the L4 nerve, which emerges from between the fourth and fifth lumbar vertebrae. "This is rare," says Dr. Tile, explaining that of the ten per cent of back pain patients who have clear evidence of nerve root compression, less than five per cent of those have a problem with the L4 nerve root.

More commonly affected, he explains, is the nerve below, the L5 nerve. To test the L5 nerve root, he examines the power of the dorsal flexor muscles in the foot, which are the muscles used to elevate the toes and move the foot from side to side. First you try to elevate the big toe of each foot against the pressure that the examiner applies. Then you try to elevate the other toes. Next, again against the pressure applied by the examiner, you try to evert the foot, or turn it out. Finally, you try to invert the foot, or turn it in. "I prefer to do this test while the patient is sitting rather than lying down, because I can detect subtle differences in strength between one foot and the other," says Dr. Tile.

On its way down the leg, the sciatic nerve runs close to the body's surface just at the back of the knee. "If the back of the knee is tender when pressed," says Dr. Tile, "this is a further indication that one of the nerves which make up the sciatic nerve may be involved." Often, there will also be tenderness in the muscles on the outside of the leg. If those on the *inside* of the leg are tender, it likely indicates a problem with the L5 nerve root; weakness in the muscles higher up in the leg will indicate a problem with the second, third and fourth lumbar nerve roots, conditions which are extremely rare.

While still sitting, the patient is next asked to pull each leg back in toward the chair against the force that the examiner applies. This test will show weakness in the hamstring muscles, which again indicates a problem with the most commonly affected nerve, S1.

The final portion of the examination is conducted while the patient is lying down.

The test that most back pain sufferers have heard of is performed with the patient lying supine, or face up. Called the SLR test (Straight Leg Raising), it will indicate if any of the nerves which merge at the hip to form the sciatic nerve are being irritated, most likely by a herniated disc. With the knees straight, first one leg is raised by the examiner to a 90-degree angle, then the other is raised the same amount, stretching the sciatic nerve. Severe pain between 35 and 70 degrees is an indication of nerve irritation. By the time the leg has been raised 70 degrees, however, the sciatic nerve will have been stretched to its full capacity; pain between 70 degrees and 90 degrees may be an indication of a joint problem – either a facet joint, the hip joint or the sacroiliac joint. "By bending the knee and rotating the foot outward, the examiner can test the hip joint," says Dr. Tile.

The Babinski Sign test is performed next, with the patient still supine. The examiner strokes the soles of the feet with the pointed end of a reflex hammer. "Normally, this test will cause the toes to curl downward. If they spread upward and outward, it is a sign that the spinal cord itself is being compressed," says Dr. Tile, "or that another neurological disease is present such as multiple sclerosis."

With the patient in the side-lying position, the examiner will next test for sacroiliac joint problems by pressing down on each hip; rotation of the hip joints will stress the sacroiliac joints.

Finally, while the patient is lying prone, or face down, several tests will be performed. One is the prone knee-bending test (femoral nerve stretch test), which will cause pain if either the L3 or L4 nerve roots are the source of the problem. The second, which is another test for the L5 nerve root, is the contracting of the gluteus maximus muscles of the buttocks. "I want to see if one side is flatter than the other and if there is the same amount of muscle tension on each side," says Dr. Tile.

If the patient is male and over the age of 45, a rectal examination to check the prostate gland for swelling, or a tumour, will likely be performed.

If your physician finds some evidence of neurological deficit, he or she may decide to proceed with some diagnostic tests to pinpoint the problem more closely. The most frequently used tests are the myelogram, the discogram and the CT Scan. Or, a period of conservative treatment may be prescribed, either a combination of bed rest and physiotherapy or bed rest alone. "At the best of times, surgery is not perfect," says Dr. Tile, "and many people with evidence of disc herniation do get better with conservative treatment."

More than likely, however, you will fall into the huge group of back pain sufferers for whom surgery will never be a wise option.

Nevertheless, if you ask the right questions, you can learn quite a few things. If your doctor tells you that there is nothing wrong, be direct. Ask if there is nothing wrong or if he or she really means that there is nothing that makes you a good surgical candidate. If you have had X-rays taken, ask if there are any visible degenerative changes and, if there are, ask your physician to point them out. (If there are no degenerative changes, your back pain could be due to lax ligaments caused by chronic poor posture, a condition which can be compensated for by exercise and good posture.) If your back hurts when you bend forward, ask about a bulging, if not a herniated, disc. If your back hurts with extension, ask about your facet joints, or the possibility of spinal stenosis.

But keep in mind that if you are not a candidate for surgery, it may not be necessary to pinpoint your back problem precisely. If your back pain is exacerbated by extension, and your doctor suspects that a worn facet joint or mild spinal stenosis is at the root of the problem, does it really matter if that worn joint or narrowed canal is at the L4 or L5 level? Probably it doesn't. If, on the other hand, bending forward exacerbates your pain and your doctor feels that a bulging disc is the culprit, does it really matter if it's the L4-L5 disc or the L5-S1 disc? Again probably not.

My experience is that many people who suffer from back pain have driven themselves and their doctors half crazy trying to pinpoint a problem whose conservative treatment would be the same regardless of where in the lumber spine it was. If you are not a candidate for surgery, a better solution would be to accept that fact of life and get on with the job of finding the treatment which will offer you relief.

7

The CT Scanner: Revolutionary Radiology

In the fifth floor radiology department of Toronto's Mount Sinai Hospital, 42-year-old structural engineer John Milford is being prepared for a Computerized Tomography Scan, a procedure which he hopes will confirm his surgeon's diagnosis of a herniated disc. For the procedure, no needles will be necessary. Nor will there be a need for a period of complete bed rest following the Scan as there would be if John Milford were having a myelogram test. (See Chapter 8.) Even more comforting is the fact that the CT Scan, unlike the myelogram or the discogram, will involve no pain, indeed not even an amount of that dubious sensation doctors love to call "discomfort."

The CT Scan's computer program has been accessed. John Milford's is ready to go! Positioned comfortably on his back, a thin pillow under his head and a blanket to keep him warm, he is slid soundlessly — lock, stock and barrel — through the doughnut-shaped "gantry," the tube-shaped outer housing of this $850,000 machine. Forty-five minutes later, he is withdrawn. Twenty seconds after that, the more than 20 million readings that the Scanner has taken have been interpreted by the program, and the clinical diagnosis can be confirmed: a large piece of disc herniating into the spinal canal at the L5-S1 level, as suspected. Clear, cut and dried. In addition, the radiologist has picked up the beginnings of spinal stenosis (which he will note for future reference) two levels above.

Dr. George Wortzman is radiologist-in-chief at Mount Sinai. He speaks about the CT Scanner in the way Leo Buscaglia speaks about love.

"The CT Scanner is a whole new area of technology. Its advent has changed everything. Suddenly you've got computers that do more than just keep records; they show views [of the spine] that are impossible by other means. It is commonly accepted now that a neurosurgeon can't really practise adequately in a hospital that does not have a CT Scanner. They are the biggest breakthrough in radiology since Wilhelm Roentgen first developed the X-ray back in 1895."

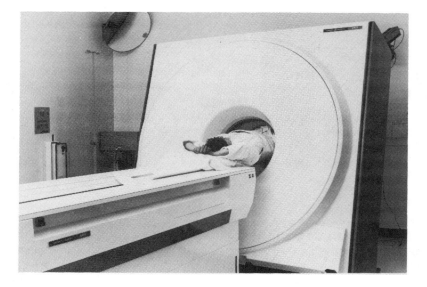

A CT Scanner and its gantry.

Describing *how* the CT Scanner provides such views of the spine is like trying to explain Einstein's formula $E = MC^2$. In fact, even when they are staring you in the face, the X-ray pictures themselves defy belief. Cross-sections of the spine, called transaxial slices, each reveal an area no more than one-fifth of an inch thick. From their appearance, you might think that to get them, the radiologist has had to slice up the patient's body like a lumberjack slices up a felled tree.

A conventional X-ray of the spine is little better than a shadow, telling no more about the *interior* of the spine than the shadow of a building tells about its occupants. With the CT Scanner, the interior can be viewed. The computer reconstructs the data provided by rotated sequences of minutely thin X-ray beams into two-dimensional slices, along any plane that is of interest to the radiologist. If you had a deck of cards stacked one on top of the other and you pulled out one from the middle, holding it upright to study its face, you'd basically be doing what the CT Scanner does.

Dr. Wortzman gives a rudimentary explanation of the CT Scanner's technical prowess. "First you select the particular level of the spine that you're interested in. You then shoot a thin beam of radiation through the body, and at the other end, a sensor measures the amount of radiation that is left." As with a conventional X-ray, the denser areas such as bone will absorb more radiation than the less dense areas such as disc. But

100

here the similarities end. "With the CT Scanner," Dr. Wortzman explains, "each X-ray beams an area approximately 1 millimetre wide and from 1.5 to 10 millimetres high. The beam then moves one degree clockwise to take the next reading." This continues, all the way around the body, until you've completed 360 degrees.

In reality, this rudimentary explanation is missing one important detail — the CT Scanner is capable of gathering such vast quantities of information so quickly because it can take hundreds of readings at once. When the patient is moved up, or down, to the next level of interest, these same readings are repeated. What you end up with is millions of calculations, which the Scanner's computer program can combine and recombine to provide particular information of any particular plane.

Like conventional X-ray techniques, a CT Scan involves the use of radiation. Because a scan of a lumbar spine can take up to 45 minutes, many people worry that the amount of exposure is so high that they will virtually light up. Not so. Taking these million readings will expose a patient to less radiation than a myelogram, or five or six conventional X-rays. "With a conventional X-ray," says Dr. Wortzman, "you're radiating a whole section of the spine at once and, generally, multiple views are necessary. With the CT Scanner, only a tiny area of the body receives radiation from any one beam. There are, in fact, no attendant dangers with the CT Scanner. No negative side effects at all."

With press like this, you have to wonder why uncomfortable, if not downright painful, tests such as the myelogram and the discogram have not been ditched completely in favour of the CT Scan. A few studies have shown that in certain instances, a myelogram can be a better tool for diagnosing a herniated disc. And the CT Scanner, which can only look at "slices" of the spine's lumbar area (not the thoracic or cervical spine), will miss the very rare circumstance where a tumour above the second lumbar vertebra is the cause of the patient's symptoms. But these are not the reasons why only two spine patients per day are being slid through the gantry of Dr. Wortzman's beloved CT Scan machine and the rest are still being diagnosed with myelograms, discograms and conventional X-rays.

The answer is a simple one: dollars and cents. "Right now," says Dr. Wortzman, "the Mount Sinai's CT Scan is almost fully booked up every day diagnosing head injuries and other medical problems that can't be diagnosed by other means. A spinal scan takes about 45 minutes — three, even four times as long as it takes to scan a brain. On a CT Scanner, time is money. Not only is there the huge capital investment of between $850,000 to $1.2 million, but CT Scanners are expensive to operate and service as well."

At the moment, there are 97 CT Scanners in Canada, one machine for approximately 250,000 people. "If all the spinal scans that are sought were done, the machines that could do them would be booked up with four, five or six patients a day. All the Scanners we have in Canada right now that are capable of doing spines would be doing nothing else.

"While I'd rather see a back pain patient with a clinical diagnosis of a herniated disc go through a CT Scan than a myelogram, I would not like to see a head injury go unscanned because of a back. With spine work (other than in the case of a severe stenosis where it can be hard just to introduce a needle to inject the myelogram dye), there are alternative methods available. And they function to a high degree of accuracy. Unfortunately, they are invasive, which means that there is some element of risk involved, however small. And, of course, there can be discomfort."

John Milford waited for three months to get his 45 minutes on the Scanner. "And I really pushed for it," he says. "I told them, 'Look, I've been through a myelogram two years ago. [At that point, the diagnosis was negative but Milford's symptoms didn't improve.] I've had the headache and the whole bit with that test. I deserve a date with the Scan'."

The Development of the CT Scanner

In 1972, Dr. Geoffery Hounsfield (who later won a Nobel Prize in Medicine for his work) installed the first CT Scanner in the Atkinson Morley Hospital in London, England. That machine, however, could not have replaced the myelogram because it was designed to take pictures of the head only. It took nine days to process the data it collected from just one "slice" of the head. Today, the models which collect data representing well over a million readings accomplish this amazing feat in less than half a minute.

Perhaps that is one of the reasons why E.M.I., the company that was first to manufacture CT Scanners, didn't realize the gold-mine that they had. Says Dr. Wortzman, "When CT Scanners first went on the market in 1973, they expected to sell between 12 and 24 in the world market. As of last year, there were more than 6,900 Scanners in operation worldwide, more than 2,500 in the U.S. alone."

By 1975, the design of the original Scanner had been improved upon substantially. The new models had "gantries." These large, doughnut-shaped structures housed curved banks of sensors which surround the patient. Because these gantries could tilt, the new Scanners became good diagnostic tools for spines; it is this additional maneuverability that allows the new CT Scanners to peer between the vertebral bodies to show the shape of the discs, as well as the normally heart-shaped canal. When the canal has become narrowed, as in spinal stenosis, the radiologist can see the altered shape with a Scanner far more readily than with a myelogram.

Since 1975, improvements have continued. In some models the speed and clarity have been increased so substantially that hospital officials are clamouring for the money to replace their "antiquated" machines. The first CT Scanner that was installed at the Mayo Clinic spent five years on the floor and has been languishing in the clinic's historical museum ever since!

CT Scanners can also be upgraded. Says Dr. Wortzman, "For $78,000, we could equip the Mount Sinai's $850,000 machine with a device that would shorten the time it takes to scan a spine from 40 minutes down to 20." In theory, those extra 20 minutes could give Mount Sinai the freedom to scan two additional spines per day. In practice, it doesn't quite work out that way. The stickler is that the amount of operational funding allotted for CT Scanners by the government is fixed. "You don't get more money just because you do more cases," says Dr. Wortzman. "The Scanner is part of the hospital's global budget, which remains the same no matter how many cases we do.

"This is a brand new major 'thing' that has suddenly frightened governments in both Canada and the U.S." he says. "Since they became available in 1974, everybody wants one." With the cost of some of the new units as high as $1.2 million, not every hospital is successful with its bid.

John Milford is adamant. "If I had to choose between a hospital that would give me a CT Scan and a hospital that wouldn't, there would be no contest. I'd take the Scan any day. If my problem was not acute and I had to choose between a myelogran today and a Scan a month down the road, I'd seriously consider waiting. As I say, I've had both. The myelogram wasn't all that *painful*, but the difference in the amount of stress they provoke is phenomenal. Psychologically, I feel I was far better prepared for surgery after my CT Scan than I would have been had my myelogram test been positive two years ago."

Two days after his CT Scan, John Milford underwent surgery to remove his herniated disc. Today, three months later, he is back at his structural engineering job full time, his leg pain completely gone.

"It's fashionable today to go on about how there is too much technology and how hospitals are spending too much," he says. "In this case, however, it's not true, at least not in my opinion. . . . At the moment, it's those of us with back pain who are getting short shrift."

8

Myelograms and Discograms

There comes a time during the course of treatment of many back pain sufferers – usually after bed rest, time and a myriad of other conservative treatments haven't worked – when a decision must be made. Are you, or are you not, a possible candidate for back surgery?

Fewer than ten per cent of back pain patients have a condition that warrants back surgery. Unfortunately, the amount of pain you are in, or the degree to which you are disabled, has little to do with whether or not back surgery is likely to be a technical success.

Surgery is useless if you are suffering from back pain because of general wear and tear at many different levels of the spine. It works when a person has a specific problem, most frequently a herniated disc at one, or perhaps two specific levels.

The most common diagnostic test for determining if a herniated disc is at the root of the problem (and which disc it is) is an X-ray called a myelogram. (Spinal stenosis will also be revealed with a myelogram test; however, many radiologists feel that a CT Scan is a far better indicator for this condition.) A less common test is the discogram. Both tests are a frequently used and frequently useful prelude to spinal surgery, although in some hospitals the CT Scan has begun to take the place of both.

The myelogram and the discogram are based on the same principle: when a radiopaque (ie., impervious to X-rays) fluid is injected into the spinal canal, the resulting picture will reveal more about a disc's condition than a conventional X-ray. Bones show up on regular X-rays, but discs, which are classified as "soft tissue," do not. Sometimes a radiologist can get an inkling of a disc problem from an ordinary X-ray, because the disc space between two vertebrae looks narrower than normal. But an actual disc herniation cannot be confirmed by a regular X-ray.

For a myelogram, radiopaque fluid is injected through the dura mater (the protective sheath which surrounds both the spinal cord and the nerve roots) into the spinal canal. For a discogram, radiopaque fluid is injected into the suspect disc itself.

The myelogram is chosen when the physician wants to examine the whole spine, or at least a certain section of the spine. The discogram, which provides information about the condition of just one disc per injection, is sometimes used if the myelogram produces no useful results. As well, a discogram is sometimes performed after a successful myelogram; if the results of the myelogram lead the surgeon to suspect that more than one disc will have to be included in the surgery, additional specific information about the exact condition of these discs may be useful.

The discogram is performed much less frequently than the myelogram. At Toronto's Mount Sinai Hospital, for instance, radiologist-in-chief Dr. George Wortzman says that his team conducts about 20 to 30 myelograms for every discogram. At other hospitals, the ratio is much less, as little as 3:1.

The Myelogram

Going to the radiologist for a myelogram is a lot like going to the dentist for root canal work. Nobody looks forward to it and nobody enjoys it.

"It's not fun, not something you would choose to do on Sunday afternoon," concedes Dr. Richard C. Holgate, director of neuroradiology at the University of South Carolina. "On the other hand," says Dr. George Wortzman, "the abject fear with which a lot of people face the myelogram is truly not justified."

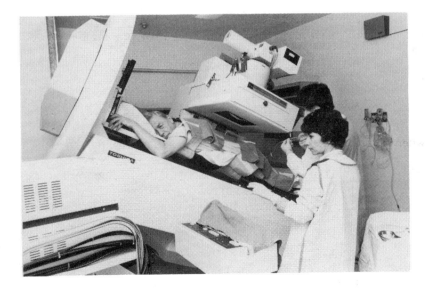

A myelogram test.

If you were to speak to several people who have undergone this diagnostic test, you would in all likelihood get as many different descriptions. Rosemary Maringold, a 21-year-old seamstress, underwent a myelogram several years ago and didn't feel a thing. "I was also surprised that I had no disturbing after-effects," she says, confirming that a friend who had had a myelogram the previous year had suffered from severe headache for two days. "I had just a slight headache and a touch of dizziness that went away after a day."

Paul Kahn, a 38-year-old engineer who considers himself a "pretty tough guy," had quite a different response to the myelogram test. "The procedure required me to lie in a position that aggravated my back pain, which was already intense. And for me, the after-effects included a terrible headache that lasted several days."

Obviously, the myelogram creates more discomfort, or pain, in some patients than others. But Rosemary Maringold and Paul Kahn agreed on one point, however grudgingly in his case: the myelogram can serve its purpose well. For each of them, it enabled the surgeon to pinpoint the source of the back problem and to perform an operation to alleviate it. The results, they admit, were well worth the aggravation.

A patient who is going to have a myelogram, is positioned face down on a tiltable table. In some hospitals, patients are sedated prior to the test. In other hospitals, no sedation is used. Dr. Holgate, for example, says that in his experience, sedated patients faint or vomit more often than those who are calm but fully alert. He also maintains that his unsedated patients rarely complain about pain.

First, the radiopaque fluid is injected into the spinal canal, usually through the intervertebral foramen between the third and fourth lumbar vertebrae. Next, the table is tilted back and forth, head to toe. This causes the fluid to flow slowly up and down the spinal canal, filling the space around each nerve root. Meanwhile, X-rays are taken from various vantage points. The whole test takes about 15 to 25 minutes, depending upon whether an oil-based or water-based fluid is used. That decision is based on the personal preference of the radiologist who is doing the test.

If the radiologist has chosen to use an oil-based fluid, it must be removed, or "aspirated," when the test is finished. The needle that is used to introduce the fluid is left in place and then used again to draw it out. The entire test can be completed in about 25 minutes. The water-soluble fluid can be left in the system to be excreted in the urine. In this case, 15 minutes is usually sufficient time for the test to be completed.

Either fluid, being radiopaque, appears on the X-ray plates as a white mass. The discs, on the other hand, allow X-rays to pass through them and show up as dark blotches. If a disc is bulging severely, or has herniated completely, the outline of the bulge or herniation will show up as a dark blotch impinging into the "white" spinal canal. If the patient is suffering from spinal stenosis, the spinal canal will appear abnormally narrow.

The myelogram test is not 100 per cent foolproof, however. In one study, 24 per cent of patients who had never experienced sciatic pain had a positive myelogram test nevertheless. "It is essential that the myelogram test be correlated with the clinical diagnosis," says Dr. Wortzman.

In the majority of cases, however, an experienced radiologist can generally tell by the shape of the outline if a disc is pressing against a nerve root and which disc it is. "In this sense," explains Dr. Wortzman, "a myelogram provides a road map for surgery."

Both Dr. Holgate and Dr. Wortzman feel strongly that as radiologists, it is they who must make sure that patients understand beforehand what a myelogram will entail. Ideally, the referring surgeon will have already given the patient a thorough briefing. However, some doctors communicate better than others and to be fair, some patients, being under unusual stress, don't listen as carefully as they should. Consequently, it's not unusual for a patient to walk into the radiology department either uninformed, or badly misinformed, about what to expect.

"Some patients," says Dr. Holgate, "come in expecting just a needle and a couple of X-rays, and it's not that simple."

"On the other hand," says Dr. Wortzman, "the greatest problem we have is the patient who has heard exaggerated stories of pain and tales of woe. We get people coming in for myelograms who are absolutely petrified."

To reduce the patient's apprehension and to improve the chances for a successful test, a good radiologist will outline the procedure, discuss the possible after-effects, and mention the risks involved, remote as they are.

"People who are relaxed, confident and unafraid are easier to position, more co-operative, and are better able to lie perfectly still," Dr. Holgate explains. "Plus you don't get into that feedback-loop situation where their nervousness and anxiety produce nervousness and anxiety in the radiologist."

During a pre-test briefing, Dr. Holgate makes it clear to his patients that discomfort is likely, although not inevitable, both during and sometimes after a myelogram. "But many of our patients say, 'I thought this was going to be excruciatingly painful,' and they're surprised when it's over as soon as it is."

Dr. Holgate also feels obliged to mention, for ethical and legal reasons, that the myelogram is an *invasive* medical procedure and, as such, inherently carries a small element of risk. In the next breath, however, he likes to point out that statistically, a myelogram is far safer than flying on a commercial airline, or driving a car on the highway.

"In terms of risk," he says, referring to the discogram as well as the myelogram, "both tests are very, very safe."

Many people suffer from headache for two or three days after a myelogram, and some say that they experienced nausea and vomiting as well. The way to prevent these symptoms is to rest in bed for 18 to 24 hours after the test.

If you are having a myelogram with the oil-based radiopaque fluid, bed rest means flat on your back, without raising your head even once. You can eat and drink whatever you like, but only by turning your head sideways. Sitting up increases the pressure on the spine, and a small amount of spinal fluid will leak out through the hole made by the injection needle. It is the loss of spinal fluid that brings on headache and/or nausea.

If you are having a myelogram with a water-soluble injection, bed rest is also recommended. In this case, however, you will be advised to lie with your head slightly raised. You should lie still to keep your body from absorbing the fluid too quickly, and you should also prop your head up slightly to keep the fluid from entering the cranium where it can irritate the brain lining and cause headache.

Hilda Tauger, a 37-year-old retail store owner, can testify to the effectiveness of this post-myelogram routine. She had a myelogram with the water-soluble solution and, afterward, remained in bed for 24 hours in the approved position. "It worked out far better than I expected," she said. "I'd heard that people have terrible migraines for two or three days after their myelogram, but I didn't experience anything like that."

In Dr. Wortzman's experience, patients who are sent home for bed rest will often ignore his instructions and suffer accordingly. To prevent this, he generally prescribes at least 24 hours of supervised bed rest in hospital.

Dr. Holgate is generally more permissive, leaving it up to the patient to follow, or ignore, his advice. "If a patient chooses to ignore the warnings and ends up with headache, nausea or vomiting, that's their choice," he says. He points out, however, that patients who get out of bed are not actually harming themselves. They are merely inducing unnecessary pain and prolonging their recovery period.

For many patients, however, bed rest becomes inescapable because they stay in hospital to undergo back surgery within a day or two. Other patients – for whom a closer look at one or more particular levels of the spine is advisable – go on to have a discogram.

The Discogram

A patient who is going to have a discogram will be positioned flat on the stomach. The radiologist, watching the outline of the spine on a fluoroscope screen, will first insert a short, stout needle into the disc in question.

The needle has a removable core, and once satisfied that the needle is in the right position, the radiologist will remove this core. Then, using the stout needle as a guiding sleeve, a much slimmer, longer needle is inserted. It is through this longer needle that radiopaque fluid is injected into the disc.

(Some radiologists have recently introduced a slight variation in the positioning of the patient. Instead of lying flat on the stomach, the patient lies on one knee and an elbow to raise one side of the body 45 degrees. When any of the three lowest lumbar discs are to be tested, some radiologists prefer this position because they find that it is easier to insert the stout needle.)

The conclusions drawn from a discogram depend upon two observations. The first is the way the fluid behaves once it has been injected into a disc. The second is whether the act of injecting the fluid duplicates the pain the patient has been experiencing from the chronic back condition.

If the fluid remains in the central portion of the disc, appearing as an almond-shaped white blob on the X-ray, the disc is normal. If, however, the fluid has moved to the outer confines of the disc, the conclusion will be that there is either a large bulge, or a herniation, in the disc. When this happens, the fluid generally presses against a nerve root, causing severe pain.

In fact, patients undergoing a discogram are asked whether the pain induced by the test is identical to the pain they normally feel. If it is the same (and some people report that it is in the same location but far worse) the needle has indeed found the offending disc.

Painful though it is, the discogram has some consoling features. For one thing, the test is fairly brief. As Dr. Wortzman observes, "The pain lasts only about a minute, although to the patient, a minute can seem like a long time." Another positive aspect to the discogram is that patients usually are able to get up from the table right away, with no need for a recovery period.

Few patients could be better qualified to make comparisons between the myelogram and the discogram than Margaret Delaware, a 40-year-old bookkeeper. Although most people do not undergo these procedures more than once, she has had two myelograms (one with the oil-based fluid; the second with the water-soluble fluid) and three discograms. According to her, the myelogram was easier to take the second time around because she knew what to expect. The discograms, however, felt increasingly worse. "When I had the last discogram," she says, "the pain was so intense that I almost hit the roof!"

The consoling factor in every case cited here is that these "road maps for surgery" led to apparently successful operations.

After her two myelograms and three discograms, Margaret Delaware finally had a discotomy and went skiing the following winter.

Hilda Tauger underwent a spinal fusion and, with the aid of a back brace, has been steadily mending.

Rosemary Maringold, who could barely put on her own shoes before surgery, had a discotomy and has since resumed her favourite pastime — dancing.

Paul Kahn also had a discotomy and has since gone back to gardening and taking his young daughter ice skating. "I can lift her up now," he says, "and she's almost five. Before my surgery, I couldn't lift up a garden trowel."

9

Surgery: Only the Chosen Few Need Apply

Marianne Singer remembers what it was like several years ago when she tried to perform even the simplest personal routines.

She was 38 and had lived with a severe back problem for almost two years. Merely getting dressed in the morning was a chore rather than a taken-for-granted act. Easing herself out of bed, she would put on a single garment. Then, she would wait for ten minutes until the pain, which was surging down both legs, subsided. Next, she would manage to get herself upright once again and, with a second garment, she'd repeat the whole process.

When she tried to walk, she could feel the pain that originated in her lumbar spine all the way to her toes. The pain in her right leg would be more severe than the pain in her left, but both legs would be more painful than she could possibly describe.

"By this time, I had tried total bed rest for three months, traction, hot packs, cold packs, you name it. Nothing worked. When I rested, the pain would subside but as soon as I was up again, it would return. I thought I was going to lose my mind."

Evelyn Weston's case was similar, at least in certain superficial ways. At 35, she, like Marianne Singer, was suffering from severe back pain and excruciating leg pain. For a number of years, her "attacks" would flare up for a month or two and then, with rest and exercise, subside. But this time was different; she had been suffering constantly for almost a year. Like Marianne Singer, she also had trouble getting dressed in the morning. And out of that misery was emerging a feeling of increasing desperation as one form of treatment after another produced no relief.

Remarkably, Marianne Singer and Evelyn Weston were suffering from two distinctly different types of back problems.

Evelyn Weston's complaint centred on that old villain familiar to so many victims of back pain — disc trouble. In her case, the problem was an acute herniation of the L5-S1 disc. The disc was pressing against the nerve root that emerges from between those two vertebrae and joins with other nerve roots to form the sciatic nerve.

Marianne Singer, on the other hand, had nothing wrong with the discs of her spine. By coincidence, her problem also centred at the L5-S1 level. But hers was a case of spondylolisthesis (see page 56), a rare mechanical condition in which one vertebra, because of a crack in its posterior section called a spondylolysis, slips over the one below it. This slipping action produces a simple rubbing action that can cause excruciating back and leg pain.

Given these marked differences in their conditions, Marianne Singer and Evelyn Weston would not seem to belong in any single group of back pain sufferers – except for one point in common. Both women were suffering from specific, *localized* back conditions that could be corrected by surgery.

For Evelyn Weston, the surgical remedy was a procedure that comes under the general heading of *decompression*; either disc material, or bone, that is pressing against a nerve root is removed. In Evelyn Weston's particular case, the operation involved a discotomy (the removal of the herniated disc itself) as well as a laminectomy (the removal of part of the bone which forms the lamina). The laminectomy was performed so that the surgeon could gain access to the herniated disc.

For Marianne Singer, the surgical remedy was a procedure that comes under the general heading of *stabilization*: specifically a spinal fusion at the L5-S1 level. Its objective, as you might suppose, is to stabilize (by rendering it motionless) one or more levels of the spine where painful movement is taking place.

Other than the extremely rare instances when back operations are performed because of trauma, an infection in the area of the spine or to remove a spinal tumour, decompression and stabilization are the only types of operations that surgeons perform to relieve back pain.

In the back of their minds, most people who suffer from chronic back pain harbour a mollifying belief: that if the pain gets too bad, goes on for too long or ultimately fails to respond to a diligent regimen of conservative treatment, there is always a final out – surgery. Unfortunately, nothing could be further from the truth.

For approximately 90 per cent of people who suffer from back pain, surgery will never be an option. The amount of pain you are in, or the degree to which you are disabled has, unfortunately, very little to do with a surgeon's decision to operate. For either a decompression or stabilization operation to be potentially successful, a back pain patient must be suffering from a specific, localized condition which is evident during the clinical examination and can be verified by a myelogram, discogram or CT Scan. No matter how skilled a surgeon may be, it is not possible to surgically repair "mechanical" back problems caused by general wear and tear at various levels of the spine.

Robert Moyer, a 40-year-old banker from Vancouver who has suffered from back pain off and on for ten years, knows the truth of this statement only too well. "I had always thought that surgery was an option I could choose if and when I wanted to," he says. "A couple of years ago, when I had had a particularly bad winter, I went to an orthopaedic surgeon and said, 'Okay, it's time. I've had enough. Let's operate.' I guess I was lucky in the sense that he was one of those doctors who takes the time to explain things thoroughly. He ordered a CT Scan and showed me the results. 'Look here,' he explained, using both the CT pictures and ordinary X-rays, 'I can show you general wear and tear at several levels of your spine, but I can't show you anything *specific* that I can go in and fix.' I'm now resigned to living with a certain amount of chronic pain and bad bouts from time to time."

Decompression Surgery

There are several specific variations to the type of surgery that comes under the general heading of decompression:

1. As was the case for Evelyn Weston, the most common decompression operation (discotomy) involves the removal of a herniated disc that is compressing a nerve root. This often requires the removal of a small

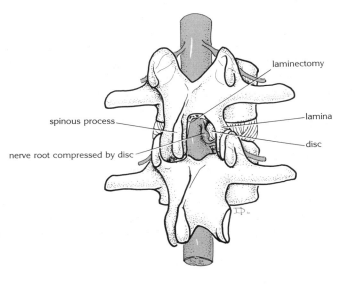

Diagram 23   Decompression Surgery

section of the lamina in order to gain access to the offending disc. In most cases, the herniated nucleus will still be attached to the rest of the disc. In rare cases, the nucleus of the disc will have sequestrated, or broken off completely, from the rest of the disc (see Diagram 14, page 39).

2. In most cases, discs herniate along the rear portion where the annulus tends to be congenitally weak, thereby making the removal of a piece of the lamina essential for access. In some cases, however, a disc will herniate more toward one side, and it is possible for the surgeon to perform a discotomy without first performing a laminectomy to gain access to the disc.

3. In some instances, a nerve can be compressed by a piece of bone rather than a piece of disc. In cases like this, a laminectomy (to remove the offending piece of bone) will be performed without a discotomy. Sometimes, because of osteoarthritic changes, a bone spur, or osteophyte, grows on the anterior section of a vertebra. If this bone spur happens to have developed near the intervertebral foramen (the space between the two vertebrae out of which the nerve root exits from the spinal canal), the exit space will become abnormally narrow. As the nerve root tries to exit, it will be pinched by the bone spur, a condition called lateral spinal stenosis. In other cases, a bone spur growing on a facet joint impinges into the spinal canal itself, compressing a nerve root.

4. In still other cases, there is no bone spur. The problem is that the spinal canal itself is abnormally narrow in either a small area or over an extensive area. This condition is called central spinal stenosis. Although a laminectomy can sometimes correct this condition when it is severe, the surgery must usually be extensive and is very difficult to perform.

Evelyn Weston's discotomy took slightly less than an hour. Having pinpointed the source of her problem by means of a myelogram, her surgeon knew exactly where to make the necessary two-inch incision in her lower back. Moving through, or around, the various layers of muscle, bone and ligament, the surgeon gained access to the vertebra in question. To gain access to the disc itself, he removed a small portion of its bony "roof." In so doing, he completed the laminectomy portion of the procedure.

Peering through the hole he had created in the lamina, the surgeon pushed aside the nerve root and reached his destination, the herniated disc. After enlarging the ruptured hole in the disc, he used a tiny scoop to remove what was left of its nucleus, thus eliminating the source of the nerve compression. Over the next several weeks, this nucleus would become partly and painlessly occupied by scar tissue.

Having completed the second part of the operation – the actual discotomy – the surgeon replaced the nerve root, muscles and ligaments he had pushed aside, then sewed up the incision.

When Evelyn Weston regained consciousness later that morning, she was dismayed to discover that hospital attendants had positioned her on her back, which, not surprisingly, was painfully tender from the surgical incision. What she didn't know at that time, or at least didn't remember being told, was that patients recovering from spinal surgery are routinely placed on their backs. The weight of the patient's body provides pressure that keeps the wound from oozing.

But not many hours had to pass before Evelyn Weston began to realize that her operation had provided her with a welcome trade-off. Certainly she was still feeling a lot of pain, but now it was a different sort of pain, the kind anyone might feel from a severe bump or bruise. She was no longer experiencing those horrible surges of pain down her leg.

Encouraged by the nurses to get up and walk around the hospital only a matter of hours after she came to, she was surprised at how quickly even that temporary pain was subsiding.

Two and a half weeks later, after an uneventful period of recovery, she marched confidently into her surgeon's office for a post-op checkup. And after only a month of physiotherapy, Evelyn Weston discontinued her treatments and started to exercise on her own, three or four times a week. A month after that, she returned to her full-time job as a computer programmer.

Spinal Fusion

There are several different situations when a spinal fusion is performed:

1. As was the case for Marianne Singer, a fusion will be performed for a severe case of spondylolisthesis which does not respond to conservative treatment.

2. In approximately 25 per cent of decompression operations, a decision is made by the surgeon to stabilize the area as well. It could be that a herniated disc has caused the space between two vertebrae to narrow so much that there has been a great deal of wear and tear to the corresponding facet joints; if this is the case, the surgeon will want to prevent further movement. Or, if the laminectomy has necessitated the removal of a substantial amount of bone, the surgeon may decide to fuse that level of the spine to give it additional stability. The decision to fuse is a judgement call made by the surgeon.

Marianne Singer remembers the snowy February day when she underwent her spinal fusion. Having pinpointed the problem at the L5-S1 level, her surgeon cut an incision about three inches long in her lower back and began pushing aside muscles, ligaments and flesh, as he made his way down to the bone.

Once he reached the pair of worn facet joints, he did something that

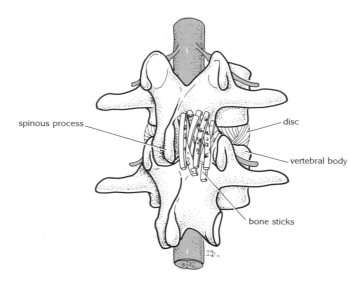

spinous process

disc

vertebral body

bone sticks

Diagram 24   Stabilization Surgery (Spinal Fusion)

would surprise any layman unfamiliar with the standard technique of surgical fusion; with an instrument resembling a double-bevelled chisel, he deliberately damaged the surface of the two little bones. The object was to activate their healing response, an essential process in any successful fusion operation.

Next, through a separate incision, the surgeon gained access to the back of his patient's pelvis. Gently and carefully, he carved off strip after tiny strip of bone, each about an inch long and scarcely thicker than a matchstick.

Once he had collected a dozen or more of these little bone sticks, the surgeon began packing them on either side of the two vertebrae to be fused. Positioned somewhat like tiny splints, the little pieces of pelvic bone were now tucked snugly against those deliberately damaged surfaces of the vertebrae. That roughening up process was a trick played on the body to make it react as though a fracture had occurred. In response, the body's healing mechanism would treat the little bone sticks as though they had broken away from the vertebrae. It would fuse all three elements – the two vertebrae and the surrounding "splints" – into a single, and mercifully stable, portion of Marianne Singer's spine.

With that deed done, the surgeon closed the incision and sent his patient to the recovery room.

Marianne still remembers how painful it was, at first, whenever the

116

attendants found it necessary to lift her. But on the third day after her operation, she managed to get out of bed and move around the hospital room with the aid of a stabilizing hip brace. Two weeks after surgery, still wearing the brace, she went home to begin four months of slow but steady recovery.

The Success Rate for Spinal Surgery

Each year in North America, approximately 200,000 back operations are performed. About 150,000 of these surgeries involve the decompression of a nerve root and about 50,000 involve fusions, either alone or in addition to a decompression.

According to most surgeons, the success rate for spinal surgery involving a decompression alone and at one level only is about 90 per cent. A fusion performed without a decompression operation, or a decompression with a fusion at one level only, is estimated by surgeons to be successful 80 to 90 per cent of the time. The chances for success when the spine is fused at two levels rather than one, however, go down to 75 per cent and to less than 50 per cent when three levels are fused. No more than three levels of the spine can be fused except in the case of severe scoliosis (see page 259).

Having a "successful" spinal operation, however, does not mean that your back will be restored to what it was when you were 16 and could dance till dawn without thinking twice about the state your back would be in the next day. Dr. Hamilton Hall explains the meaning of "success" when applied to back surgery in his book *The Back Doctor* " . . . no back operation can be unconditionally guaranteed," he says. "And even if it could, your back problems would not necessarily be over for all time. Some disc or joint that never caused trouble before could start hurting next week or next year. In any case, spinal surgery can't really cure a bad back – at least not in the sense that an appendectomy can cure appendicitis . . . . [Spinal surgery] will leave you with a back that is something less than normal . . . . In fact, the alterations that take place in your spine during surgery may even cause or contribute to new back trouble at some time in the future . . . . The fact is that when you are left with a less-than-normal back, you will have more reason than ever to keep it in condition with exercise and proper living habits."

About spinal fusion in particular, Dr. Hall has this to say, "[The patient] must realize that fusion won't make his spine normal. He must acknowledge the importance of post-operative care – indefinitely. He must be prepared to accept a degree of post-operative discomfort, if not pain. If he comes to me with a mild backache and wants fusion so that he'll have no backache at all, I can't help him."

A year after surgery both Evelyn Weston and Marianne Singer remain fearful that another attack of back pain might somehow occur. They avoid any sort of heavy lifting, even groceries, and Marianne Singer doubts whether she'll ever resume her favourite pastime – bowling. "I'd be afraid to pick up a bowling ball," she admits.

But like Evelyn Weston, Marianne Singer is thrilled that she can now go through a normal daily routine and even sit for several hours without suffering any back or leg pain.

"I think a person's attitude is very important," she says. "I believe in my surgeon. I told myself that the operation was going to be a success and that I would get better. But I have never forgotten how disabled I was, and I don't expect my back to be 100 per cent. Within certain limitations, I live an almost pain-free life. After what I went through during that last year before surgery, that's as good as 100 per cent for me."

10

Discotomy by Microsurgery: A Morsel to Ponder

In simple terms, a discotomy by microsurgery — technically called a microdiscotomy — is the surgical removal of a disc, or a portion of a disc, with the aid of an operating microscope. It is not all that dramatically different from the traditional discotomy. But because a smaller incision is made to access the disc, less bone and muscle have to be cut, and fewer nerves must be pushed aside. According to the surgeons who routinely perform microdiscotomies, these subtle differences usually mean: 1. less time under the knife; 2. less loss of blood; 3. less post-operative pain; 4. a shorter period of post-operative hospitalization; 5. a more rapid return to normal activities, even jobs that are physically demanding; 6. and less scar tissue, which can sometimes lead to post-surgical complications.

When a traditional discotomy is performed (see page 113), an incision of approximately two inches must be made. In the majority of cases, a portion of the "roof" of the posterior section of the vertebra — the lamina — must be cut away in order for the surgeon to gain access to the disc. This cutting of bone is called a laminectomy and, strictly speaking, a disc removal operation that involves this cutting away of bone should be called a laminectomy-discotomy. Most surgeons, however, just use the shorter term *discotomy*, the laminectomy portion of the procedure being implied.

With a section of the lamina gone, the surgeon will then push aside any nerve roots that are obstructing the view. At this point, the offending disc, and the surrounding structures, become visible to the naked eye. The surgeon, using normal operating room illumination, can actually see the source of the problem.

Usually, the surgeon will see that the disc in question has indeed herniated as shown on the pre-surgical diagnostic tests. The annulus of the disc will be torn; the nucleus will be leaking out (or in some cases will have sequestrated completely from the disc) and will be pressing against the nerve root. At other times, the disc will not actually have herniated but will be bulging sufficiently to be compressing the nerve root. In a few cases, the surgeon will find that the disc which was thought to have herniated is, in fact, intact, and the pressure on the nerve is being caused solely by bone. When the problem has to do with compression due to bone rather than disc material, the laminectomy will suffice. In addition, while all these possibilities are literally being looked into, the surgeon will also be able to examine the nearby facet joints and make an additional decision: are they worn enough to warrant an additional procedure called a spinal fusion to stabilize the area? Fusions for the purpose of stabilization are also sometimes performed when a large amount of bone must be removed during a laminectomy.

When the standard procedure is finished, the surgeon will replace any nerve roots, ligaments or muscles that have been pushed aside, and the incision will then be stitched up.

The average time for the standard discotomy procedure is one hour to one and a half hours. The average length of stay in hospital is about a week to ten days, the first few days of which are often quite painful. Most patients are able to return to their jobs anywhere from about six weeks to several months, depending upon the type of work that they do.

The Microdiscotomy

When a surgeon uses an operating microscope, the internal areas are illuminated and magnified. A smaller field of vision is adequate and, for this reason, a smaller incision (about one inch) will do. The laminectomy part of the laminectomy-discotomy is unnecessary, and there is less surgical trauma and less loss of blood during the operation. The length of time for surgery is reduced to between 30 and 45 minutes. Usually there is less pain and earlier movement after the operation. The patient is generally able to leave the hospital in about five days, and in some cases a mere two days on the ward will suffice. Most microdiscotomy patients are able to return to work in a couple of weeks to a month.

However, it is important to consider that fewer decisions can be made during this type of surgery. Because the surgeon's vision is restricted to such a small area, it is not possible to examine the discs above and below for the possibility of an additional herniation that the pre-surgical diagnostic tests did not pick up. If there is a bone spur, it will probably be missed. As well, with such a small field of vision, there is no opportunity for the facet joints to be examined for severe wear and tear.

Marci MacBain, a 37-year-old surgical nurse, underwent microsurgery a couple of years ago for a herniated L5-S1 disc, which was causing extreme sciatic nerve pain in her left leg. Her problem had begun five years before and was caused, she felt, by the heavy lifting required in her job.

The first time she experienced an acute bout, conservative treatment – three weeks of bed rest followed by a month of physiotherapy – did the trick, and four years passed before the disc again became a problem.

Then Marci MacBain's sciatic nerve pain returned, got better and returned again several times, becoming increasingly worse with each new "attack." A strict regimen of exercise and bed rest did little good, and she began to feel that surgery was her only alternative.

As a nurse, she knew of the possibilities of complication with the traditional discotomy procedure, as well as the length of time it could take to recover. She was also, as she put it, "terrified of surgery." But a friend had had a successful microdiscotomy during this period and was back at work after only two weeks. This convinced Marci MacBain to seek out the same kind of procedure.

"Before surgery I was in terrible shape," she says. "My L5-S1 disc was so badly herniated that the outline of its bulge was *clearly* visible on the myelogram X-ray, the diagnostic test which I had had the day before. But when I woke up in the recovery room, the only pain I experienced was a slight headache, which many of my own patients have felt after a myelogram."

The operation had taken place on a Wednesday morning. That same evening, Marci MacBain was up and around. By Saturday, she was out of the hospital, and four weeks later she was at work doing all the normal duties of a surgical nurse. "I could have returned to work a week sooner," she says, "but I chose to wait until I had regained all my strength." She spent the extra time at home getting back into gear by walking (over a mile a day) and strengthening her back with exercise.

"I think microsurgery is wonderful," she says. "Of all the [surgical] alternatives, I think it's the best." But she is quick to add that it's important to be as certain as possible that a single herniated disc – not worn facet joints or bone spurs for example – is at the root of the back problem. "It's also important to be in good shape for surgery, both physically and mentally. When I finally decided that microsurgery was the answer for me, I was up for it. I think that helped shorten my recovery time."

The Future of Microdiscotomy

The question begs itself: Why hasn't the microsurgery procedure superceded the traditional discotomy in cases of herniated discs? Even if the success rate reported by surgeons for the traditional procedure is as high as 90 per cent, surely a shorter hospital stay, reduced pain and a shorter convalescence time would be enough to warrant a greater interest in the microdiscotomy procedure.

The answers to these questions vary, depending upon whom you ask.

One answer has to do with the conservative attitude of the medical profession and its disinclination toward change. Pioneered in the mid-1960s by American neurosurgeon Dr. Thomas Speakman, and only performed by a handful of surgeons until the early 1970s, the microdiscotomy is still considered a relatively new technique.

But in sorting through the comments on microdiscotomy made by various surgeons, another angle begins to emerge: orthopaedic surgeons seem to have more doubts about the developing field of microdiscotomy than neurosurgeons. Upon reflection, these divergent attitudes make sense.

The training that orthopaedic surgeons receive, as well as the experience they gain over the years, concentrates on the area of big bones. The training and experience of neurosurgeons, on the other hand, is more delicate. Neurosurgeons routinely use operating room microscopes when they perform surgery on other areas of the body, the brain being just one example. It could be that when a surgeon is already familiar with a surgical tool, making the transition from the brain to the back is not so difficult a task.

Orthopaedic surgeon Dr. Hamilton Hall comments briefly on microsurgery in *The Back Doctor*. "There is nothing wrong with this technique," he says, "but I believe a good surgeon can do his job just as well with a conventional pair of magnifying glasses or with the naked eye."

Dr. Marvin Tile, deputy surgeon-in-chief at Sunnybrook Medical Centre in Toronto, is stronger in his opinion of microdiscotomy. In his experience, the post-operative recovery period is not even significantly reduced with microsurgery. He also questions the technique in terms of the difficulty involved in performing surgery in such a restricted space.

Dr. Tile himself has undergone the standard procedure. "You can be up and out of hospital in four days with the traditional discotomy," he says. He also blames the media for the recent surge of interest in the microdiscotomy procedure saying that it sells new procedures to back pain sufferers.

"The media buys into anything that's sensational," he suggests, adding that the technique is gimmicky, especially in the United States where they are doing thousands each year. In his opinion, the indications for microsurgery on the back are very small.

Dr. Hart Schutz, a Toronto neurosurgeon, has performed microsurgery on more than 100 back pain patients at Toronto Western Hospital over the past several years. His feeling is that the success rate with microdiscotomy is "at least as good" as with the traditional procedure and that it is less traumatic. However, he warns that microsurgery should not be looked upon as a panacea for back pain, but as one alternative that is only indicated for a properly diagnosed herniated disc.

Dr. William O'Callaghan, an Edmonton, Alberta neurosurgeon, has reviewed the cases of his approximately 1,800 microdiscotomy patients. He says that only 15 per cent have had recurrent problems due to facet joint instability. Of this 15 per cent, he says, less than 7 per cent eventually end up having to have a spinal fusion.

Dr. Michael Schwartz, a neurosurgeon at Sunnybrook Medical Centre in Toronto, is even more conservative. He points out that of the two major causes of post-operative problems, only one – scarring on or around the nerve as a result of the incision – is likely to be reduced with microsurgery. The other major cause of post-operative trouble – ineffective relief of nerve compression – is not, in his opinion, necessarily lessened with microsurgery. "I also question whether total relief can be achieved with certainty when the surgeon is working through the tiny incision and has such a narrow field of vision," he says.

More extensive research on microdiscotomy has been conducted in the United States. It seems to indicate that the pluses of microsurgery outweigh the minuses. Dr. Harold Goald, a neurosurgeon from Virginia, studied 425 of Dr. Robert Williams's patients; Dr. Williams is a Las Vegas, Nevada neurosurgeon, who began using the microdiscotomy technique in 1972. The average post-operative hospital stay for these patients was only 3.1 days, and the success rate after five years of follow-up was 92 per cent.

Dr. Goald also studied 147 of his own patients and published his results in the June 1972 issue of the internationally renowned medical journal *Spine*. The post-operative hospital stay for these patients was less than three days and the success rate 96 per cent. A year after surgery, *all* of the patients not on worker's compensation were back at their jobs. As well, 80 per cent of those who were on compensation were back at work.

American research studies also report that after the microdiscotomy technique, patients usually return to their usual activities within four to six weeks, unless heavy labour is involved. When the patient's job is labour intensive, the convalescence time can increase to a couple of months, which is not all that different from the standard procedure.

Perhaps the most interesting comment, however, comes from one Canadian neurosurgeon, and the most interesting thing about it is that the doctor making it refuses to be identified. "In cases of well-diagnosed acute disc herniations," he maintains, "microsurgery is better for the patient. I am convinced that it will be the technique of the future and that neurosurgeons will be doing more back surgery and orthopaedic surgeons less."

For the moment the controversy will likely whimper on.

11

Chymopapain: Myth or Miracle?

While one group of doctors argues with the other over which surgical procedure is better for patients with herniated discs, yet another group contends that in many cases, surgery is not necessary at all. These are the proponents of the chymopapain injection, the enzyme that simply *dissolves* the offending nucleus of a herniated disc.

Chymopapain has been legal in Canada since 1972 even though the U.S. Food and Drug Administration did not approve the drug until a decade later. This situation is unusual. For one thing, chymopapain was first synthesized in the United States. For another, in matters such as the approval of drugs, Canada is usually far more conservative than her southern neighbour.

To date, about 10,000 North American doctors have taken courses and attended seminars to learn about the technique, which is invasive but still less radical than even microsurgery. Once they have tried it on patients of their own, most of these doctors swear up and down that if the candidate is well chosen, and the technician adept, the results are almost always superb.

A good candidate for chymopapain is someone who has a herniated disc which is compressing a lumbar nerve root. That person will have the classical clinical symptoms of a disc herniation: a Straight Leg Raise test that causes severe sciatic pain; a myelogram or CT Scan test that shows a definite disc protrusion; and at least six to twelve weeks of conservative treatment, including bed rest, without any results. (Some physicians question whether a person who has had severe sciatic pain for more than two years can benefit from chymopapain. By this time, they believe, adaptive changes such as adhesions (see page 39) may also have occurred, making the problem more complex than the original herniated disc.)

Dr. J.C. (Carl) Sutton, Jr., is director of orthopaedic surgery at St. Mary's Hospital in Montreal. Since 1973, a year after the drug was approved in Canada, he and his fellow orthopaedic surgeons at St. Mary's have used chymopapain on almost 2,000 patients with herniated discs. If it weren't for this technique, all of these patients would have undergone disc surgery – either the standard procedure or microdiscotomy.

Dr. Sutton has followed his chymopapain patients in two studies. The first study, which was completed in 1980, was encouraging – a success rate of 78 per cent. "By 'successful,' I mean excellent to good results (as opposed to fair results or no relief at all) as reported *by the patients themselves*, rather than their surgeons," says Dr. Sutton.

Few physicians are surprised when they are told that chymopapain is successful over the short term. What they want to know is whether or not the results will endure. In Dr. Sutton's 1984 study were 228 long-term chymopapain patients; they had had their injections between six and eleven years earlier, and the success rates were exactly the same. "But not only are the success rates as good as, or better, with chymopapain as compared with traditional surgery," says Dr. Sutton. "Because there is no cutting with chymopapain, there is the added advantage of no scar tissue, which has been known to lead to complications down the road. As well, there is usually a faster, and often a less painful, recovery period with chymopapain than with surgery."

The lay press has described the chymopapain enzyme as having the same effect on the nucleus of a herniated disc as meat tenderizer has on a tough pot roast. Chymopapain breaks down the protein material that is normally contained within the nucleus of the disc, but does not affect the disc's annulus, or outer ring, which is made up of cartilage. Basically, chymopapain reduces the nucleus to a consistency that can be absorbed by the system and ultimately excreted through the urine.

Says Dr. Sutton, "There are five orthopaedic surgeons here at St. Mary's. None of us has performed 'primary' disc surgery since 1979. We all believe that it makes sense to try chymopapain first.... And only a small percentage of our patients have ended up having to have spinal surgery because of a failure with chymopapain."

The Chymopapain Procedure

The chymopapain procedure is not terribly complex. An experienced orthopaedic surgeon who has performed diagnostic discogram tests, or a radiologist, can become proficient at performing chymopapain injections after a few days of practice.

The procedure is performed either in a standard operating room or radiology suite with the patient under general anaesthetic. (A few centres perform chymopapain injections with the patient under local anaesthesia.) Patients are positioned on their side with their legs bent at the hips and the knees. Throughout the procedure, the surgeon uses X-rays, which can be watched on a fluoroscope screen, to ensure that the position of the needle, which is critical, is correct.

In most centres, at St. Mary's for example, a two-level discogram is routinely performed prior to the chymopapain injection as a final diagnostic measure. Says Dr. Sutton, "The discogram is just one more failsafe procedure we go through, although by this time we're almost certain that we've got a true disc herniation from the other tests – the clinical diagnosis and either a CT Scan or a myelogram."

For the discogram, Dr. Sutton inserts a single, six-inch, 18-gauge needle into the nucleus of the L4-L5 disc and then another needle into the L5-S1 disc, checks the position of both needles on the fluoroscope screen and then injects radiopaque dye. (Because he is gaining entry to the nucleus laterally – the patient is positioned on his or her side – Dr. Sutton uses a single needle technique, rather than the double needle technique described on page 108.) If there is a herniation, and in almost all cases there is, the way the dye flows into the disc will confirm the diagnosis. Most of the time there is only one herniation, but sometimes he will find two. "One of the beauties of chymopapain," he says, "is that the chances of success when you inject two levels are just as good as they are when you inject one; when you use the surgical technique, the chances of success diminish when more than one level is involved."

Using the same needle (or needles if two levels are being treated), he will then inject approximately 1.5 cc of chymopapain into the disc. At this stage, he and the anaesthesiologist will be particularly on guard for an anaphylactic, or allergic, reaction to the drug. Although rare (occurring in less than .5 per cent of patients), anaphylactic reactions can be fatal if not responded to immediately. To reduce the chances of this type of reaction, many doctors routinely give their chymopapain patients antihistamine medication for three days before their procedure is to take place. "Since we started taking this extra precaution at St. Mary's," says Dr. Sutton, "we have not had a single anaphylactic reaction."

After the chymopapain has been injected, the needle (or needles) is withdrawn, the small injection site is covered with a bandage, and the patient is wheeled into the recovery room.

Dr. Sutton's typical chymopapain patient can be seen walking the halls of St. Mary's Hospital unaided on the second day after the chymopapain procedure. Moreover, he or she is usually free of their disabling sciatic pain after only two or three days. In most cases, patients can return to work after four to six weeks, which in Dr. Sutton's experience is about the same number of weeks as the patient who has undergone the standard procedure. In some instances, however, chymopapain patients have gone back to work in two weeks or less.

Robin Ward, a 34-year-old elementary school teacher, underwent a chymopapain injection of the disc between the L4 and L5 vertebrae last summer. "My doctor said I was the perfect candidate. I had had nagging backache and a bit of sciatic pain for about four or five years. It was the "on again, off again" type of chronic back pain until one day, bam! The pain running down my left leg was so severe I saw stars. At that point I didn't really have much back pain, or perhaps I just couldn't feel any through the madness that was surging down my leg."

Prior to his chymopapain injection, two months of bed rest — during May and June — accomplished nothing for Robin Ward. Anxious to be back in shape again before the school year started in September, he tracked down a doctor who had been performing chymopapain injections for several years. "I had read about the technique and it was what I wanted," he says. "I figured there was always time for surgery and why not try this first. I was given a myelogram test, which was positive, and I stayed in hospital for the next three days. I had my injection on a Wednesday morning, the second week in July."

When he woke up from the anaesthetic, Robin Ward was experiencing extreme discomfort. "*Discomfort* is the word my doctor used! My back was killing me. I felt as if I had a vise grip around my waist and I thought, 'Oh boy, Ward, have you ever bitten the biscuit this time'." The nurses, however, assured him that this was not an abnormal occurrence and had no bearing on whether his injection had been a success.

"For two days I took pain-killers and felt sorry for myself, and then the back pain began to subside. It was only then that I realized that my leg pain was all but completely gone."

For the next month Robin Ward took it easy, sitting as little as possible and letting his wife carry the groceries. In September, on schedule, he made it back to school, and although he still tries to avoid excessive sitting and does back exercises daily, life has more or less returned to normal.

"I wouldn't go so far as to say it was a *good* summer," he says. "But I have a few friends who've gone through back surgery, and believe me, the stories they have to tell about pain and suffering and recuperation were a heck of a lot worse than mine. I can't imagine anyone who is a good candidate not preferring chymopapain to the knife."

The History of Chymopapain

The chymopapain enzyme was first used experimentally in the late 1950s. Its use was pioneered by Dr. Lyman Smith, an orthopaedic surgeon from Elgin, Illinois. Dr. Smith had read about the dissolving properties of papain in a paper published by Dr. Lewis Thomas, Chancellor of Memorial Sloan-Kettering Cancer Center and author of *Lives of a Cell* and *The Youngest Science*.

Ironically, the actual discovery had been pure serendipity; Dr. Thomas, an oncologist, was not the slightest bit interested in herniated discs when he isolated papain (a less refined version of chymopapain) from a papaya fruit and injected it into a group of rabbits. On the contrary, Dr. Thomas was trying to see if various enzymes could alter the concentrations of certain proteins in the blood. When he returned the next morning, he was surprised to find that his rabbits had their ears literally to the ground. He quickly figured out that the gelatinous protein of the cartilage in the rabbits' ears had been dissolved by the enzyme, and he published his paper the following year.

Realizing that the protein of the cartilage in a rabbit's ear is much like the material that composes the nucleus of an intervertebral disc, Dr. Lyman Smith began to experiment with papain on herniated discs.

Soon after, he sold his patent rights for the drug to Baxter-Travenol, an American drug company whose Canadian branch is called Travenol Canada. Baxter-Travenol refined papain into chymopapain, named the product Discase and, in 1963, obtained U.S. Food and Drug Administration approval to use it as a human investigational drug. Dr. Smith initiated the first clinical studies using chymopapain and coined the term *chemonucleolysis* to describe the operative procedure by which a disc's nucleus can be dissolved by chemical means.

For 12 years, the route to final FDA approval seemed to be progressing smoothly; some 15,000 patients were treated with chymopapain injections and, in most cases, the sciatic pain caused by their herniated discs was relieved without any need for decompression surgery. In 1972, Discase was approved in Canada. Then, in 1975, a Baxter-Travenol study – whose technique and validity have since been assailed on numerous fronts by several notable researchers – ground the quest for the approval of chymopapain in the United States to a halt.

The study suggested that Discase was no more effective at dissolving the nuclei of herniated discs than the placebo against which it was measured. (The irony was that the placebo itself was later found to have dissolving properties of its own and became the only placebo in history to be patented as a potentially useful medicine!)

In any case, Baxter-Travenol, perhaps feeling that it had expended enough effort on chymopapain research for the time being, withdrew its FDA application and stopped producing the drug. That left a situation with a number of unusual, and certainly interesting, characteristics.

For one thing, the drug Discase, which had been used for three years here in Canada, was suddenly unavailable in the United States; in almost every case, with drugs that are developed in the U.S., it's the other way around. For another, studies on the use of chymopapain being conducted by notable researchers in Australia and Europe were coming up with highly positive results. This threw the Baxter-Travenol study into question.

128

In 1976, a group of Americans – comprised of both doctors and lay people – formed CADUCEUS (Committee Advocating the Development and Use of Chymopapain to Eliminate Unnecessary Surgery). The sole aim of the committee was to see chymopapain made available in the U.S. A couple of years later, through CADUCEUS's efforts, the drug was legalized at the state level in Texas, Indiana and Illinois, although only the Lone Star State had the legislative processes needed to license a drug not federally approved, as well as the environment to grow the papaya trees to provide the fruit. But access to American physicians using chymopapain was limited and many Americans with sore backs – thousands by some estimates – flocked to Canada for chymopapain injections. During those years, there was such a frenzy of activity and so much misinformation floating around about "Chymopapain the Wonderdrug" that many Canadian doctors were afraid of giving interviews to the lay press. Every time such an article appeared, it would bring crowds of back pain sufferers. Most of them were not candidates for chymopapain but hadn't read the fine print.

"It's true," says Dr. Sutton, "during the years that chymopapain was not accepted in the U.S. but recognized in Canada, Americans flowed over the border in droves whenever there was a lot of press about the drug. They all wanted the new miracle drug for back pain . . . . Many of them didn't realize that chymopapain is only good for the same type of patient who would benefit from disc surgery. The problem is, chymopapain can't do a lot of other things that hopeful patients ask it to do. It can't dissolve bone spurs that are pressing on nerves. It can't dissolve emotional problems, and it can't dissolve general wear and tear mechanical problems that account for at least 90 per cent of all back pain."

During the remainder of the 1970s, while American citizens continued to journey to Canada for chymopapain injections, CADUCEUS continued its efforts in the U.S. They distributed information on how to be referred to Canadian physicians for chymopapain treatment. They lobbied for public hearings before the Senate Subcommittee on Health and Scientific Research and the House Subcommittee on Health and Environment. The effort brought to light what kind of impact a consumer group can have on health issues when its objectives are clear and its members undaunted.

Then, in July 1979, Dr. Lyman Smith's nephew, general surgeon Dr. W. Scott Smith, formed Smith Laboratories to pursue the potential of chymopapain in the U.S. Smith Laboratories developed a new chymopapain product, an even more purified version than Baxter-Travenol's Discase, and named it Chymodiactin.

Early in 1981, Smith Laboratories began two large American studies using the new drug. The results of both studies were positive, and in November of 1982, Chymodiactin was approved by the FDA. In Canada, Chymodiactin was licensed by Smith Laboratories to Ayerst Laboratories, and the drug was approved in the fall of 1984. Since the efficacy of chymopapain was no longer disputed, Discase was also approved in the U.S. during 1984.

Says Dr. Carl Sutton, "In my opinion, chymopapain is the procedure of the future for herniated discs. I wouldn't be surprised if, in a decade, chymopapain — at least as the *primary* procedure — does replace the knife."

Considering that approximately 200,000 decompression operations are performed in North America every year, a statement like that could do a lot for papaya fruit futures as well as the scarless back.

12

Orthopaedic Physicians: Manipulative Medicine

Ned Franklin's back problem was one of those cases that makes orthopaedic surgeons wring their hands and roll their eyes upward for divine intervention. An active man who had always lifted weights, jogged, played hockey and baseball, Franklin injured his lower back in the late 1970s while on the job as a dog catcher in Rochester, New York. He was in such pain that he could hardly walk. His physician ordered a myelogram (see page 105) hoping to find that a disc herniation – for which surgery would be indicated – was at the root of his back trouble. Unfortunately, the results revealed nothing. Ned Franklin was told that there was nothing an orthopaedic surgeon could do.

A short while later, he consulted Dr. Donald Fraser, one of a small number of North American physicians who specializes in orthopaedic medicine as opposed to orthopaedic surgery. As a result of Dr. Fraser's treatment, Franklin is now mobile. "I've never been able to resume an active sports life," he says, "but at least I'm somewhat human again. That's the main thing. And it's been a great help to me psychologically."

Dr. Donald Fraser of St. Catharines, Ontario, had taken only a mild interest in orthopaedic medicine until he found himself in hospital with a severely bulging disc. For almost a week, he lay in agony, unresponsive to conventional treatment and, like Ned Franklin, an inappropriate candidate for back surgery. Finally, figuring he had nothing much to lose, Dr. Fraser talked his own attending physician into trying out one of the techniques frequently used by practitioners of orthopaedic medicine. That evening, Dr. Fraser underwent a caudal epidural block. Within days, he was able to walk unaided. A few weeks later, he returned to his busy family practice.

"That was in 1971 and I haven't looked back since," says Dr. Fraser, referring to his own back problem. Impressed by the results, he began to involve himself in the speciality, and several years ago, he gave up his family practice to pursue orthopaedic medicine full-time. In August 1983, he was appointed clinical assistant professor of orthopaedic medicine at the Rochester, N.Y. Strong Memorial Hospital. Dr. Fraser commutes to Strong from Canada, once a week.

Orthopaedic physicians, as they call themselves, are a distinct breed, not to be confused with orthopaedic surgeons. Their founder Dr. James Cyriax, now in his nineties, began to lay out the speciality's credo in 1929 while training to be an orthopaedic surgeon at St. Thomas's Hospital in London, England. Dr. Cyriax was aware that soft tissue does not show up on regular X-rays, one of the diagnostic mainstays of the orthopaedic surgeon; the only thing that shows up on regular X-rays is bone. As a result, injuries of the discs, muscles, ligaments, tendons, joint capsules and other soft tissue of the back cannot be pinpointed easily. Instead, they are treated generally rather than specifically. The entire area receives such treatments as heat, exercise and massage to relieve the symptoms. The hope is that this generalized application will hit the right spot.

Dr. Cyriax, however, was not satisfied with the concept of *hoping* to hit the right spot. All pain has a source, he reasoned, and to be properly treated, this source has to be identified accurately. On the basis of this concept, he developed orthopaedic medicine, which he defines as "the nonsurgical management of soft tissue disorders of the musculoskeletal system." According to Dr. Fraser, these disorders comprise 20 per cent of the complaints seen in a general practitioner's office. Surgery for ailments of the musculoskeletal system, he believes, should remain within the domain of the orthopaedic surgeon.

The most common back ailments that Dr. Fraser treats are disc problems and joint problems. He also treats backache caused by strained ligaments, which in his opinion is more rare.

The Orthopaedic Physician's Diagnostic Examination

To determine the source of a back problem, Dr. Fraser puts the patient through a series of movements called Selective Tissue Tension (STT), the diagnostic kingpin on which the entire body of orthopaedic medicine rests. The initial diagnostic session can take up to half an hour.

First, the back is put through its six major movements: flexion, extension, right rotation, left rotation, right side flexion and left side flexion. The patient is first asked to perform each of these movements unaided; when performed actively, the physician can get an indication of the patient's range of motion and the area of pain.

Next, the same movements are repeated, but this time the patient remains passive. In this sequence, the muscles do not contract and, according to orthopaedic physicians, it is possible to detect if the pain is coming from structures such as the dura mater, the spinal canal or nerve roots.

Finally, the movements are repeated *against* resistance, and this, according to orthopaedic physicians, indicates if the pain is originating from a muscle or a tendon.

"With this kind of examination," says Dr. Fraser, "the source of referred pain to the leg can also frequently be pinpointed.

"If all six movements intensify the patient's pain, then the problem is likely due to traumatic arthritis, a fracture or even a tumour," says Dr. Fraser. "If five, or fewer, of the movements cause pain, we begin to look for a protruding disc."

When they talk about disc problems, however, orthopaedic physicians are not speaking about the operable, true disc herniations which orthopaedic surgeons are looking for when they order a myelogram. Instead, they are talking about two distinctly different types of protruding, or bulging, discs. One they refer to as a hard disc problem. The other they call a soft disc problem.

What Dr. Fraser refers to as a soft disc is the condition where the outer layer of the disc — the annulus fibrosus — has cracked slightly. As a result, a portion of the disc's nucleus oozes out through the crack. "This is the kind of disc problem that often produces a backache when you are spending hours in a bent over position such as gardening, or typing while hunched over a desk," says Dr. Fraser.

With a hard disc, a section of the annulus, usually the rear portion, has lost its strength. "The annulus has become weak, but there is no actual crack. The pressure of the nucleus against the annulus causes the annulus to bulge," he says. While there are few pain receptors in the annulus itself, a bulging annulus can come into contact with a nerve root, or one of the other pain-sensitive structures, such as a ligament or the dura mater. "This is the condition that is usually affecting the person who bends over, hears a click, and finds himself stuck, unable to get back up," says Dr. Fraser.

In both instances, says Dr. Fraser, there is a great range of severity, from the minor condition to the extreme case.

Orthopaedic physicians believe that if the situation is not serious enough to cause any neurological deficit (no loss of sensation or muscle strength) the soft disc condition can frequently be successfully treated with traction. If this is the diagnosis, the orthopaedic physician will generally turn the patient over to a physiotherapist who will apply the treatment. Basically, during traction, the upper and lower parts of the body are pulled in opposite directions and, according to orthopaedic physicians, this can reduce stress on a soft disc condition sufficiently to enable the disc to heal. Usually, traction for a disc problem is applied continuously for 15 to 30 minutes. The hard disc condition, on the other hand, is generally treated with manipulation. Dr. Fraser, however, is quick to point out that in contrast to most chiropractors, orthopaedic physicians do not manipulate almost every patient they see.

Says Dr. Fraser, "Many chiropractors will also continue to manipulate a patient even if there are no results over the short term. In contrast, manipulation is only a *small* part of the roster of orthopaedic medicine, one remedy for carefully selected, well-diagnosed injuries. As well, in our opinion, manipulation works almost immediately or not at all. If, after two or three sessions of manipulation, either the range of motion has not increased or the pain has not subsided, then the diagnosis or the choice of treatment must have been wrong. As well, we do not believe in repetitive manipulation. If there is any amount of joint instability – there frequently is when a hard disc problem is involved – then it doesn't make good sense to wiggle it about too much." As with traction, Dr. Fraser often refers patients in need of manipulation to a physiotherapist who has been trained in the technique.

The Caudal Epidural Block

When a disc protrudes far enough to produce some amount of neurological deficit, however, manipulation and traction are both useless, according to orthopaedic physicians. At that point a patient sometimes becomes a candidate for a caudal epidural block, the treatment Dr. Fraser himself tried in 1971. Dr. Fraser has also tried the caudal block technique on some of his patients who have not responded to traction or manipulation and says he has had a good deal of success.

The caudal epidural injection is a technique that Dr. Cyriax stumbled on by accident decades ago. Cyriax was trying to diagnose a particularly difficult case and used a procaine injection as a diagnostic tool, rather than as a method of treatment. His theory was that if he injected procaine (which is an anaesthetic) into a specific spot in the back and the patient's pain temporarily disappeared, then he could assume he had found the source of the problem. What astounded him was that a week later, the patient returned and stated categorically that her back pain had disappeared completely, and, what's more, had not returned.

After many years of experimentation, Dr. Cyriax developed the caudal epidural injection technique, which he has now used on thousands of patients. He injects a procaine solution into the caudal aperture, the small opening in the sacrum, or tailbone. (This is the same opening into which an epidural anaesthetic used to be injected during childbirth; in recent years, doctors have been using a different technique.) The procaine rises up in the spinal canal just to the third lumbar disc level. Generally, that is far enough, because it is the two lower lumbar discs that account for most protrusions, or herniations.

134

Why caudal epidurals work is still theory, rather than fact. The explanation that orthopaedic physicians use is that the procaine desensitizes the nerve root and can also hydraulically separate a protruding disc from a nerve root or the dura mater, if it happens to be adhering to one or both of them. Dr. Fraser, who has performed more than 1,200 caudal epidural injections since 1974, says that the technique is also frequently effective on patients who have chronic backache caused by scar tissue after disc surgery.

The caudal epidural injection takes about ten minutes to perform. Strictly speaking, it is not painful because the area where the long needle is inserted is first desensitized by an injection of local anaesthetic. The feeling is most often described as "uncomfortable pressure."

"It's not only the pressure that I remember," says Jean Williams, a 34-year-old teacher from New York, who had a successful caudal epidural block in 1983. "It's the fear. You can't actually say that it's painful, but it's frightening, and it's really awfully hard to relax knowing that such a long needle is in there. Still, it was worth it. It's not perfect. My back still aches a lot of the time. But I no longer get that sort of nerve pain, as if someone was twanging a nerve at the base of my spine. I had tried everything by the time I heard about Dr. Fraser and so far it's given the best results."

In Dr. Fraser's case, a single injection did the trick. In other cases, Ned Franklin's for example, more than one injection is necessary. Since 1978, Franklin has had 12 caudal epidural blocks. Usually, he feels fine for between three and six months, after which a gradually increasing backache tips him off that it's time for another injection.

"Without this treatment, I don't know what I would have done," he says. "I don't think I could have endured going on indefinitely knowing that there was nothing that could be done for my case."

Sclerosing

Another technique that orthopaedic physicians use is still somewhat controversial in North America, although it has been used in England for more than 20 years. It is called sclerosing, and it is used when ligaments in the area of a problem disc have become lax, usually due to chronic poor posture. Normally, stretched ligaments will not become tight on their own, even if the posture is corrected and the patient exercises diligently. If a ligament *tears*, however, the area will become inflamed and the inflammation will cause the ligament to contract.

To tighten up lax ligaments, Dr. Fraser injects a ligamentous thickening agent — a mixture of phenol and glucose — into the ligaments which have stretched. The result is a sterile inflammation, which causes the stretched ligaments to thicken and shorten.

"Sclerosing is useful for ligaments in the lumbar area," says Dr. Fraser.

"It's also useful for the ligaments around the sacroiliac joints. That's where I use it a lot, especially on people who've been in car accidents."

Depending upon how loose the ligaments are, or how much heavy work the patient does afterward, a booster injection might be needed every few months or years.

One of Dr. Fraser's "prize sclerosing patients" is 44-year-old Roger Endicott. Endicott first came to Dr. Fraser in 1975 and was diagnosed as having a strained sacroiliac joint. After his treatment, Endicott was able to return to his job as a warehouse stockman.

If a patient fails to improve after any of these methods, an orthopaedic physician will refer him or her to an orthopaedic surgeon – often one who specializes in chymopapain injections. Although chymopapain is an invasive procedure, it is still more conservative than surgery and preferred for this reason by Dr. Fraser. Only if chymopapain fails, or the patient is simply not considered to be a suitable candidate for the injection, will surgery be considered. "But only about five per cent of back pain patients should end up with surgery," Dr. Fraser insists. "The rest we can carry back to functioning again with these more conservative methods."

Like other practitioners with other methods, Dr. Fraser does not try to imply that orthopaedic medicine is a magic solution for all back pain. Once the initial crisis is over, Dr. Fraser ensures that his patients are taught body mechanics – both proper posture and movement – to reduce the chances of recurrence. For some patients, Dr. Fraser recommends a light nylon lumbar back support to prevent them from bending forward, which causes excess pressure on the posterior portion of the discs. In fact, Dr. Fraser and his colleagues disagree with many other physicians who feel that most back pain is caused by worn facet joints rather than disc problems. "We feel that discs contribute more than they are given credit for," says Dr. Fraser, "and for someone with a disc problem, a slight amount of lordosis is a good thing. Lordosis puts pressure on the anterior portion of the disc so that if it does bulge slightly, it will bulge toward the front of the body rather than the back, where it is more likely to irritate a nerve root."

While it has certainly become recognized in recent years, orthopaedic medicine has not exactly taken the world by storm. The International Society of Orthopaedic Medicine has only 800 members. Approximately half are physicians and half are physiotherapists, many of whom work with orthopaedic physicians. The society conducts instruction courses across North America and England, but only one medical school, the University of Rochester's Strong Memorial Hospital, has an entire department dedicated to orthopaedic medicine. While at least 500 North American physicians and physiotherapists have completed the eight-day orthopaedic medicine instruction course over the past decade, only a handful of physicians actually practise orthopaedic medicine full time.

"Part of this may be due to the fact that our methods of diagnosis and treatment are so time-consuming," says Dr. Fraser by way of an explanation. "Because of the way health insurance plans are set up, physicians are reimbursed for the volume of patients they see, rather than for the length of time they may spend with each one.

"Orthopaedic physicians are certainly not in competition with orthopaedic surgeons," he adds. "In fact, we complement each other. Ideally, the orthopaedic physician can help the orthopaedic surgeon with the soft tissue problems that don't require surgery. Most surgeons can scarcely keep up with the load of trauma patients who do require surgery that keeps coming down the road."

If you would like more information about orthopaedic medicine and a list of physicians who practise it in your area, write to: The Secretary, The North American Society of Orthopaedic Medicine, c/o 145 Queenston St., St. Catharines, Ontario, Canada, L2R 2Z8.

13

Acupuncture: Pinning It Down

It is a damp, cloudy day in Northern China; the year is 2000 B.C. A soldier who has suffered from sciatic pain in his right leg for two decades is fighting for the sanctity of his homeland when he is struck in the hip by a Mongol's arrow. As he is lugged off the battlefield on a stretcher, he notices a curious phenomenon. While his hip hurts like hell, his leg pain is gone! Even more interesting (and still a mystery to those who know that in the heat of battle, people's perceptions of pain are often altered) is that months later, after the hip wound has healed, the leg pain is still gone.

An apocryphal story? Perhaps. Nonetheless, it is the one that is most often recounted when someone asks how acupuncture was first discovered to be an effective method of treating chronic pain.

Almost 5,000 years pass. It is 1971, and *New York Times* columnist James Reston is recovering in a Chinese hospital from an emergency appendectomy. When he is practically overcome by gas pain, a frequent phenomenon after abdominal surgery, the Chinese physician does not pass a tube into Reston's stomach, which is what a North American doctor would have done. Instead, with Reston's permission, the Chinese physician inserts a few paper-thin, stainless steel, two-inch acupuncture needles into Reston's leg and, for several minutes, twirls them around. Miraculously, the gas pain disappears.

This time, however, the story is definitely no apocrypha. Reston writes about his acupuncture treatment in the *New York Times*, the column is syndicated, and the western world, receptive in any case to all things eastern during this turbulent decade, responds with alacrity. Acupuncture, some headlines say, is the best medical discovery since doctors began to reduce patient mortality by washing their hands! Acupuncture is the long-sought-after panacea that is going to cure everything! Acupuncture is the best damned invention since sliced bread!

Like most fads, acupuncture did not live up to its snake oil image, and within a few years its use — and the amount of publicity it was receiving — diminished. Many doctors dismissed it as a load of mystic hokus-pokus, rejecting all claims that sticking needles into strategic points of the body could provide long-term relief from chronic pain.

But quietly, first a handful, and then more doctors, began to pursue the technique. At first, they used the classical Chinese approach, which divides the body into meridians, or pathways, and names hundreds of acupuncture points that correspond to different organ systems. Then they began to transpose the eastern methodology into a western version, which meant that anyone who had studied anatomy in a western medical school could learn the acupuncture points.

Dr. Linda Rapson is Director of Education for the Acupuncture Foundation of Canada, which trains doctors and dentists to use the technique. "In the early years," she says, "I saw no reason why acupuncture shouldn't be approached as a good additional tool to be used. I had a lot of patients with chronic pain, and so I began to study it and incorporate it into my general practice." She disagrees vehemently with those who rejected acupuncture as useless when it didn't alleviate pain completely. "Ironically," she says in defence of her discipline, "those same people didn't expect instant and complete relief from other treatments such as massage therapy, physiotherapy or even drugs."

Several years later, Dr. Rapson was finding acupuncture so useful that she gave up her busy family practice to become an acupuncturist full time. Today, she treats approximately 400 new patients each year, many of whom suffer from back pain. While she cannot exactly say that public interest in acupuncture has come full circle since its fiery arrival in North America and subsequent decline, Dr. Rapson has witnessed a slow but steady resurrection. In 1975, the Ontario Medical Association came out strongly against the technique, saying that there was no scientific proof that it did any good at all. By the end of the decade, however, many physicians had seen their patients go for acupuncture treatments and get positive results. In 1980, the association changed its position to accept acupuncture as a valid modality of treatment in the management of pain. It surveyed 450 of its members who had had some acupuncture training from the Acupuncture Foundation. Of the approximately 150 physicians who responded, 97 said that they were using the technique. They also reported that they had given 6,200 separate acupuncture treatments during a three-month period, although the number of patients who were treated was not specified, and the survey did not inquire about the success these doctors were having, or the lack of it.

Around the same time, however, several studies that did deal with the efficacy of acupuncture received some press. One, which had been conducted by the Workers' Compensation Board of British Columbia during

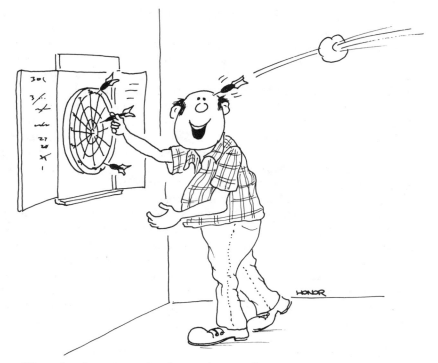

"Gee, thanks . . . my back pain's gone!"

1976-77, compared 29 people who received the standard therapy regimen of the WCB clinic *plus* acupuncture with 27 people who got the regimen *without* acupuncture. At the final follow-up – about six months after the patients were discharged – the group that had received acupuncture was found to be "clearly and significantly" better off than the group that had not.

A larger study conducted by the Acupuncture Foundation on 91 back pain sufferers (who had suffered back pain from a variety of musculo-skeletal and degenerative disc disorders for an average of ten years) also got positive results. It found that almost three-quarters of the over-all group had "significant relief" from their pain. Some got total relief. Others still had "mild" pain and some had what they called "good relief with some continuing discomfort."

Maureen Dawson, a 47-year-old secretary, was one of those 91 patients. She sought acupuncture treatments from Dr. Rapson, like many chronic back pain patients, "as a last resort." "Over the years," says Maureen Dawson, "I had used many strong drugs to relieve my back and leg pain.

Nothing worked very well. Now that I have acupuncture, I lead an almost pain-free life."

Patients who come to Dr. Rapson for chronic pain normally receive acupuncture treatments once a week, although if someone is suffering from severe acute pain, she will sometimes treat them daily for up to, but not longer than, one week. She does not promise immediate relief, but she at least does not hold out the prospect of endless treatments without results.

"If acupuncture is going to work for someone, then in my experience, you begin to get an improvement rather quickly," she says. This, according to her records, means sometime between the first and second of an initial series of seven or eight visits. "Of course, I don't treat people with acupuncture in isolation," she explains, "I also make suggestions regarding changes in posture, work habits and exercise." She advises her patients to continue with their acupuncture treatments until their back pain is gone or until it stops improving. Some people find that once their pain either stops completely or improves to an acceptable level, it stays that way. Others find that they must return for acupuncture treatments from time to time to maintain their pain-free or reduced pain status, or that using a TENS machine at home, which works on a similar principle (see page 148), will suffice.

Does Acupuncture Hurt?

To the uninitiated, acupuncture, with its many needles seems to make use of pain to get rid of pain. What really happens during an acupuncture session and how stressful a treatment is it to endure?

"When I first heard about acupuncture," says Maureen Dawson, "I was too scared to try it. I'm terrified of needles. The thought of having a bunch of them stuck into my back all at once was just too much. It took me a couple of months, and a few stories from some friends who had had good results, to work up to it."

But when she actually did try it, she found that acupuncture was not particularly painful. "I was amazed," she says. "There was a slight sensation, like a pinprick, as each needle went in and then nothing much at all during my half hour of treatment. Once or twice, when a needle was slightly off target, there was a feeling like a nerve being pinched, but without the sharp pain. It was more like a slight prickling that hurt for an instant. After a few weeks, my doctor learned which points worked best for me, and I lost my fear completely."

One of the main reasons why acupuncture doesn't hurt is that the needles used for the technique are different from the needles with which most of us are familiar. The acupuncture needles that Dr. Rapson uses for back pain, for example, are one to three inches long but much finer in diameter than hypodermic needles. "A hypodermic needle is a cutting needle," she explains. "The ones we use for acupuncture have rounded tips. They're not designed to slash through tissue. As well, when you get an injection, it's not just the needle that causes the pain, since there is really no sensation of pain once you break through the skin; mostly what you feel is the stuff they're injecting. Penicillin, for example, hurts like the dickens. It irritates the tissue."

Maureen Dawson's treatment for sciatic pain involved the use of ten needles of various sizes. Two were placed on each side of the spine just below the point at which the L5 nerve roots exit from the spinal canal. The next two were placed at the S2 level, again one on each side. The other six were placed down her right leg, the one in which Maureen Dawson had her sciatic pain, from the thigh to the ankle.

After the needles were in place, Dr. Rapson's nurse would hook them up to an electrical stimulator, which is part of the treatment. When she first began to practise acupuncture, Dr. Rapson would twirl the needles by hand. Hooking them up to a stimulator – in which case the treatment is technically called electroacupuncture – makes hand twirling unnecessary. "It also enables us to use different currents and different intensities, and to stimulate the patient uniformly," says Dr. Rapson. "Electrostimulation doesn't hurt. It's simply a pulsating feeling."

How Acupuncture Works

Just what is going on while the acupuncture needles are vibrating? The answer depends upon whether the acupuncturist believes in the classical, Chinese explanation for the technique's efficacy, or the westernized version which is more scientific.

Proponents of the classical approach explain acupuncture as part of a complex theory of medicine in which all disease is due to an imbalance, or disharmony, between the yin and the yang, the equal and opposite life forces. Ancient Chinese practitioners of acupuncture studied the body and identified 26 meridians, pathways or channels through which the vital energy force (called ch'i) flows. Along these meridians are about 800 points where energy and blood supposedly converge. When the ch'i becomes blocked, an unhealthy state results. By feeling the pulse at the wrist, skilled classical acupuncturists first choose the point, or points, of obstruction and then insert an acupuncture needle into each one. Some classical theorists say simply that acupuncture stimulates the body's own regenerative powers.

When western physicians like Dr. Rapson began to study this classical technique, they quickly realized that virtually all of the 800 acupuncture points corresponded to western neural structures. For example, the classical points on the back correspond to the pathways of the spinal nerve roots as they exit from between two vertebrae. Once this was realized, it meant that western physicians could learn acupuncture without studying the classical methods; it also meant that they could incorporate acupuncture into the framework of western medical principles, choosing points on an anatomical basis.

Once acupuncture began to be described in western terms, the explanation for why it worked became westernized as well.

In the 1970s, most people began to explain acupuncture through world-renowned researchers Ronald Melzack and Patrick Wall's Gate Control Theory of Pain. Large fibres, say Melzack and Wall, conduct sensations like touch and temperature to the brain while smaller fibres conduct the sensation of pain. According to the Gate Control Theory, acupuncture needles stimulate the large fibres to the point of overload. At that point, the "gate" that controls the small fibres is shut down. Once a small fibre gate is shut, so this theory goes, pain sensations can no longer get through. This is the same "overload" theory that is often used to explain why techniques such as massage and just plain rubbing often work to alleviate back pain. The beauty of acupuncture, however, is that it is more specific. The stimulation goes directly and precisely to the nerve in question, and the correct pain gate is more likely to be shut down. If massage and other similar techniques could be more specific, say proponents of the Gate Control Theory, the results would probably be more dramatic.

The Gate Control Theory of Pain has remained a theory, however, because no gate mechanism has ever been physically identified. Nevertheless, it did generate a new way of looking at pain and a tremendous amount of research. One of the major breakthroughs was the discovery, in 1975, of endorphins and enkephalins, which are powerful opiates that the human brain itself is capable of producing (see page 67). If the source of the pain can't be found – or if it can be found but due to the current state of the art of medicine, it cannot be cured – perhaps the pain itself can be modified by stimulating the production of these natural pain-killers.

Today, the endorphin/enkephalin concept is more popular than the Gate Control Theory for explaining why acupuncture works. Studies, some done at the University of Toronto by world-renowned neurophysiologist Dr. Bruce Pomeranz, have conclusively shown that acupuncture stimulates the brain to produce endorphins and enkephalins. Dr. Richard Cheng, who worked under the direction of Dr. Pomeranz, has also shown that the pain-killing effects of acupuncture can be blocked by naloxone, a chemical which blocks the effects of endorphins and enkephalins. In addition, Scandinavian studies have shown that chronic pain patients often have low levels of endorphins in their spinal fluid and that these low levels rise after treatments with acupuncture.

"Ironically, the endorphin/enkephalin theory has made a treatment with such ancient roots more sophisticated and more scientific than almost any other you can name," says Dr. Rapson. "We now believe that acupuncture can stimulate the brain to produce microdots of endorphin which get sent, via the nervous system, to the precise site of injury where they turn off pain . . . . This type of pinpointing is certainly far better than blasting the entire body with a shot of morphine."

Although acupuncture is still viewed as a last-ditch maneuver by many of her colleagues who deal with back pain, Dr. Rapson remains undaunted. "Unless there is some emergency situation and you have to operate right away, I don't think it's unreasonable to suggest that virtually everyone with chronic back pain should have a trial of acupuncture," she says without hesitation. "I have seen such excellent results regardless of what some doctors still say. In any case," she adds, listing some of the more radical types of treatment she was forced to resort to in the past, "acupuncture certainly can't do anybody any harm."

Legislation regarding the practice of acupuncture varies from province to province. For more information or a list of doctors and physiotherapists in your area who have been trained by the Acupuncture Foundation of Canada write: The Secretary, The Acupuncture Foundation of Canada, 7321 Victoria Park Avenue, Suite 201, Markham, Ontario, L3R 2Z8.

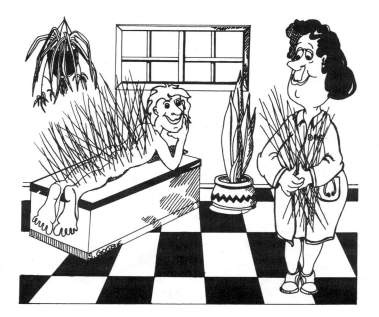

14

Physiotherapy: Treatment to End All Treatment

There has been a fair amount of confusion about the physician's role in the conservative, or non-surgical, management of back pain. While physicians sometimes offer prescriptions for bed rest, or drugs, to help a patient get through an acute episode of back pain, most doctors do not actually *treat* back pain in a "hands on" way. They diagnose back pain. They assess back pain. And, because of their extensive clinical experience, they are better equipped than any other type of professional to eliminate the rare but more serious causes of back pain such as an infection or a tumour. But once they have determined that physical therapy, exercise, better posture and education are what a back pain patient requires, most doctors delegate him or her to their "right-hand man" who, in 90 per cent of cases, is not a man at all but a woman – a physiotherapist.

The physiotherapist's goal is two-fold. It is to assist a patient back to a state that is normal in terms of function and then to teach that patient what he or she has to know in order to remain in that normal state without further help from a professional. Says Judy Flaschner, a Toronto physiotherapist in private practice, "Once a patient is on the road to recovery, getting that patient *off* treatment becomes our next goal. The philosophy of physiotherapy is to teach self-reliance – whatever it is that a person needs to know in order to get by on his or her own rather than becoming dependent upon a professional."

To achieve the first part – normal function – physiotherapists use a wide roster of treatments. These include: massage, heat, deep heat, ice, TENS, traction, mobilization, and, on occasion, manipulation.

To achieve the second part of the goal, physiotherapists teach patients anatomy, physiology, proper postural habits and exercises that take the specific nature of their back problem into account. In doing all this, they combine the global goals of the holistic-type practitioners with the specific knowledge they have as a result of their medical background. This makes them unique, rendering the whole they have to offer greater than the sum of its parts.

The profession evolved as a result of the need to rehabilitate soldiers who had been wounded in World War I. Prior to 1914, the professional status of those practising massage and what was then called "remedial gymnastics," was well established in Britain; in North America, however, very few people had been trained in these various techniques. During World War I, most of the Canadian and American soldiers who had been wounded in battle were, by necessity, kept in French and English military hospitals; no one in North America was trained to rehabilitate them.

Toward the end of the war, a group of 28 men and women were trained in rehabilitation medicine at the Ontario Hospital in Whitby, Ontario. Soon after, the Military School of Orthopaedic Surgery and Physiotherapy was opened at the University of Toronto. Finally, in 1929, the university began a two-year degree course in physiotherapy. Some years later, the course was lengthened and today, all qualified physiotherapists follow a four-year university program as well as a five-month clinical internship in a teaching hospital.

Many of the people Judy Flaschner treats suffer from back pain. "My first goal," she says, "is to reduce pain and the stiffness that usually goes along with it. At that point, I can teach my patients about posture, exercise and better ways of going about their activities of daily living, all of which can help them deal with their chronic back problem. (Physiotherapists generally refer to activities of daily living, which include both household chores and leisure activities, as "ADL.")

Judy Flaschner also tries to help people learn the warning signs of an acute attack before it is too late to prevent it. But unlike some therapists of other persuasions who promise long-lasting cures and permanent relief, she is realistic in her approach. "The hardest thing to get people to realize is that they probably won't ever be *totally* pain-free," she says. "Someone who has had an injury or is suffering from a first episode of back pain can often recover from it completely. But the majority of people who come to physiotherapy have had more than one incident. They have a chronic problem, and it's unlikely that they'll be able to completely avoid an occasional acute episode in the future. What we hope to do with treatment and education is increase the time between those acute episodes and decrease their severity."

Some physiotherapists group patients into one of three categories, which were developed by Australian physiotherapist Robin McKenzie. Judy Flaschner explains: "If I find no exacerbation of pain, or loss of mobility, upon assessing the joints of the spine, then I'd most likely place the patient in the first group: 'postural' problems. I'd attribute the person's pain to overstretched ligaments due to faulty posture while sitting or standing."

Most people in this category, she says, are 35 and under. They have had no particular injury. They have become aware that they have a back problem over the years; they have pain when they spend long hours sitting at a desk, standing behind a counter or engaging in activities – for example, housework or sports – that strain the spine. Typically, their pain subsides fairly quickly if they lie down for a while. They may, or may not, have some amount of *secondary* muscle spasm, which means that the spasm is a result of the strained ligaments, the *primary* cause.

"For these people," says Judy Flaschner, "correcting poor posture and learning an exercise program is usually enough."

Unfortunately, most back pain sufferers are not aware of the cumulative effects of poor posture and lack of exercise and do not opt for intervention at this early stage. Their pain continues intermittently until, after five or ten years, they realize that they are in pain, or at least discomfort, more often than not. When lying down for a couple of hours fails to relieve their back pain, they show up at the doctor's office and are referred to a physiotherapist.

"By this time," says Judy Flaschner, "degenerative and adaptive changes have usually taken place and they have moved into the second of McKenzie's three stages: 'dysfunction'."

For example, the person who slumps over a desk eight hours a day for a couple of decades may have adaptive shortening of the anterior, or front section, of the facet joint capsules of the lumbar spine (see page 161). The person who stands behind a counter in a position of hyperextension may also have adaptive shortening, but in this case the posterior, or back portion, of the capsule will have shortened.

"By the time a person has reached this stage of a back problem," says Judy Flaschner, "one or more facet joints may have lost some of their range of motion, and there will be pain toward the end of the range. In some cases, a disc whose annulus has frayed slightly may be bulging. In other cases, one or more facet joints may be hypermobile, or unstable, and this is the source of the pain."

Unfortunately, a person in one of these categories will sometimes be diagnosed as normal by a physician who is looking for a true disc herniation. And these are the people who make up the bulk of the physiotherapist's practice.

In Robin McKenzie's third group – called 'derangement' – are the very few people who are suffering from a true disc herniation. "Some of these people have surgery right away but in other cases, a physician will give physiotherapy a try. Some patients with a true herniated disc do respond to conservative treatment," she says, excluding those who have a herniated disc that is also sequestrated. "Those who do not respond often go on to have surgery or a chymopapain injection."

The Treatments Used by Physiotherapists

Once a patient is assessed by the physiotherapist and the origin of the problem has been established, the next step is to determine which treatment, or treatments, is appropriate to alleviate the problem. "But no matter which modality is chosen," says Judy Flaschner, "the effectiveness of the treatment will depend to a large extent upon the physiotherapist/patient rapport. The therapist who is able to motivate the patient will have a greater chance of success. At the same time, the patient who is willing to take an active role in his or her treatment will improve far faster than the person who remains passive."

ULTRASOUND • Ultrasound delivers high frequency sound waves – over a million cycles per second – to the tissue to which it is directed. (The frequency used for diagnostic ultrasound is the same but the wattage, which delivers the heat, is lower.) The result is a micro, as opposed to macro, massage effect. Instead of moving a mass of tissue, which is the aim of a "hands on" massage, each single cell is vibrated by ultrasound in a similar way that each cell of a pork roast vibrates while cooking in a microwave oven. Ultrasound affects tissue in two ways, one mechanical, the other chemical. It is also thought to reduce pain by stimulating the input to the large sensory fibres, so that the relatively few pain messages travelling along the small fibres are no longer perceived (see page 67).

From the mechanical perspective, ultrasound helps to break down scar tissue and stimulates the cells of new connective tissue to be laid down symmetrically rather than asymmetrically. The advantage of symmetry in cell formation is elasticity; the new tissue has more flexibility than it otherwise would have.

From a chemical standpoint, ultrasound changes the permeability of each cell wall. With heightened permeability, waste products can be expelled and nutrients can be absorbed more efficiently. Where an area is inflamed, healing can take place more rapidly.

TENS (TRANSCUTANEOUS ELECTRICAL NERVE STIMULATION) • Using electricity to reduce pain is as old as the Roman empire, although back then, electric eels were attached to arthritic joints making electrical stimulation natural in the literal sense. The modern use of electricity in the treatment of pain was honed in the late 1960s when electrodes were surgically implanted into painful backs. This led to the development of machines called TENS, sometimes called TNS, which are worn externally. TENS machines are battery-powered and deliver an electric current to nerves via electrodes that are first covered with a water-soluble conducting gel and then taped to the skin. The method is similar to acupuncture except that with TENS, no needles are used and the skin is not pierced.

Most TENS machines have two currents. One feels like a buzz, the other like a gentle, completely painless electric shock. By a process of trial and error, the best location for the electrodes must be found for each individual along with the appropriate current.

The efficacy of TENS – which, according to American pain expert Dr. John Bonica provides long-term relief for about a third of chronic pain patients – is explained in the same way as acupuncture. The higher frequency is thought to stimulate the large sensory fibres, thus lessening the perception of pain sensations travelling along the smaller sensory fibres. The lower frequency is thought to stimulate the production of endorphins and enkephalins (see page 67).

COLD AND HOT PACKS • Cold packs are generally used to reduce the swelling from an episode of acute pain whose onset was not more than 48 hours prior to treatment. It works by reducing circulation to the injured area, thereby decreasing swelling. If a cold pack is left on an area for more than about 15 minutes, however, the effect begins to reverse. The blood vessels dilate, and circulation increases. In this situation, an ice pack will have the same effect as a hot pack; ice is chosen over heat when, for one reason or another, a patient finds heat painful rather than soothing.

In most cases, however, heat is soothing rather than painful. By increasing circulation to an area, heat increases the blood (and therefore the oxygen) supply which, in turn, can decrease muscle tension. Heat will also stimulate the large sensory fibres (see page 67), thereby decreasing the perception of pain.

SHORT WAVE DIATHERMY • The waves sent out by a short wave diathermy machine are longer than ultrasound waves. Two electrodes are placed on the body, one at each end of the painful area; the extremely deep heating effect increases circulation and relaxes muscle tension. Short wave diathermy also has the same chemical effects on tissue as ultrasound. It is used less frequently than ultrasound, however, because it requires a lot of space. This is due to the fact that the waves a short wave diathermy machine produces can interfere with the functioning of pacemakers, hearing aids, some watches and other physiotherapy modalities such as Interferential Current and TENS; patients must therefore be treated in a separate area.

INTERFERENTIAL CURRENT • The patient having interferential current applied to the back looks a bit like a hot-cross bun with the four electrodes arranged in the shape of an X. Two of the electrodes are wired up to one frequency and the other two to another frequency. Where they cross, which is just over the painful area, an "interference" is created, hence the therapy's name. The interferential current alleviates pain in much the same way as a TENS machine. It also reduces swelling by stimulating a part of the nervous system which, in turn, causes blood vessels to constrict thus reducing blood supply to the area.

MASSAGE • While massage therapists use massage in a generalized way, physiotherapists tend to use localized massage for specific problems. For example, the scar tissue that forms after surgery sometimes adhers to normal tissue and massage can be used to free it up. Soft tissue – muscles, tendons and ligaments – that has shortened and/or tightened due to injury, or chronic poor posture, can be stretched back to its normal length with "localized soft tissue massage." When muscle fibres, ligaments or tendons tear, the scar tissue that forms generally lacks adequate flexibility and a type of massage called "deep transverse frictions" can be used to mobilize these fibres. (For more information about massage, see Chapter 20.)

TRACTION • Traction – during which joint surfaces are separated intermittently by mechanical means – is used for disc problems and also to mobilize a spine that is stiff due to degenerative changes at many levels. There are many different ways of applying traction and different amounts of weight are used for different purposes; anywhere from 20 pounds to 150 pounds of pull can be used. The routine may also vary. For a bulging or herniated disc, static traction is usually applied for 15 to 20 minutes. Intermittent traction is usually more effective for generalized degenerative changes; one common method is to apply traction for 15 seconds, then release it for five seconds, repeating this regime for approximately 15 minutes.

MOBILIZATION AND MANIPULATION • For a description of mobilization – which is similar whether used on the cervical or the lumbar spine – see page 268. For a description of manipulation and what it accomplishes, see page 193.

Most physiotherapists prefer to improve joint mobility by using mobilization rather than manipulation, if possible. They believe that when you manipulate, a minor trauma is created, and when they can achieve the same end with mobilization, which is less traumatic, they prefer it.

Mobilization produces movement in a joint. With a joint that is stiff, the goal is to return the range of motion to normal. With a joint that is inflamed, the goal is to decrease the pain which, in turn, will increase the range of motion. Very gentle oscillatory mobilization in the beginning of the range will lower the patient's perception of pain in the same way as TENS. With the stiff joint, a stronger form of mobilization performed at the end of the range of motion of that joint will stretch the capsule and ligaments which surround the joint. This can be done with either an oscillatory movement or a sustained stretch. The increased range of motion gained by this technique will also help to alleviate the pain.

A number of biomechanical studies have shown that if you mobilize a joint over a period of time, it is less likely to return to its shortened position than if you stretch it beyond its normal physiological range for a brief moment as is done when a joint is manipulated.

To mobilization treatments, Judy Flaschner always adds daily stretching exercises that her patients can do at home, between treatments. If these two modalities do not restore movement to a stiff joint, she will sometimes elect to manipulate. "But physiotherapists do not believe in manipulation over the long term," she says. "You may not get complete relief of pain with one or two manipulations, but you should see some change in the person's range of motion. If there is no change in either range of motion or pain, I will not continue to manipulate a joint. My philosophy is that if a treatment is not working then either the assessment was incorrect or the choice of treatment was wrong and should be changed."

15

Psychiatry: If Your Back Hurts, Try Using Your Head

"It's normal not to be normal when you're in pain," says Dr. Stanley Greben, psychiatrist-in-chief at Toronto's Mount Sinai Hospital. Dr. Greben himself ought to know. In the early 1970s, the lean, athletic physician was playing a game of tennis when, as he puts it, "my back went out and didn't come back." After ten weeks of bed rest, physiotherapy and a permanent life-style change which emphasizes good posture, swimming and walking as regular activities, Dr. Greben is relatively pain-free. But he still remembers how helpless he felt when he could barely get out of bed. His greatest fear was that his back condition would *never* go away. "There's nothing more demoralizing than chronic pain," says Dr. Greben. "It can cause depression in an otherwise cheerful person . . . and it's amazing how quickly the depression can lift when the pain subsides."

Dr. Greben believes that a great deal of back pain has to do with lack of exercise and poor posture, rather than psychiatric imbalances. But he believes that long-term back pain can drive a person to see a psychiatrist. "Chronic pain can affect your self-esteem and confidence, disrupt your normal pattern of activities, and undermine your relationships," he says.

"Back pain is so all-encompassing," says Linda Davis, a 34-year-old television researcher. Used to living her life in the fast track, Linda saw herself as a "doer," not a victim. As her back pain became progressively worse, she made the usual rounds: a general practitioner, various specialists, a physiotherapist, a massage therapist and a chiropractor. "Because of my profession, I was used to digging for answers and finding them. Not being able to come up with a single solution for my back problem was infuriating and demoralizing at the same time.

"I put a lot of energy into discovering *the cure*," she says. "Finally, a massage therapist I was seeing said to me, 'Linda, you're doing part of this to yourself. Your anger about this back pain is making it worse.' There was a ring of truthfulness to this, but what was I supposed to do? Was I supposed to ignore it? My back pain was the last thing I thought about at night and the first thing I became aware of each morning. It was all I could do to keep up with my work. Fun was out of the question. I'd have been crazy if I hadn't been upset!"

According to Toronto psychiatrist Dr. Jerry Friedman, it's well documented that people with chronic back problems are more prone to depression than people with other chronic ailments. "You can't control a back problem as easily as diabetes, for instance, where the solution is pretty straight forward; you take insulin. As well," he adds, "there's always the fear which goes along with knowing that back pain can strike at any time." Dr. Friedman has lectured on the emotional components of back pain and acts as a consultant to orthopaedic surgeons whose hospitalized back patients sometimes require the help of a psychiatrist.

Studies have shown that many patients recovering from back surgery suffer from anxiety and even disorientation. "Being immobilized over a period of weeks," explains Dr. Friedman, "can even cause distortions in perception. There is also a high incidence of what is known as 'postoperative delirium' in people recuperating from back operations."

Generally, these feelings subside when the patient leaves the hospital and returns to normal activities. For most back pain sufferers, however, there will never be a magic solution such as surgery. For them, the realization that their condition is chronic can lead to feelings of anger, frustration or depression, which must be resolved.

"Having to give up normal activities," says Dr. Friedman, "can heighten those emotions." In one group of back pain sufferers that Dr. Friedman lectured to, a woman described how she became depressed because she had had to give up playing tennis. "It wasn't only because she enjoyed the game so immensely," he explains, "but that part of her identity was tied up with being able to be a competitive person." Some people react by getting angry or anxious. Others tend to retreat into a depression, feeling that their entire reason for existing has been undermined by their back problem.

Men, more so than women, tend to talk about the loss of self-esteem. "You feel less of a man if you're not as powerful as you once were, if you can't shovel snow anymore, or take out the garbage," says Dr. Friedman. In this instance, he candidly admits that he is talking about himself; back pain is a common occupational hazard among psychiatrists who sit attentively for hours, often on badly designed chairs. Dr. Friedman's experience was not unlike Dr. Grebin's. "When I had to stay in bed because of my back pain, I was afraid I'd never work again. I pictured myself lying on the couch."

For both sexes, chronic back pain can affect relationships. Linda Davis recalls a period in her life when she wondered if she could even think about beginning a relationship with a man. "For a year I kept asking myself how I could even consider beginning a relationship when I had to do weird things like get out of bed in the middle of the night to sleep on the floor. And it wasn't simply a fantasy. When I finally did start to spend a lot of time with one man, he was surprised – and I think a bit disappointed – that I couldn't do 'ordinary' things like play squash or jog. I also worried about the fact that on particularly bad days, it takes a lot of energy not to be irritable and sometimes, hard as I try to be cheerful, I fail."

How do you get it across to someone that you are in a lot of pain without sounding like a chronic complainer? How do you ask for help? Says Joan Bilton, who has had a chronic back condition for more than three decades, "Quite frankly, back pain is boring to everyone but those of us who suffer from it. I try not to say to my family too often 'I can't do this,' but on the other hand, if you say nothing, they forget that you have it. They make a few cursory gestures and think they are helping. What is hard for them to understand is that four or five times a year, for weeks on end, I'm thinking about my back almost every waking moment. How do you tell someone that without sounding as if you're a nag?"

Psychiatrists can sometimes help back pain sufferers find answers to questions such as these.

Dr. Friedman maintains that *clear communication* is essential. "Often people try to communicate non-verbally. They put their hands on their backs, or they sigh, or close their eyes to exemplify the intensity of their pain. From these sorts of gestures, back pain sufferers often expect others to respond."

"Women," Dr. Friedman adds, "are often so used to looking after others that it's hard for them to express their needs and ask their families to look after them for a while. Hence the martyr syndrome: 'Nobody can wash the floor like I can.' But often all this is done unconsciously until someone – often a psychiatrist who can be objective – points it out."

Communicating with their children is another area that back pain sufferers sometimes neglect. "Parents frequently don't realize that their illness, or pain, can evoke fantasies in a child which vary depending upon the child's age," says Dr. Friedman. "A three-year-old child," he explains, "might worry that a parent who is bed-ridden for ten weeks is dying. It's so important to truthfully explain the condition in a way that's appropriate to the child and can alleviate his or her fears."

Dr. Klaus Minde is a professor of pediatrics and psychiatry at Toronto's Hospital for Sick Children. He points out that children learn how to communicate their own discomfort from the role models presented to them by their parents. In his opinion, the best way to ensure that your children are communicating clearly when it comes to their own ailments is to set a clear example and to express your back pain realistically. Children of hypochondriacs, for example, often grow up to be hypochondriacs themselves. On the other hand, children whose parents act completely stoic, never mentioning their physical ailments, often grow up to act the same way. "They don't mention their problems or seek help when they should. This is no more a healthy type of attitude than being a hypochondriac."

For some people with a chronic back problem, back pain can also be an unconscious metaphor – a way of expressing the need for attention, love or kindness. "Often," says Dr. Minde, "it's easier to ask the people around you for these things if you are in physical pain." At times, these people (whom Dr. Minde calls somaticisers) may dwell on a relatively minor backache to get attention, and because they are focusing on it, the pain actually becomes more intense.

According to Dr. Minde, somaticisers usually have a difficult time perceiving things in a psychological way. "These people don't express their emotions. For example, they don't cry. The only way their emotional suffering can come out is in a physical way." Back pain, however, which is less obvious than a broken leg in a cast, is not a great ailment to use as a sympathy ploy. At work, a person in a cast will get far more attention than someone who is suffering from an "invisible" back problem.

Can a psychiatrist help a somaticiser learn to express emotions? And can learning to be emotional help someone to avoid back pain?

"I would hope that if someone learns to express their emotions, an acute episode of back pain would happen less often," is how Dr. Minde puts it. But he emphasizes that with the relatively recent discovery of endorphins and enkephalins (see page 67), the already fine line between emotional and physical states has become even more blurred. "We don't yet know enough about endorphins and enkephalins," says Dr. Minde. "What we do know, however, is that we shouldn't disconnect physical problems from emotional states. The same back pain can be far less troublesome to someone who is feeling focused emotionally."

Linda Davis did end up seeing a psychiatrist for a period of several months. She gives him credit for helping her to develop a fresh perspective and renewed hope. "First of all, I began to realize that I'm not the only person who has become depressed because of back pain. I stopped feeling like such a failure for not always being able to be strong. What I also really needed was an outlet, someone to pour out my frustrations to. What I learned to recognize was *how* and *when* I was playing into that vicious circle of pain leading to anger, leading to more pain, leading to more anger. My massage therapist had pointed out that I was doing it. My shrink helped me learn my trigger points, how to fall into this pattern less often and, more importantly, how to forgive myself when I failed."

After several months, Linda also began to see that she was focusing on her back pain and allowing her entire life to become consumed by it. "When I couldn't find *the cure*, I started to concentrate on the crummy physiotherapist, the crummy chiropractor, the crummy massage therapist. It was entirely *their* fault that my back hurt so much; they didn't know their job. When I began to do the same thing with my psychiatrist, however, he helped me recognize the pattern. Ironically, when I began to concentrate on the more pleasant aspects of my life, rather than on the stressful parts, my back started to get better, very slowly.

"It's a complicated process. I mean, I do have a disc problem, and my back still really bothers me at times. But at times, it doesn't bother me. You have a choice about which to focus on. This, however, is a very simple version of what happened after a lot of introspection and a lot of emotional pain."

Says Dr. Minde: "Being in touch with your back pain and understanding how and when it acts up can help you learn to deal with stress in general. Pain – as long as it's not so severe that it disables you – can be used as a barometer to tell you where you are at with your body and your feelings."

Barometer is exactly the word Linda Davis eventually came to use. "My back problem tells me when I haven't been sleeping enough, when I'm overworked, or when something about my relationship with my husband is wrong and we're not dealing with it. [She was, in the end, able to have a lasting relationship!] Now, in some ways, I'm actually glad that I learned at a fairly young age to take good care of my back. It taught me to take good care of the rest of me as well. I swim regularly. I do relaxation and stretching exercises to reduce stress and stay flexible. And once in a while, I go back to talk to my psychiatrist!"

"Back pain," says Dr. Friedman, "prompts many people to start dealing with other conflicts. Problems in a relationship are only one good example. It can also teach people how to compromise. Many back pain sufferers start off by taking the 'all or nothing approach.' If they can't find a miracle cure, they give up completely and resign themselves to misery."

Most people with chronic back pain find that they don't have to give up everything. Linda Davis had to stop planting her garden. The stooping and shovelling were too strenuous on her back. But she found a viable compromise. "My neighbour puts the plants in and I do a lot of the weeding for both of us, as well as all of the pruning. I get a lot of pleasure from that, perhaps more because I've learned to handle what used to be a negative aspect of my life in a positive way."

When it comes to your back, it sometimes makes sense to work on your head.

16

Traditional Exercises: Margaret Duffy's Twenty-Minute Workout for the Back

"I was shocked!" says Susan Horne, a 42-year-old teacher, who had been doing back exercises daily for 18 months with no noticeable improvement. "I mean, every book you read on back pain tells you to exercise to strengthen the abdominal muscles, and I had been devoted to my morning regimen for a year and a half. Then I learned that I'd been doing most of the exercises incorrectly. Boy was I mad. But what did I know? I'd picked up a few tips here and there, you know, from magazines and books. Meanwhile, I was probably doing my back more harm than good. Just for openers, I thought a good way to strengthen my abdominal muscles was to do *full* sit-ups, the more the better. I was pretty smug about knowing to keep my knees bent rather than straight, and I thought that was all there was to it!"

Margaret Duffy is a senior physiotherapist at Toronto Western Hospital. "Many people who suffer from back pain learned to do back exercises in school, years ago," she says. "What they often don't realize is that we have learned a lot about body mechanics over the past 20 years. Most people now know, for example, that doing sit-ups with both legs straight, or even hooked under a sofa, not only stresses the lower back but also works the hip flexor muscles as much as the abdominal muscles. Very few people, however, realize that almost all of the abdominal strengthening value from a sit-up comes from the first 30 degrees. Once your shoulders leave the ground, the hip flexor muscles take over."

In fact, most people don't realize a lot of things about doing back exercises. A few tips are:

• When exercising, you should warm up your muscles *before* you stretch. If you try to stretch "cold" muscles, they cannot lengthen sufficiently to do you much good. If you *force* them to lengthen when they're cold, you may strain or even tear them.

• Strengthening (contracting) exercises cause a build-up of lactic acid in the muscles, which can cause pain. Stretching (lengthening) and cool-down exercises increase the blood flow into these muscles, which, in turn, enables the lactic acid to be dissipated from the muscle. Therefore, after you work at strengthening a muscle, you should stretch it out during your cool-down period.

• It's useless to try to learn the pelvic tilt with the objective of correcting a sway-back posture if your back and/or hip flexor muscles are chronically tight. These shortened muscles must be stretched out first so that you can do a proper pelvic tilt.

• To stretch a muscle, you must anchor one end and stretch the other. If you do not pay attention to technique, you'll frequently end up stretching the wrong muscle. *Never* bounce during a stretch; this may tear the muscle. Instead, maintain a steady stretch for a minimum of ten seconds.

• To strengthen a muscle you must work it to its maximum capacity. Working within a muscle's mid-range will maintain the muscle's strength but will not increase it, unless you *continually* increase the number of repetitions.

• There are two ways to strengthen a muscle: isotonically and isometrically. An isotonic contraction – a sit-up, for example – involves shortening the distance between the two ends of the muscle. An isometric contraction – a pelvic tilt, for example – is a static contraction that does not involve shortening. On days when you are in pain, you can frequently find an isometric variation of an exercise that will achieve the same goal with less stress and less chance of exacerbating your pain.

Says Susan Horne: "Finally, in desperation, I went back to my doctor. He suggested that I see a physiotherapist, and I figured I was up for some traction or something like that. Instead, I got an exercise program with specific instructions on how to do each exercise correctly.... What a difference! Within six weeks, I began to realize that I was sleeping through the night most of the time. After three months, I would say I was among those people who consider their back problems to be more or less 'under control'."

What follows is a general but detailed exercise program for the chronic back pain sufferer, designed by Margaret Duffy. The "hows" and "whys" of each exercise are described as well as potential pitfalls to watch out for. There are several ways to perform various strengthening and stretching exercises for the back. You can choose an easier or more difficult variation, depending upon the severity of your back problem and the current state of your condition. The program begins with a few basic rules of thumb.

How Often Should You Exercise?

To be effective, a back exercise program should be done a minimum of three times a week, 20 minutes each time. Some people prefer to exercise daily, setting aside 15 or 20 minutes at a certain time of the day. They find that if they vary from a strict regime, they have a tendency to get out of the habit of exercising and their good intentions fall by the wayside. Other people find it too difficult to exercise daily. For them, a strict regime is impossible to adhere to and trying to keep to a daily program simply sets them up for failure. "You don't have to exercise every day," says Margaret Duffy. "Three times a week for 20 minutes is fine. You may also find that you don't have time to do every exercise every time and that's okay. Just double the repetitions the next day."

A general recommendation is to do an exercise a minimum of ten times. (In the case of left and right muscle groups, this means ten times on each side!) If you find an exercise to be particularly helpful, you can work up to 30 repetitions. Use your own judgement and don't try to advance too quickly.

Should You Stop Exercising If It Causes You Pain?

In theory, pain is a warning sign. If doing an exercise causes pain, you should either alter the way you do it or not do it at all. In practice, however, trying to adhere to this philosophy can be more difficult than reducing the federal deficit.

For one thing, chronic back pain sufferers come in different varieties. Some people experience a bad bout of back pain two or three times a year. It lasts for a couple of weeks, or a month, but between bouts, they are more or less pain-free. If you are this type of chronic back pain sufferer, the rules about pain are fairly easy. While coping with an acute stage of back pain, avoid exercising completely. (Two exceptions to this rule of thumb are exercises 3 and 5, which are described at the end of this chapter; the pelvic tilt and the low back stretch can be done while you are in pain.) As the pain subsides, do some of the easier variations, and when the pain is gone, add some of the more difficult variations.

Far more difficult is deciding how to proceed if you have constant low-grade back pain. The advice to wait until your back pain subsides completely before you exercise is not very helpful for those people who have a certain amount of pain most of the time. "If exercising does not *exacerbate* their pain at all, I tell them to go ahead," says Margaret Duffy. However, many chronic back pain sufferers in this group find that exercising does increase their discomfort. "In a case like this, I tell them that if they have *increased* pain for more than 15 or 20 minutes after they have finished exercising, then they have done too much. Any pain that exercising *provokes* should subside within 20 minutes. This means that if you have constant low-grade pain, then within 20 minutes, the *level* of that pain should return to what it was before you began to exercise," she says.

There are also some general rules of thumb for specific types of pain. "First of all," says Margaret Duffy, "you have to distinguish between soreness and sharp pain. If you are stretching a tight muscle, you'll feel it pulling, but this is different than if an exercise provokes the kind of pain that makes you wince. Sciatic pain is one example.

"If you suffer from intermittent sciatic pain," says Margaret Duffy, "you should forgo the exercises for stretching the hamstring muscles on the days that your sciatica is bothering you because hamstring exercises also stretch the sciatic nerve. Those are good days on which to concentrate on pelvic tilts and abdominal strengthening exercises and perhaps some back extension exercises."

If extension exercises – arching the back – cause pain, you're best off to consult a physician or physiotherapist. If it turns out that you have worn facet joints, extending your back will just irritate these joints by jamming them together, and you should eliminate extension exercises from your program completely. However, a certain amount of lordosis is normal and, in fact, necessary. If you lack a normal amount of lordosis, the pain could be caused by the stretching associated with increasing that curve, and you should continue with your extension exercises very slowly. It may take a professional to help you decide.

What Is the Best Way to Warm Up?

There are two ways to warm up before you begin exercising: actively or passively.

If you are pain-free, or suffering from minimal pain that is not easily exacerbated, then an active warm-up is fine. Five minutes of fast walking or bicycling, either on a stationary or regular bicycle, should do the trick. The objective is to increase the heart rate moderately and to loosen up the muscles, which will enable them to be stretched without strain.

If you are experiencing pain, especially sciatic pain, an active warm-up is likely to do you more harm than good.

"In that case, take a hot bath or shower," says Margaret Duffy. This applies whether you are in the middle of an acute bout of back pain or just having a bad day. The hot water will warm up the superficial muscles sufficiently to loosen them, and this is why so many people are first given a hot pack when they arrive for a physiotherapy session. Ironically, most people take a shower *after* they exercise rather than before, even though a 20-minute back exercise program is not enough to make you perspire. "You're better off taking that hot shower first," says Margaret Duffy.

What Are You Trying To Accomplish?

If you suffer from chronic back pain, a back exercise program can help you accomplish several things: 1. It will strengthen muscles which, in turn, can help compensate for lax ligaments that cannot be strengthened or tightened; 2. It will make your body more flexible and increase your range of movement to normal; 3. It will stretch a tight lumbar spine back to normal, which is essential before attempting exercises to correct a sway-back, or hyperlordosis.

1. WHY STRENGTHEN? • If the ligaments in your back have stretched due to chronic poor posture, it is impossible for them to become taut again. "Only *torn* as opposed to *stretched* ligaments can become taut again," says Margaret Duffy, "and in order for this to happen, they pretty well have to heal in a shortened position over a period of time. This is why people with torn collateral knee ligaments are put in a cast with the leg bent; the idea is to get the ligaments to heal in the shortest position possible."

This is where the muscles of the back and abdomen come into play. If you can no longer depend upon your ligaments to help you maintain proper posture, you have to turn to the structures that still have a contractile element to them – that is, the muscles. "If you have misused your back for many years, you are more dependent than ever upon your abdominal and back muscles to prevent further degeneration," says Margaret Duffy.

2. WHY BECOME FLEXIBLE? • Most chronic back pain sufferers are less flexible than normal. It's logical. If you suffer from back pain, you are likely to stiffen up out of fear of doing yourself harm. Stretching exercises will help lengthen contracted muscles. This will make you less vulnerable to injuries when you move slightly beyond that range.

3. WHY STRETCH BEFORE YOU STRENGTHEN? • While poor posture over many years will cause some ligaments to stretch and sag, it will also cause other structures to contract and shorten in order to take up the slack. The term professionals use is *adaptive shortening*. For example, if you walk around in a sway-back posture for many years, the anterior longitudinal ligament will stretch but the posterior section of the facet joint capsules, as well as the erector spinae muscles, will shorten. The hip flexor muscles (which run from the lumbar spine through the pelvis and attach to the top of the thigh bone) will shorten as well. Before you can correct a sway-back posture, it is first necessary to stretch out these shortened muscles and capsules.

The Program

The basic back exercise program includes both stretching and strengthening exercises. Altogether, there are seven exercises plus their variations: I. The Hamstring Stretch; 2. The Hip Flexor Stretch; 3. The Pelvic Tilt; 4. The Sit-Up; 5. The Low Back Stretch (Knee to Chest Stretch); 6. The Low Back Extension Stretch; 7. The Small Muscle Group Strengthener.

If you suffer mainly from a facet joint problem, concentrate on exercises I to 5 inclusive.

If yours is mainly a disc problem (with or without sciatic pain), concentrate on I, 3, 6 and 7. Add exercise 4 provided it does not exacerbate your pain and do exercise 5 within your pain-free range.

If you suffer from both problems, try to concentrate on I to 5 inclusive, avoiding any exercises that exacerbate your pain. You will likely find that I and 3 provide the most effective relief.

First do five to ten minutes of warm-up exercises, or have a hot bath or shower. Always read through the entire section describing an exercise so that you can become familiar with the different variations and can choose the one that is most suitable for you.

I. THE HAMSTRING STRETCH • The hamstring muscles start at the buttocks, run down the back of each leg and attach to the back of each knee. The bone you sit on is where the hamstring muscle starts. If you place your hand under a buttock, you will feel a round bone, which is the lower end of the pelvis. This is the spot where the hamstring muscle begins.

If your hamstring muscles are flexible, the pelvis will be free to move when you bend over. If your hamstring muscles are tight, then your back will have to absorb all the stress associated with bending. With tight hamstrings, the back is stressed even when you bend over slightly.

You can test the flexibility of your hamstring muscles by lying on the floor on your back with both legs extended. Keeping both knees straight, lift one leg. If your hamstrings are flexible, you should be able to lift your leg to a full 90 degrees. If you can do this, then you can begin by doing a full hamstring muscle stretch. If you feel a tightness – but not the sharp pain of sciatica – when you raise your leg more than 60 degrees, you should begin with a modified hamstring stretch.

Stretching the hamstring muscles also stretches the sciatic nerve. Therefore, if you suffer from intermittent sciatic pain, you too should do a modified hamstring stretch even on the days when you are pain-free.

The last hamstring stretch described will allow you to stretch your hamstrings statically without stretching the sciatic nerve at all. If you frequently suffer from sciatic pain, or you are just recovering from an acute bout, always stretch the hamstrings statically. Many people find that this variation actually helps them to resolve their sciatica. When you have been free of sciatic pain for six months, you can proceed *cautiously* to a more difficult variation of the hamstring stretch.

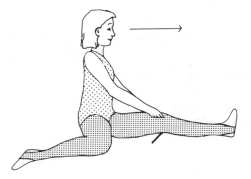

FULL HAMSTRING STRETCH (HURDLE STRETCH) • Sit on the floor with your left leg extended and your right leg bent at the knee. The gap between the legs should be 90 degrees. Place both hands on the knee of your left leg and press it into the floor to fix the lower end of the muscle. Some people find that placing a pencil under the left knee prompts them to keep it pressed down. If the knee bobs up while you are performing this exercise, press it down again with your hands. Focus your eyes on the wall straight ahead. Keeping your back straight, stretch forward, moving toward the spot on the wall straight ahead. Do not bend your back or bring your head down toward the left knee. (If you do, you will stretch the lower back as well as the hamstrings, putting stress on the discs and muscles of the lumbar spine.) Hold for a minimum of 20 seconds. Do not bounce. Relax and repeat a minimum of ten times. This will stretch the left hamstring muscle. To stretch the right hamstring, change legs and repeat the exercise.

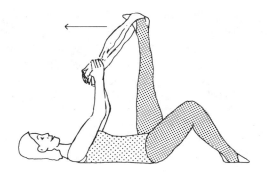

MODIFIED HAMSTRING STRETCH • Lie on your back with both knees bent. Holding a towel, one hand at either end, place the sole of your left foot in the centre of the towel. Using your arms only, not the leg or back muscles, pull the left leg up toward your face and hold for a minimum of 15 seconds. Do not allow the leg to bounce. Relax and repeat a minimum of ten times. To stretch the right hamstring muscle, switch legs. After you have done this modified hamstring stretch for a few weeks and are feeling comfortable with it, you can increase the stretch by doing the exercise with the free leg straight instead of bent.

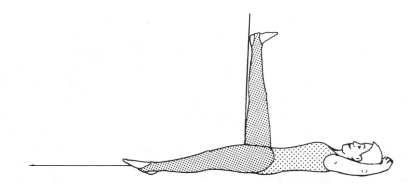

STATIC HAMSTRING STRETCH • Lie on your back, positioning the buttocks in line with the jamb of a doorway so that the left leg can extend through the doorway. Prop your right leg up on the door jamb and let it hang there for several minutes. Your buttocks should be as close to the door jamb as possible, but the knee of the right leg should not bend; if it tends to bend, you are too close. As the stretch becomes comfortable, you can increase it by moving your buttocks closer to the door jamb.

Once your acute sciatic pain has subsided substantially for six months, and you are able to do this exercise comfortably with your buttocks right up against the door jamb, you can progress to the modified hamstring stretch.

2. THE HIP FLEXOR STRETCH • There are several hip flexor muscles: the iliacus, the psoas and the rectus femoris. The iliacus and psoas muscles are side by side and are sometimes referred to together as the ilio-psoas muscle. They are attached at one end to the inside, or gut side, of the vertebrae of the lumbar spine and run through the pelvis where they attach to the top of the upper leg bone, or femur. The rectus femoris muscle is attached at one end to the top of the hip joint and runs to the kneecap. Technically speaking, the rectus femoris muscle is one of the four quadraceps muscles whose function is to extend the knee. But because it also crosses the hip joint, the rectus femoris is involved in hip flexion as well.

If your hip flexor muscles are shortened, the top of your pelvis will tend to rotate counter-clockwise when you stand or walk. The effect will be a sway-back posture. This posture, in turn, will place additional stress on the facet joints of the lumbar spine. As I've already mentioned, if the hip flexors are tight, it is pointless to practise pelvic tilt exercises alone, since the pelvis will be too tight to rotate clockwise into the pelvic tilt position. You must stretch those tight hip flexor muscles.

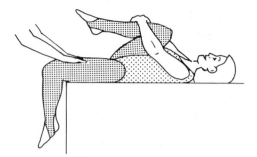

HIP FLEXOR STRETCH WHILE LYING DOWN • The advantage of stretching the hip flexors while lying down, as opposed to standing, is that it is unnecessary to worry about inadvertently assuming a sway-back position which can exacerbate your back pain. However, in order to stretch the hip flexors while lying down, it is necessary to find a solid table edge to lie on; the surface of a bed is not hard enough. The only other practical possibility is to lie at the top of a stairway and let one leg dangle over the edge of the top step.

Lie flat on your back and bring both knees up to your chest to flatten the spine against the table or floor and anchor the top end of the hip flexor muscles. Using both hands, hold the right leg tight against the chest. (If this results in discomfort in the groin area, placing a rolled up towel between the groin and the right leg should relieve the discomfort.) Let the left leg drop over the edge of the table, or top stair, being careful not to let the right leg move. Have a friend press down on the thigh of the left leg to increase the stretch or place a weight on the thigh, such as a thick book. Hold this position for a count of 20 seconds. Relax and repeat a minimum of ten times. Then return to the original position of both knees pressed up to the chest and stretch the hip flexors of the opposite leg.

166

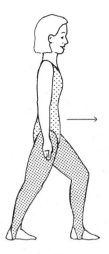

HIP FLEXOR STRETCH WHILE STANDING • It is far more difficult to stretch the hip flexors while standing. If you have not yet mastered the pelvic tilt, which is described next, don't try it because you'll likely end up increasing your sway-back without achieving any hip flexor stretching at all.

To stretch the flexors of the right hip, stand with your left leg approximately one foot in front of your right leg and do a pelvic tilt. Next bend the left knee, ensuring that your body is erect and your right knee is straight. Don't allow your back or pelvis to sway. Your pelvis must be in line with your shoulders and you must be able to maintain a good pelvic tilt the entire time. Hold the stretch for 20 seconds. Relax. Repeat a minimum of ten times and then switch legs to stretch the left hip flexors.

3. THE PELVIC TILT • The pelvic tilt is considered the bastion of back exercises. If you can learn to maintain the pelvic tilt while you are standing and walking as well as lying down, you will have no trouble correcting a sway-back posture. For many people who suffer from back pain due to facet joint problems, the pelvic tilt is *the* answer.

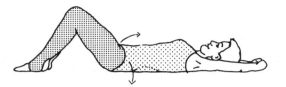

PELVIC TILT WHILE LYING DOWN • Learning the pelvic tilt properly involves a progression of positions. Start by lying on your back with your knees bent, your feet flat on the floor. Do not tense the muscles of the feet and legs. It is also important to breathe normally. Press your lower back down into the floor by tightening your abdominal muscles; the hip joint will thus roll clockwise toward your face. Hold this position for ten seconds.

To see if you are doing the tilt properly, ask someone to insert three fingers into the space between the small of your back and the floor before you do the tilt. When you tilt, your contraction should be strong enough to prevent him or her from removing these fingers. Some people find it helpful if they visualize moving the pubic bone toward the nose. Another important tip is to be sure to use *only* the abdominal muscles, not the buttock (gluteal) muscles or the hamstring muscles. If you contract either of these other muscle groups, you won't be able to hold a strong pelvic tilt when you attempt to do it while walking.

When you become more confident with the first of the pelvic tilt exercises, try extending the legs, one at a time, while maintaining the tilt. The third stage is to extend the legs, one at a time, and then bend them up again without losing the tilt. When you have mastered this version, try doing the pelvic tilt with your legs straight to begin with rather than bent. Some people find it helpful to concentrate on the muscles below the navel rather than the ones above. Always hold a pelvic tilt position for ten seconds and then relax. Repeat a minimum of 20 times.

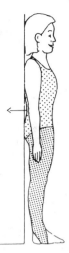

PELVIC TILT WHILE STANDING • The next stage in the progression is to do a pelvic tilt while standing. Stand with your back to a wall, the heels approximately two inches away from the wall to allow for the shape of the buttocks. The back of your head should touch the wall and your face should be vertical; you can check your position by making sure that your eyes are focused straight ahead, rather than at the ceiling or the top of a window. Do a pelvic tilt by pushing your lower back in toward the wall, concentrating on reducing the hollow in your lower back. Don't tighten the buttock muscles or hold your breath. Some people find it helpful to have someone try to insert several fingers into the small amount of space that will still remain between your lower back and the wall. With a good standing pelvic tilt, a person should be able to insert several fingers up to the middle knuckle, but not the entire hand or the wrist. Again, some people find it helpful to visualize the pubic bone moving toward the chin. Remember also to concentrate on your lower abdominal muscles rather than the ones above the navel.

If you have trouble doing a pelvic tilt while standing, it may be because your hip flexors are tight. If you find that you are tending to bend your knees, this is most likely the reason, and it would be a good idea to spend additional time on hip flexor stretches.

PELVIC TILT WHILE WALKING • After a couple of days, you should feel comfortable doing a pelvic tilt while standing. The next stage is to walk away from the wall and around the room. Then come back to the wall to recheck your posture. This is where you will run into trouble if you have been tightening your buttock muscles. If you find that you are walking like a tin soldier, contracted buttock muscles are most likely the reason. But even if your technique is faultless, learning to walk with a controlled pelvic tilt takes a lot of practice. Be patient.

4. THE SIT-UP • You can strengthen your abdominal muscles sufficiently with pelvic tilt exercises alone. Says Margaret Duffy, "I've had patients with excellent abdominal strength who've never done a single sit-up. They are, however, very serious about their pelvic tilt exercises."

If you are interested in superb abdominal strength, you might want to add some sit-ups to your exercise regime. If so, consider several important points. First of all, sit-ups done with the legs extended and the knees straight are not recommended. If you do them this way, you will be working the hip flexor muscles more than the abdominal muscles and undoing all the effort you spent stretching the hip flexors.

Furthermore, lying on the back with the legs extended tends to encourage a sway-back posture; doing sit-ups in this position will strain the lumbar spine, possibly exacerbating a chronic back problem rather than alleviating it. Similarly, if you do full sit-ups rather than half sit-ups, you will be working the hip flexors as well as the abdominals. While there is no reason to *avoid* working the hip flexors, most people (especially those who suffer from chronic back pain) would be far better off expending this effort on their abdominal muscles, which are almost invariably too loose.

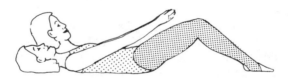

NORMAL HALF SIT-UP • Lie on the floor with the knees well bent and the arms either resting loosely on the abdomen or stretched toward the knees, whichever is more comfortable. First do a pelvic tilt. Then proceed with the sit-up, tucking in your chin gently and lifting only the head and shoulders off the floor to get the maximum abdominal contraction. If the shoulders don't clear the floor, the contraction won't be full, but if you raise yourself any higher, you will begin to lose the maximum abdominal contraction as the hip flexors take over. Hold for ten seconds and lower your shoulders and head to the floor very slowly. Over several weeks, try to work your way up to a minimum of 20 repetitions.

THE ROTATED SIT-UP • The normal sit-up described above mainly works the outermost abdominal muscle, which is called the rectus abdominis. There are, however, two other sets of abdominal muscles: the obliquus internis and the obliquus externis; and the transversus abdominis. While it is not essential to strengthen these abdominal muscles specifically, you can if you are really keen about abdominal strength. As you are lifting your head and shoulders off the ground, reach your right hand toward your left knee and hold. Alternate sides with each repetition.

ISOMETRIC ROTATED SIT-UP • This variation of the rotated sit-up is recommended if the normal rotated sit-up exacerbates your back or neck pain. Start by doing a pelvic tilt while lying down as described above. Bring the left knee about halfway to the chest while stretching the right hand toward it. Push your left knee up while pushing down against the knee with the right hand for an isometric contraction of the oblique abdominal muscles. Hold the contraction for ten seconds and relax, remembering to maintain the pelvic tilt until you have returned your left leg and right hand to the resting position. Repeat a minimum of five times to begin with, working your way up to twenty repetitions. Then repeat, changing sides.

5. THE LOW BACK STRETCH (KNEE TO CHEST STRETCH) • The knee to chest stretch exercise is excellent if you've recently exacerbated a chronic back problem by twisting awkwardly or lifting something incorrectly. It will stretch out the lower portion of the erector spinae muscles, which run from the middle of your back to the sacrum along each side of the spine. These muscles extend (arch) your spine when they work together and bend your spine sideways (to the side that is being contracted) when working unilaterally.

You do not have to be afraid to do this exercise when you are in pain; simply do it within the range that is comfortable and do not strain to the point of exacerbating your pain further. If you have muscle spasm in your lower back, you can first reduce it by lying on an ice pack for five minutes. Start with a single stretch and then, as you feel comfortable and your pain begins to subside, progress to the more difficult variations. If you are pain-free, start with the second variation which includes a dural stretch.

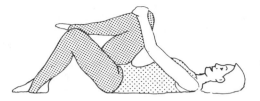

KNEE TO CHEST – SINGLE STRETCH • Lie on the floor on your back with your knees bent. Using both hands, pull the right knee up to the chest, stretching the muscles of the lower back only to the point at which you feel pain. Hold this stretch for five seconds and relax. Repeat a minimum of ten times and then switch legs. As your back pain begins to subside, increase the range of your stretch.

KNEE TO CHEST WITH DURAL STRETCH • When the single stretch no longer exacerbates your back pain and you are able to bring each knee all the way to the chest, you can progress to the next variation, which stretches the dura mater in addition to the low back muscles. The dura mater is the thick, fibrous, outer layer of the various layers of tissue that cover and protect the spinal cord within the spinal canal.

Having first stretched the knee to the chest, raise your head off the floor tucking in your chin gently. Do not raise the shoulders. Hold for five seconds. Then relax, lowering your head to the floor first and only then lowering your leg to the floor. Repeat a minimum of ten times and then switch legs.

KNEE TO CHEST STRETCH WITH ISOMETRIC CONTRACTION • If you are having difficulty increasing the range of your stretch, try adding a variation which includes an isometric contraction to this exercise.

Do not raise your head with this variation. Stretch one knee to its pain-free limit and hold the stretch for five seconds. Then, while the knee is still in position, use both hands to resist as you push the knee isometrically – that is, without moving it – toward the feet. Hold this contraction for three seconds, being careful not to allow the lower back to wobble. Then relax completely before pulling the knee up again. This isometric variation will cause the small muscles of the back to contract. When you relax them, the range of your next stretch will be greater because the muscles, having just contracted, will be tricked into relaxing completely. Repeat a minimum of five times and then switch legs.

KNEE TO CHEST – DOUBLE STRETCH (WITH OR WITHOUT ISOMETRIC CONTRACTION) • Repeat the knee to chest stretch but stretch both knees to the chest at the same time. To increase the range of your stretch, add the isometric variation described above.

6. THE LOW BACK EXTENSION STRETCH • Although most people who suffer from chronic back pain have a greater than normal lordosis, or hyperlordosis, in their lumbar spine, some people lack lordosis, having what is sometimes called a "poker" spine. While a hyperlordosis will put excess stress on the facet joints of the back, the normal spine should be curved slightly in order to absorb stress when you walk and run. (Most people who lack normal lordosis have inherited the posture rather than developed it.) If you lack a normal amount of lordosis, your anterior spinal ligaments will likely be abnormally short, and it is important to stretch them out.

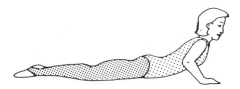

FULL EXTENSION STRETCH • If you have a normal amount of lordosis, you should be able to do a half push-up without feeling pain. Lie on the floor on your stomach and rise up on your hands to arch the lower back without lifting the pelvis off the floor. Hold this position for ten seconds. Relax and repeat a minimum of ten times. If this exercise does cause pain, refer again to the section on exercising and pain.

MODIFIED EXTENSION STRETCH • If you have a worn facet joint, this exercise may exacerbate your back pain by jamming the joints together. Try a simpler variation: instead of pushing yourself all the way up onto your hands, push yourself up onto your forearms only. This is a passive stretch into extension, and you should be able to hold this position for five minutes. If doing this variation still causes back pain, and that pain does not subside within 15 to 20 minutes after you relax, eliminate this exercise from your program and consult an exercise specialist, preferably a physiotherapist. Chances are, however, that if you do have a facet joint problem, you will have *more* lordosis than is normal rather than less. If this is the case, extension exercises are unnecessary for you. Eliminate this exercise from your program and spend the extra time on pelvic tilt exercises to decrease your lordosis.

7. THE SMALL MUSCLE GROUP STRENGTHENER • There are hundreds of pairs of small muscles in the back. The shortest ones are no longer than the little finger and run from one vertebra to the next. Others run from one vertebra to another several levels below.

Millions of years ago, when these small muscles were designed for an animal that walked on all fours, their function was to aid the body in side-bending and rotational movements. They were never intended to bear weight. Like the delicate muscles of the hand, they were meant to perform fine movements and contract for short durations only. Now that man has evolved to the upright posture, however, these muscles are required to perform tasks for which they were not designed. When you bend over, even to pick up something as light as a Kleenex, it is these pairs of muscles which help pull you back up into the upright position.

This is the main reason why you should always bend your knees and use your strong leg muscles when you want to pick up any object. In practice, however, it is impossible to always bend with the knees, and it is therefore important to strengthen these small muscle groups as much as possible.

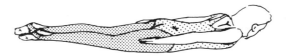

SMALL MUSCLE GROUP STRENGTHENING EXERCISE (EASY VARIATION) • Lie flat on the floor on your stomach, arms by your sides, your head to whichever side feels more comfortable. Do a pelvic tilt but be careful not to tighten the buttock muscles. Lift the shoulder blades, but not the head, off the floor, pinching the shoulder blades together to create a furrow. Your hands should come off the floor about an inch, and your head should lift up just high enough so that you can now turn it to face the floor. Be sure that your face is horizontal to the floor rather than tilted. If it is tilted, tuck the chin in slightly. Hold this position without letting the shoulders drop and count to ten. Relax and repeat a minimum of ten times. This will strengthen all the small muscle groups of the spine, especially the muscles of the thoracic spine, which are so often neglected by exercise programs.

LOW BACK MUSCLE STRENGTHENING EXERCISE (DIFFICULT VARIATION) • If you have rounded shoulders, you can add a variation to the above exercise that will help correct this problem. Lie on your stomach, but place your arms so that the elbows are at a 90-degree angle to the body. When you lift the shoulder blades as described above, lift the elbows as well, turning the head so that your face is horizontal to the floor. Hold for ten seconds. Relax and repeat a minimum of ten times. Be patient with this variation. It is difficult, and you may find that you must start off with only four or five repetitions and work your way up.

174

17

Posture: The Best for Your Back

"The effects of poor posture don't usually start to bother people until they reach their late thirties or early forties. When you think about it, the resilience of the human body is amazing. What other piece of machinery could withstand 40 years of misuse?"

Margaret Duffy, Senior Physiotherapist,
Toronto Western Hospital

Many professionals who treat back pain sufferers believe that the contribution of poor posture to back pain is seriously underplayed. They blame this on the fact that until recently, few world-class researchers considered the role of posture a worthy topic to address. Professionals had many general ideas about posture but few were specific and none had been documented scientifically.

One of the first researchers to tackle the subject of posture and its relation to back pain was Dr. Alf Nachemson, a world-renowned Swedish orthopaedic surgeon. Dr. Nachemson first published the results of his research on posture as it relates to disc stress in the mid-1970s. (See Diagram 16, page 42.) One of his studies demonstrated that sitting at a desk in an unsupported posture puts more stress on the discs and muscles of the lumbar spine than any other posture, including standing.

Quantifying this information was a major breakthrough. It also had the effect of influencing other researchers to become interested in the challenges of posture. West German professor Dr. Hanns Schoberth, for example, has since completed extensive research to work out the optimum dimensions of a chair at a desk. (See Diagram 25, page 180.) Others, including Canadians Paul Waitzer, John Lama and Frank Roberts, have designed postural aids. Paul Waitzer's Milburn's Backeaser footrest, John Lama's Lama Orthopedic Chair, and Frank Robert's Obus Forme Backrest, which are sold at surgical supply outlets and retail stores, have helped tens of thousands of North Americans who suffer from back pain. In recent years, enough products have been developed that entrepreneurs in both Canada and the United States have found it economically viable to open retail stores devoted *entirely* to the back pain sufferer, the best being The Back Store in Toronto. Most of the products these stores carry — chairs, backrests, pillows, travelling beds, extensions to pick up out-of-reach objects, to name just a few — are designed to help back pain sufferers carry out their daily activities in postures that are good for their backs.

In a perfect world, we all would have learned the techniques of good posture as youngsters, at school. How to use our bodies when sitting, standing, sleeping, working and playing would be as basic as reading,

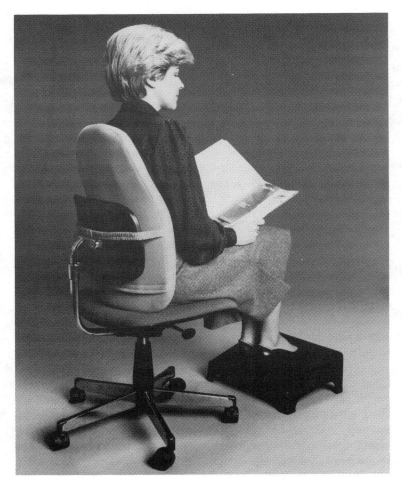

Obus Forme Backrest.

writing and arithmetic. According to professionals who treat back pain sufferers, this would significantly reduce the amount of back pain that plagues our society.

In our imperfect world, most people must learn the rules of good posture as adults. They must also undo the damage that years of bad habits have caused. To do this takes patience and diligence.

If you suffer from chronic back pain, you should be aware of proper

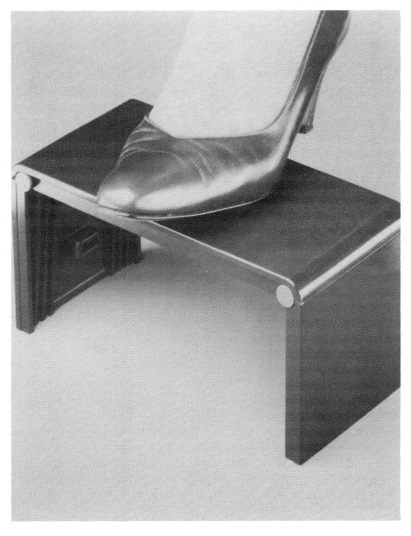

Milburn's Backeaser footrest.

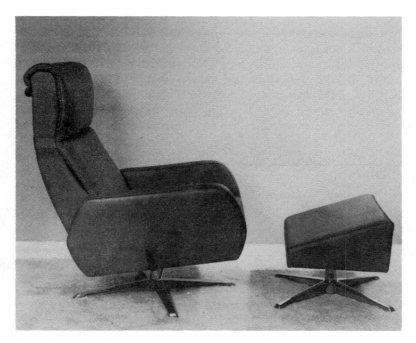

The Lama Orthopedic Chair.

posture in four specific areas: sitting, standing, lying down, and lifting. Using the body correctly in these postures will reduce strain on your muscles, ligaments, joints and bones. If you already suffer from chronic back pain due to many years of poor posture, you can stop the damage from progressing, but you cannot reverse all of the damage that has taken place. Muscles that have been strained due to poor posture can be corrected; sagging ligaments, or worn joints, cannot. In addition to correcting poor posture, it is therefore also essential to strengthen weak muscles so that they will be strong enough to compensate for worn joints or lax ligaments. How to do this through specific exercises is discussed in Chapter 16.

The Basics Of Good Posture

SITTING •

1. To take some of the strain off the lumbar spine, keep your knees raised above your hips when sitting. This posture will decrease excessive lordosis. The ideal way of doing this is to sit in a chair that tilts back slightly, an excellent position for reading. Use an ottoman to support your feet and a headrest to reduce neck strain.

178

At a desk, however, a tilting chair is impractical, unless you are in a position to have a tilting desk custom-built. (Some avant-garde designers believe that tilting desks will become commonplace in the near future.) To raise your knees above hip level at a desk, try placing a small footstool under the desk. Some people find that a slanted footstool works best, others disagree, preferring a flat one. If you are in a situation where it is impossible to find even a makeshift footrest (in a pinch, a telephone book will do), cross your legs, switching legs frequently to avoid cramping.

2. When buying a desk chair, select one that is adjustable, and easy to adjust. If the seat of your chair is too high, the normal lordosis in your lumbar spine will increase. If it is too low, the muscles of both the upper and lower back will be strained. Different tasks require different heights. When typing, for example, you will want to raise the height of your chair. If you are reading a book that you can hold in your lap, you will want to lower it. Many of the office chairs that are now being manufactured have hydraulic mechanisms for changing height, and these are recommended. A chair with five rather than four legs for its base is also preferable as it provides more stability.

3. Whenever possible, use a chair with specific lumbar support. If you sit for several hours in a chair that offers none at all, your back muscles will have to support themselves and this can lead to muscle strain. It is, in fact, harder for your back muscles to remain in a stationary, unsupported position than it is for them to be alternately expanded and contracted during rigorous exercise. When the back muscles remain in a strong contraction for several hours, the blood supply to them decreases. Less oxygen is delivered to the muscles and they become fatigued. When muscles become fatigued, they sometimes go into spasm. Research has shown that in order to sit comfortably for an extended period of time, you must support your back muscles to the extent that they contract to only 15 per cent of their maximum capacity. Many poorly designed chairs scarcely support the back muscles at all.

If you are scientifically inclined, the results of Dr. Hanns Schoberth's investigations will interest you. His design for the ideal office chair, which is completely adjustable, takes the needs and dimensions of most people into account. An illustration from Dr. Schoberth's publication *Correct Sitting at the Workplace* is on page 180.

4. Avoid chairs and sofas that you sink into. The image of "soft is comfortable" is as erroneous for sitting as it is for sleeping. Rather than allowing your muscles to relax, a soft chair causes muscle tension in the lower back and buttocks to increase; the muscles must contract to provide the support that the chair lacks.

5. If you are in the market for a new chair, try to buy one that has a curved front edge, or scroll. This will prevent the flow of blood to your thighs from being constricted.

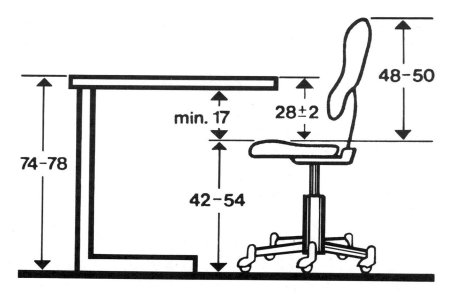

Diagram 25   Dr. Hanns Schoberth's Design for the Ideal Office Chair

6. Try to ensure that your weight can be comfortably transferred to your chair through your buttocks rather than your thighs. Some straight-backed chairs are so straight that they throw the weight of the body forward, switching the load from the buttocks to the thighs.

7. Whenever possible, choose a chair with armrests. Armrests (which should be positioned at a comfortable height, 21 to 25 centimetres/8 to 10 inches above the height of the seat) will reduce fatigue and tension in your shoulders and neck. Be aware of the position of your neck as well as the position of your lumbar spine. Slumping in a chair while watching TV, or reading with the neck craned forward, will strain the muscles of the neck and shoulders.

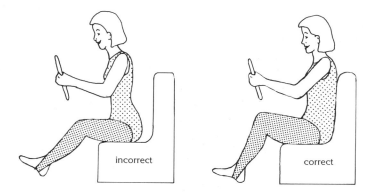

Diagram 26   Incorrect and Correct Positions for Driving

8. When driving, pull the driver's seat as close to the pedals as possible to reduce strain on the lumbar spine.

STANDING • Of all the postures we were "taught" as children, the military stance is the worst. Not only is the lumbar lordosis increased, but the head also becomes imbalanced – tipped back over the cervical spine, which strains the ligaments and the muscles of the upper back.

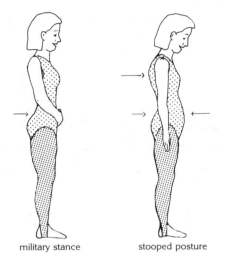

military stance   stooped posture

Diagram 27   Incorrect Standing Postures

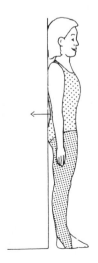

Diagram 28   Correct Standing Posture

A stooped standing posture is almost as bad. The lumbar lordosis is increased, and the abdomen sags as well.

1. To find the standing posture that is correct for you, stand against a wall with your heels about two inches away from it to allow room for the buttocks. Do a pelvic tilt, which is described in detail on page 167.

To many people, this correct posture feels uncomfortable or strange. Don't be surprised; if you have been standing incorrectly for 30 or 40 years, it will take time to get used to doing it right. Be patient and practise the pelvic tilt while lying down (see page 168). These exercises will strengthen your abdominal muscles which, in turn, will help you to maintain proper posture while standing. Remember also to avoid locking your knees.

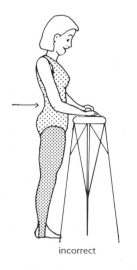
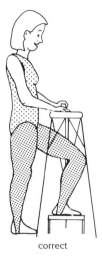

incorrect   correct

Diagram 29   Standing Posture

2. If you must stand without moving for any length of time, use a footrest to help reduce excessive lumbar lordosis (and the strain on the facet joints of the lumbar spine, which results from it). Remember to alternate the raised foot frequently.

3. Try to avoid leaning over objects to perform routine activities: for example, bending across a high table to answer a wall telephone, or reaching across a sofa to open or close a window. If you have no alternative, at least bend your knees to absorb some of the strain on the lumbar spine.

4. You'll be amazed at how much backache you can eliminate, or at least reduce, by moving household objects to eye level. The bathroom mirror and items in kitchen cabinets are two examples. Plates and other

182

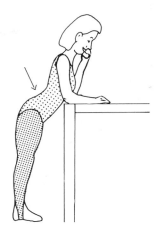

Diagram 30   Incorrect Posture

utensils that you use daily should be at shoulder level. If you are planning to redo your kitchen, keep your height in mind when planning the height of cabinets and counters, as well as the amount of space between counters and cabinets.

5. High heels increase the lordosis of the lumbar spine. Avoid them when you can. Crepe-soled or other soft-soled shoes help cushion your joints when walking.

LYING DOWN • First a few words about beds. What people who suffer from chronic back pain sleep on has as much to do with the way they feel the next day as the way they sit and stand.

If your bed is too soft, your spine will have to rely on its ligaments and muscles to keep it in its normal "double-S" shape.

If your bed is too hard (most beds aren't, of course, but the floors that soft beds drive us onto *are*) and you sleep on your side, the same problem exists. Your hips and your shoulders are much like the towers of a suspension bridge, your spine being what is suspended between them. Because of the difference in both weight and size of the shoulders and hips, a totally ungiving surface will not allow your spine to assume its natural "double-S" curve much better than a saggy mattress will.

A plywood board under a mattress is not necessarily much better. It simply provides a hard base for a soft mattress to sag into. A board is only useful when you are faced with a situation where you have a good mattress resting on a saggy metal frame, a camp bed for example.

If you have inserted a plywood board between a perfectly good mattress and its box spring in the hope of making the surface harder still, you may inadvertently be causing your mattress to wear out sooner than normal.

Mattresses and their box springs are designed to work in tandem to provide support for the body. Using a box spring, which unlike a plywood board has some amount of give, will prolong the life of your mattress; the box foundation will absorb some of the weight. If you place a board between them, the mattress will be forced to bear the entire burden.

The average well-made mattress and box spring set should last between ten and fifteen years, if treated well. That means turning it end to end and upside down every month for the first few months to ensure that it adjusts evenly and smoothly to your body weight. After that, a turn every couple of months will do.

If you're in the market for a new bed, invest wisely. Try to think of a bed as the place where you spend approximately one-third of your life and budget accordingly. Don't buy a bed without trying it for at least five or ten minutes.

Waterbeds? The people who sell waterbeds insist that they are excellent for chronic back pain sufferers, and that in many instances, they can actually "cure" a bad back. (I especially love the waterbed brochure that features a smiling gentleman in a doctor suit on the cover!) On several occasions, I have asked these retailers for copies of the research studies on which these opinions are based, but none have ever arrived. The only research on waterbeds that I've been able to find addresses the problems of burn victims and women who are pregnant. Waterbeds are considered to be helpful for both.

This does not suggest, however, that waterbeds are not good for people who suffer from chronic back pain. Many people insist that the warmth of a heated waterbed is soothing for their backs. Only a few people that I've spoken to say that waterbeds make their backs feel worse. In trying to assess who is likely to benefit from a waterbed, I have observed that people whose back pain is better with activity seem to prefer waterbeds more often than those whose back pain responds to rest.

If you're interested in a waterbed, buy it from one of the dealers who offer a money-back guarantee to customers who are not satisfied after 30 days. (Often it takes a month to get used to a new bed.) Be sure to read the fine print that goes with the guarantee. Some companies require you to complain within seven days and give the company an opportunity to make adjustments to the bed's water level.

Once you have acquired a bed with the potential to give you a good night's rest, here are some tips to follow:

1. Most people find that the best position for their backs is the fetal position. Both hips and knees should be bent equally. If you find it more comfortable, place a small pillow between the knees. A thin pillow should be placed under the head and neck, to fill the space between the head and shoulders; a thick pillow will strain the neck and shoulders.

If you find yourself in a situation where there is no alternative but to sleep in a saggy bed, try sleeping in the fetal position with a thin pillow under your hips as well as your head. By fiddling with the position of the pillow under your hips, you should be able to reduce the ill-effects associated with the sag.

2. Lying flat on your back with your legs outstretched will increase your lumbar lordosis. If you prefer to sleep on your back, however, you can support your hips by bending your knees and placing a bolster, or rolled up pillow, under them. A thin pillow should also be placed under the head and neck.

3. Lying on the stomach will increase your lumbar lordosis even when one leg is bent. Avoid this position.

4. Reading in bed is generally bad for the back unless you use a bedrest cushion.

5. Keep in mind that a soft sofa is as bad for your back as a soft bed. If you have a chance to lie down for a few minutes during the day, lie on the floor on your back with the knees well bent. Place a thin pillow under your neck and head, and place your legs across the seat of a chair as shown in Diagram 31. Many people find that if they can get themselves into this posture immediately for five or ten minutes when they feel a backache coming on, they can circumvent, or at least minimize, the pain.

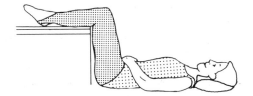

Diagram 31   Correct Posture for Relaxing

LIFTING • First a few pearls of wisdom about lifting, which illustrate the importance of doing it properly.

If you lift a 10-pound weight with the weight 14 inches from your body rather than close to it, you will be lifting the equivalent of approximately 150 pounds.

When you lift an object, the discs of the spine become compressed. Normally, this is not a problem since discs can withstand enormous amounts of stress. For example, the fibres of the annuli of the discs of the lumbar spine can withstand a compressive pressure of 3.2×10^7 newtons per square metre before they stretch to the breaking point. The meaning of this mathematical equation is less interesting to most of us than the fact that discs can withstand ten times as much compression as the vertebrae themselves. A heavy load will crush the bones of the spine before it ruptures a disc. The equation changes, however, when you lift an object and twist at the same time. If you read Chapter 1, you will recall that the annulus of an intervertebral disc is made of layers of fibres which are arranged in a criss-crossed type of pattern, much like the plies of a radial tire. Because of this construction, torsion tends to shear one layer from another, and the mathematical equation changes considerably. If you lift and twist at the same time, the compressive pressure that the same disc can withstand is reduced to 1.4×10^3 newtons per square metre. Amazing as it sounds, this is almost 23 thousand times less than the equation mentioned above!

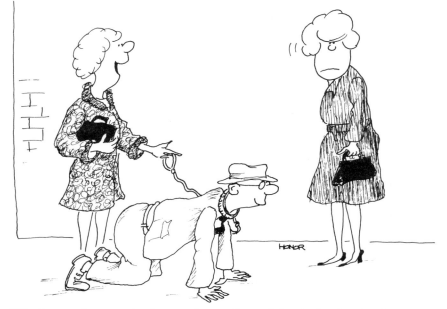

"His theory is . . . only those who walk upright get backache."

Now that you are undoubtedly convinced of the importance of learning good lifting techniques, here are some specific tips:

1. Try to carry a balanced load. Two lighter bags of groceries, one at each side, will strain the back far less than one heavy bag carried to one side.

2. Always bend from the hips and knees (rather than from the waist) when lifting an object, even one that is light. Avoid lifting objects above waist level whenever possible and *never* lift anything above shoulder level. These two postures increase the lordosis in your lumbar spine, placing unnecessary strain on the muscles, ligaments and facet joints of the lower back.

3. Avoid twisting when lifting. Instead, turn the entire body to face the place where you want to put the object you are lifting.

186

4. Avoid stooping into deep bins and constricted spaces, which make it impossible to follow good lifting rules.

5. It is often easier to push a heavy object than to pull it. Think before you lift.

6. Although people's strength varies, the maximum lifting load for women is 33 pounds. For men it is 55 pounds.

IV

The Holistic Alternatives

18

Chiropractic: All That It's Cracked Up To Be?

During a blustery February in 1975, the National Institute of Neurological and Communicative Disorders and Stroke (NINCDS) invited 58 chiropractors, osteopaths, basic scientists and physicians to meet at their conference centre in Bethesda, Maryland, down the road from the Watergate Hotel. The topic: The Research Status of Spinal Manipulative Therapy. For the first time in North America, a world-class medical and biological organization was granting chiropractors and medical experts a hearing on equal footing.

When the NINCDS conference was over, it was evident that the muddy waters which have surrounded chiropractic for nearly a century had yet to clear. Osteopath Dr. Murray Goldstein, editor of the conference's monograph, summed up: "... analysis of available data," he told the professional audience, "clearly indicates that specific conclusions cannot be [drawn] either for or against the efficacy of spinal manipulation therapy or the foundations from which it is derived ....

"Chiropractors, osteopathic physicians, medical manipulative specialists and their patients," he continued, "all claim manipulation provides relief from pain, particularly back pain, and sometimes cure; some medical physicians, particularly those not trained in manipulative techniques, claim it does not provide relief, does not cure, and may be dangerous, particularly if used by nonphysicians. The available data do not clarify either view. . . . "

Hard data or no hard data, the 1970s witnessed inroads by chiropractors into territories traditionally sacrosanct to medical doctors. By the beginning of the 1980s, North America's approximately 20,000 practitioners of chiropractic had forged what seems to be an indelible place for themselves in the health care field. In both Canada and the United States, they had lobbied for the right to render their services under medical plans and they had won.

But, in return for these privileges, both the public and the governments who are now supporting chiropractors financially are asking questions and making demands:

• Are the chiropractors who imply to their patients that manipulation may affect "visceral pathology" (diseases of internal organs) justified in doing so? Studies show that manipulation can affect such bodily functions as blood flow and heart rate, but to move from that notion to the assumption that manipulation plays any role in the amelioration of human disease is a quantum leap for which there is no concrete scientific evidence whatsoever.

• Should chiropractors limit their scope of practice to manipulating painful fixated (stiff) joints and forget about "top-me-up-once-a-month" preventive manipulations for patients when they are pain-free?

• When should chiropractors be using X-rays? While sectional films — X-rays of a *particular* area of the spine — are often important in order to establish contraindications (diseases such as cancer or a bone abnormality that would rule out manipulation as a therapy), some chiropractors are using *in addition* motion, or stress, X-rays which are taken when the patient bends to the end of his or her range of motion. Those who favour motion X-rays say they provide clear *objective* information about joints that are either fixated or stiff (hypomobile), or unstable (hypermobile). Other chiropractors disagree, preferring to rely on a clinical diagnosis in most cases. They believe that the risks from radiation far outweigh the advantages, except in exceptional circumstances, pointing out that the lumbar spine requires more radiation to X-ray than any other part of the body.

• Should patients with back pain consider a chiropractor the only necessary contact with the health care profession for that back pain; chiropractors have the right of primary contact, but might it not be wiser for back pain sufferers to also consult a medical doctor who, having been trained in a hospital setting, is more experienced in the diagnosis of disease?

• What *exactly* does manipulation, the mainstay of chiropractic treatment, accomplish? When is it helpful? And when, if ever, might it be a waste of both money and time?

Ian Coulter, Ph.D. is co-author of the 1980 book *Chiropractors: Do They Help?* He worked on the book, which is very positive about chiropractic, while he was administrative assistant to the Vice-Provost of Health Sciences at the University of Toronto. (The book was based on the results of a $500,000 research study funded by Health and Welfare Canada.) In 1981, Dr. Coulter left U. of T. to become vice-president of the Canadian Memorial Chiropractic College, Canada's only college of chiropractic. Last year, he was named president.

According to Dr. Coulter, the focus of chiropractic has changed over the past number of years. "For most of its history, the paradigm of chiropractic was really what I'd call a 'practice' paradigm . . . . The shift has been one very much into the basic sciences and research." Dr. Coulter says that chiropractic now resembles the other health care professions. "We have exactly the same basic sciences taught at exactly the same level, and usually by the same professors.... The health sciences like dentistry, medicine and ours share the same common body of knowledge in the basic sciences, the biological sciences. Then each one of us chooses another set of applied sciences.... In our area it is called spinology – the study of the spine."

What Is Manipulation?

The therapeutic mainstay of those who study spinology is manipulation. (In fact, to bill a health insurance plan, a chiropractor must perform one.) Manipulation is defined as "an assisted passive motion applied to the spinal facet joints and sacroiliac joints," meaning that the patient is passive and the manipulator assists. Dr. David Cassidy, a chiropractor who is a research fellow in the department of orthopaedics at the University of Saskatchewan's University Hospital, explains: "It's very simple. You have a stiff joint and you manipulate it and that makes it move. You're increasing the range of its motion.... We know that a mobile joint is less likely to be painful than a stiff joint. That's true for the elbow, for the ankle and for the spine."

For the benefit of those who are scientifically inclined, Dr. Cassidy talks about joint ROM (Range of Motion). Toward the end of a joint's normal physiological range of motion, he explains, is a buffer zone. At the end of that, there is an elastic barrier of resistance. This barrier, he says, has what he calls a "springlike end-feel," which is the result of negative pressure within the joint capsule. (This negative pressure is one of the mechanisms that helps to stabilize the joint. Muscles, ligaments and the capsule itself are the others.)

If the joint surfaces are forced beyond this elastic barrier by a manipulator, they move apart with a cracking sound, entering what is called the paraphysiological ROM. This constitutes manipulation. Mobilization, on the other hand, stays on the buffer zone side of the elastic barrier within the joint's normal physiological range of motion. (See page 268.)

The cracking sound, says Dr. Cassidy, results from the sudden liberation of gases that are contained in the synovial fluid of the joint's capsule. Physicists call the phenomenon cavitation. The bubbles of gas can be detected on an X-ray right after the manipulation but are reabsorbed within a few minutes. For approximately 30 minutes, however, the elastic barrier of resistance between the buffer zone and the paraphysiological ROM is absent. During this time, there is an increase in the joint space and the joint is somewhat unstable, making further manipulation unsafe. After the gases are reabsorbed, the negative pressure returns to normal. The joint space narrows and the elastic barrier of resistance between the buffer zone and the paraphysiological zones is re-established.

In some cases, the manipulative "thrust" is thought to stretch a contracted muscle, relieving spasm. In other cases, it is thought to break down adhesions, which may be restricting the joint's ability to move. (See page 39.) There is also some evidence that manipulation decreases pain itself in the same way that a TENS machine or acupuncture can reduce pain.

Says Dr. Cassidy, "When you manipulate a joint, you stimulate the large afferent nerve fibres, which then inhibit the small afferent 'pain' fibres from transmitting pain." (See Chapter 4.) A recent study conducted by the Canadian Memorial Chiropractic College's head of research Dr. Howard Vernon substantiates this view. In Dr. Vernon's controlled study, which was published in the *American Journal of Physical Medicine*, it was found that subjects' ability to tolerate pain increased for at least ten minutes following manipulation.

Chiropractors feel that considerable training and experience are necessary to perform a manipulation competently. Dr. David Drum, a Toronto chiropractor, agrees. Dr. Drum has the reputation of keeping Canada's National Ballet dancers on their toes. He also distinguished himself by being asked to present a paper at the NINCDS conference in 1975.

"Manipulation," he says, "is not particularly demanding to learn, [but] it takes about five years of constant practice to get really good, and you have to do it all the time to stay good or you lose it."

Should You See a Medical Doctor Too?

Many medical doctors believe that while chiropractors spend a lot of time learning manipulation techniques, they spend too little time, and the wrong kind of time, learning how to make a differential diagnosis. (A differential diagnosis is the list of things that might be producing a symptom or a sign.)

Because of this belief, most medical doctors advise back pain patients who are treated by a chiropractor to also consult a medical doctor for a full differential diagnosis. Certain conditions, they explain, can refer pain to the back or down an arm. Many physicians worry that a symptom such as this could be mistaken for a musculoskeletal condition by a chiropractor. Examples that doctors use are: an expanding aortic aneurysm, or angina, at the very serious, life-threatening end of the spectrum; and Paget's disease, goiter, or a thyroid problem at the less life-threatening end.

In *Chiropractors: Do They Help?*, the authors say that chiropractic students do suffer from some disadvantages by not training in hospital settings, where they would be exposed to the great range of abnormal pathologies that medical students see. Furthermore, chiropractors are not allowed to take blood tests, or urine samples. In fact, Saskatchewan is the only province which even allows them to refer their patients to labs which do. This, doctors say, eliminates the possibility of a chiropractor doing a full diagnostic workup.

While it is true, as Dr. Coulter says, that in recent years a number of medical doctors – even some eminent medical doctors – have been teaching courses at the Canadian Memorial Chiropractic College, some of these very physicians say that this does not make up for chiropractors' lack of exposure to a hospital setting. And while fourth-year chiropractic students "intern" in the chiropractic college clinic, some of these same physicians say that this does not provide the kind of patient contact necessary to make them adept at making a full differential diagnosis. The exposure chiropractic student interns get in a chiropractic college clinic, they say, is nothing like the exposure a medical doctor gets while doing a rotating internship in a general hospital.

Dr. Paul Caulford is a Toronto general practitioner who teaches a 14-hour course in endocrinology at the Canadian Memorial Chiropractic College. For a number of years he also ran the medical end of the chiropractic clinic, meaning that he was the medical doctor who took care of the patients who were referred to him by chiropractic students. This happened, he explains, when, for example, the patient was thought to need anti-inflammatory drugs for a back problem (chiropractors cannot prescribe drugs) or had other problems. Having a medical doctor in the clinic, says Dr. Caulford, was more efficient than referring patients all over town.

Dr. Caulford believes that chiropractic has a tremendous role to play in the conservative management of back pain. He doesn't think that doctors should be doing manipulation, because they don't get adequate training in this therapeutic technique. But he also agrees with many of his colleagues that, while a chiropractor really knows backs, joints and biomechanics, he or she is not adequately exposed to the full range of pathology and is therefore ". . . unable to rule out the different diagnostic possibilities that have to be ruled out before he manipulates."

In Dr. Caulford's opinion, it goes without saying that a back pain patient who decides to see a chiropractor for that back pain should also see a medical doctor, if only to rule out other disease. "Chiropractors and doctors should work jointly," he says, "no pun intended!"

Expanding on the comment from *Chiropractors: Do They Help?*, Dr. Caulford stresses that the problem is not the teaching at the chiropractic college per se but the exposure. "They're adequately *taught*," he says, "but they are not adequately *trained* because they don't intern . . . . They may miss something that's causing back pain, or assume it's something else and adjust for it."

Recalling his own experience after he graduated from medical school and entered a hospital as an intern, Dr. Caulford says, "I thought I knew everything [but] I couldn't make a diagnosis. I'd never seen it before. I had all the knowledge, but I had not yet had the patient contact. It was during that year that all the teaching began to make sense."

Dr. Drum agrees with Dr. Caulford. "I insist that every patient who comes to see me have a family medical doctor," he says. "I do not see myself as an alternative to allopathic medicine . . . . If you're coming here, your family doctor knows. I want him to know what I'm doing and I want to know what he's doing. In fact, with every X-ray I take, I insist that the patient show it to the family doctor." Dr. Drum says that as a chiropractor, he does not feel adequately prepared to make a full differential diagnosis.

The Issue of X-rays

Chiropractors say that there are ten to twenty different ways of manipulating every moveable joint in the body. Some maintain that when someone has mastered the art, they can be very specific about which joint they are moving. Dr. Cassidy is not so sure. "Chiropractors like to think they are very specific, but there is no scientific evidence to say that they are or are not. I practised for ten years and I used to think that I could manipulate L4-L5 on the right side if I wanted to. I tend to think now that when I try to do that I might also move the facet joint below or above, but I still think I can be fairly specific."

The issue of specificity becomes particularly important in the case of a patient who has an unstable joint, or joints. Just as it is unsafe to manipulate a joint during the 30 minutes after a manipulation when it is temporarily unstable, it is also unsafe to manipulate a joint that is unstable due to degenerative changes.

Joint instability sometimes occurs after many years of disc degeneration. The narrowing of the disc can cause the facet joint at the back of that disc to become unstable, or *hypermobile*, meaning that the joint moves too much. Lax ligaments, due to years of poor posture, can also contribute to joint instability. In extreme cases, the joint can actually wobble slightly when the person moves. If you repeatedly manipulate a hypermobile joint, you'll just increase the instability.

The diagnosis of unstable joints is where the issue of motion, or stress, X-rays comes into play.

To understand the controversy, it is first necessary to understand a bit of X-ray terminology. A *sectional* X-ray of the spine can be taken while the patient is standing, or lying down, but it is always taken with the spine in its normal posture – not bending in any way. It is used to look for contraindications to manipulation such as a tumour or a bone abnormality.

If there is anything suspicious, another X-ray, called a *spot* film, can be taken. Spot films zero in on a tiny area, providing more detail of the suspicious-looking area, hence the name *spot*.

Motion, or stress, X-rays, on the other hand, are taken while the patient bends to the end of his or her range of motion. To look for an unstable joint, two flexion/extension motion X-rays are taken — one while the patient flexes the spine, or arches it forward, the other while the patient extends the spine, or arches it backward. To look for fixated, or stiff, joints, two lateral motion X-rays are taken — one while the patient bends laterally, or sideways, to the right, the other while the patient bends laterally to the left.

Most chiropractors believe that they can pick up a fixated (*hypomobile*) joint by "palpating" the spine during their clinical diagnosis. To diagnose a fixated joint, you don't really need the two lateral motion X-rays. Some chiropractors believe that while it is more difficult to pick up an unstable (*hypermobile*) joint by palpation, they can still do it most of the time. For one thing, they know it is unusual to find an unstable joint in a patient who is under age 45, or who has only had back pain for a few months. So right off the top, that eliminates the need for either type of motion X-ray for many patients.

"X-rays, even motion X-rays, are not perfect," says Dr. Cassidy. "Most lay people think that the ultimate answer lies in an X-ray, but it doesn't. An X-ray is added information that you consider along with and equal with your clinical findings and your history . . . . Most people who have low back pain have stiff backs. Some of those people also have one segment that's worn out and a little bit unstable, and differentiating between them on physical examination is very difficult. The [flexion/extension] X-rays help . . . but if someone has only had back pain for a few months, chances are they don't have any instability. Instability is the result of an ongoing long history of back pain . . . . If someone has had years of back pain and a history of recurrent attacks, I start to suspect instability. If when I examine them and stress their spines in different directions and they jump and yell, well then, that also makes me suspect instability; *then* I'm also going to order motion X-rays."

Dr. Drum, who sees more people with acute back pain than chronic back pain and more people who are under 45 than over, rarely uses X-rays. "Other than to eliminate a fracture, for example, for which you'd look at an X-ray of a particular segment of the spine, I hardly ever use X-rays. With regular X-rays, the X-ray findings frequently don't correlate with the symptoms. If you do motion X-rays, you can pick up major fixations and unstable joints. But you can do that with motion palpation during a clinical diagnosis . . . . If you say that you don't have the skills to palpate and you need a film, then you're also saying that after you do what you think is going to correct it, you need another film to check. My feeling has always been that the danger inherent in repeated X-ray far outways the danger of a patient being left with some aberrant motion of a joint."

Says Dr. Cassidy, "Maybe our results, because we use X-ray, are slightly better."

But there is even more to the controversy than all this.

When Dr. Cassidy decides that a patient may have an unstable joint, he takes a flexion/extension motion X-ray *instead of* a sectional X-ray, not in addition to it; he uses the motion X-ray both to look for joint instability and for contraindications such as a tumour or bone abnormality. Other chiropractors, however, routinely take a sectional X-ray *and* motion X-rays. Some chiropractors even take a couple of sectional X-rays, *then* two flexion/extension motion X-rays, *then* two lateral bending motion X-rays for a total of six X-rays.

A few chiropractors actually do all this and then *retake* the lateral motion X-rays a month later to see if the treatment has led to any improvement in the joints that were stiff! (The chiropractors who take a large number of X-rays often use a procedure whereby the motion X-rays are "rarefied," meaning that less radiation is used. However, X-raying the lumbar spine requires more radiation than X-raying any other area of the body and so even rarefied X-rays, which use two-thirds of the normal dose, have a potential danger.)

Fortunately, most chiropractors believe that in almost all cases, if more than four X-rays at the outside are taken, the risks of radiation far outweigh the advantages that may be gained. Says Dr. Cassidy, "I would caution people to be conscious of the number of X-rays they are getting."

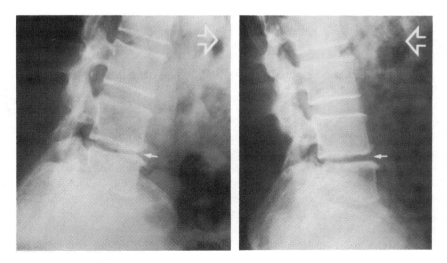

Motion X-rays of the spine.

198

Nevertheless, there are times when motion X-rays to locate an unstable joint can be useful. The two motion X-rays on page 198 illustrate how flexion/extension motion X-rays can help a chiropractor to identify an unstable joint.

In the left photograph, the patient is flexing, or bending forward. In the right, he is extending his spine, or bending backward. If you look carefully at the X-ray, you can see a number of things. First of all, the disc space between L4 and L5 looks very narrow. This, along with the history and the clinical diagnosis, would give the chiropractor a clue that there might be an unstable facet joint in the same area. Second of all, if you look at the small arrow in the left photograph, you'll see that the bottom right tip of L4 has moved slightly more than the vertebra below it. (The bottom right tip of the L4 vertebra is further to the right than the top right tip of the L5 vertebra.) This would be diagnosed by a chiropractor as an instability and manipulation of that particular joint would be avoided.

When Does Manipulation Work?

There is also some disagreement among chiropractors about just what type of back problem manipulation works best for. Dr. Drum, for example, prefers to deal with acute, rather than chronic, back pain. "I can adjust a person who has had chronic back pain for many years, and they usually feel better for 20 minutes. But by the time they go out and have lunch, they are right back where they started. (This may account for Dr. Vernon's findings. See page 194.) In many patients who have had chronic back pain for many years, the tone of the muscles, the joints, even the messages that the nerves are delivering to these structures have become so modified that anything I might do in terms of manipulation is insignificant in the overall scheme of things . . . .

"The people who respond best to manipulation are the people who have made an unguarded movement and as a result have a fixated, or frozen, joint. After the inflammation has subsided, that joint will often remain frozen. What I do is free those joints, and the results are great."

This is not to say, however, that Dr. Drum never treats those who suffer from chronic back pain. "Sometimes I will tell a chronic [back pain] patient that we can have a trial of manipulation, try it and see what happens, and sometimes it helps. But I don't make any promises. People with chronic back pain, however, do have acute exacerbations [episodes where their pain gets worse], and I believe that with manipulation I can often get them back to their normal 'dull roar.'

"People who suffer from chronic back pain need to look at their entire life-style," he says. "They need to look at how they are using, or abusing, their bodies, and they need much more than just manipulation. Otherwise, they are going to become dependent upon you and be in your office once a week for the rest of their lives."

Dr. Cassidy agrees. "I think that in a lot of cases . . . instead of trying to get patients off treatment and making them responsible for their own health, [chiropractors] try and make patients dependent."

In 1984, Dr. Cassidy completed a study with Dr. W.H. Kirkaldy-Willis, professor emeritus of orthopaedics and director of the Low-Back Pain Clinic at the University Hospital in Saskatoon. The study was "observational" as opposed to "controlled," where the design is such that bias on the part of the researcher is eliminated. Conducted on 283 patients with chronic back pain, the results showed that patients with facet joint and/or sacroiliac joint problems responded well to manipulation. Those with conditions where there were signs of neurological deficit, such as sciatic pain that extended below the knee, did not respond as well. Those who had central spinal stenosis, confirmed by a CT Scan X-ray, responded poorly.

But there was something very interesting and unusual about the procedure that Drs. Cassidy and Kirkaldy-Willis used. In their study, patients were manipulated *daily* for a period of two, and in a few cases three, weeks. "In our experience," the paper stated, "anything less than two weeks of daily manipulation is inadequate for chronic back pain patients."

"I think going once or twice a week [for manipulation] for nine months is a waste of time," says Dr. Cassidy. "I think it just reminds people they have a back problem. Here we do it for two weeks. Then we stop treatment and they have to go off and do their exercises or whatever . . . . I think a lot of chiropractors take advantage of chronic back pain patients. They don't give them exercises, and they don't give them any education. It's just come back in three weeks and we'll put it back again."

The History of Chiropractic

Whether it is for acute pain or chronic pain, manipulators have been adjusting joints for thousands of years. Chinese artifacts from as early as 2700 B.C. describe the technique. A Greek papyrus from 1500 B.C. gives instructions on how to manipulate the lumbar spine for back pain.

During the Renaissance, manipulators were known as "bone-setters" and by the middle of the 1850s, apothecaries had added the therapy to their bag of potions. It was around this time that British physicians and surgeons began a campaign to have their profession legislated. Being hospital-trained rather than apprenticed, these two groups united against the inclusion of the apothecary as a legitimate doctor. At the time, however, apothecaries were regarded favourably by the rural gentry, who had a sizable membership in parliament. As a result, when physicians and surgeons became a legal entity, they were forced to include apothecaries, who became today's general practitioners.

Had medicine decided to incorporate manipulation into its roster, chiropractic as a separate entity would in all likelihood have never developed. What happened, instead, is that the apothecaries were forced to relinquish their apprenticeship training and move into the hospital setting.

There they studied such courses as anatomy, physiology, pathology (the science of disease), and the treatment of fractures. But they had no opportunity to acquire the knowledge to manipulate bones, joints and ligaments.

Recognizing that manipulation certainly worked at least sometimes, a few physicians advocated its study. The eminent British surgeon James Paget was one. "By their practice of [manipulation]," he wrote, "bone-setters ... are held in repute. Their repute is, for the most part, founded on their occasionally curing a case which some good surgeon has failed to cure.... Learn then," he told his students, "to imitate what is good and avoid what is bad in the practice of bone setting."

Paget's advice was shunned by his colleagues, and soon his worst fears came true. In 1874, in Missouri, Andrew Taylor Still founded osteopathy, proclaiming that all diseases were caused by improper nourishment of the nervous system by the blood and could be corrected by manipulation. Twenty-one years later, Canadian-born Daniel David Palmer "discovered" chiropractic.

Oddly enough, Palmer, who operated a "magnetic healing studio" in Davenport, Iowa, claimed that when he discovered chiropractic he was totally unaware of the existence of osteopathy. The light dawned on Palmer while he was trying to restore the hearing of his deaf janitor by manipulating one of the vertebrae in the man's thoracic spine.

Palmer's theory was that he had relieved pressure on a spinal nerve that had been affecting the man's hearing for 17 years. The manipulation, he maintained, had removed the blockage, thereby allowing the body's "Innate Intelligence" to effect an instantaneous cure. What Palmer didn't realize was that the nerves associated with hearing do not emerge from between two mobile vertebrae in the thoracic spine. They don't, in fact, emerge from between any of the mobile – and therefore able to be manipulated – vertebrae at all. They are inside the head.

Nevertheless, Palmer and his followers established the basis of chiropractic: that "misaligned," "subluxated," or "displaced" vertebrae were the cause of most disease and that manipulation could cure it. However, in a study that is widely quoted as the definitive scientific investigation of the basis of chiropractic theory, American researcher E.S. Crelin found no evidence of subluxation. Using the spinal columns of cadavers, Crelin used a drill press to apply pressure, torsion, bending and twisting motions to the vertebral bodies to see if he could get the intervertebral foramen to narrow sufficiently to impinge on the nerve passing through. When he couldn't do it, he concluded that " ... the subluxation of a vertebra as defined by chiropractic – the exertion of pressure on a spinal nerve which by interfering with the planned expression of Innate Intelligence produces pathology – does not occur."

In fairness, Palmer's beliefs and doctrine were not as outrageous at the turn of the century as they sound today. At the time, some medical doctors were still using leeches, which they applied alongside the spine as a therapeutic treatment. Louis Pasteur had only recently demonstrated the existence of germs as a cause of disease. Many physicians of that era still regarded the spine as the "heart" of most human ills.

By the beginning of the twentieth century, however, medicine had abandoned such practices and begun its scientific revolution. While maintaining their focus on the use of manipulation for problems of muscles and joints, osteopaths adopted the philosophical concepts and practices of medical doctors. (Today, in Canada, there are few osteopaths; those who choose to live in Canada must practise under the same Drugless Practitioners Act as chiropractors. In the United States, osteopaths are allowed to prescribe drugs when necessary and practise in osteopathic hospitals. Most osteopaths therefore feel that their training skills are wasted in Canada.)

Modern chiropractors recognize the role of bacteria, viruses and other factors in illness. Like osteopaths, they focus on the treatment of the musculoskeletal system. But many still retain a philosophical bent toward seeing the spine as the focal point of disease.

Says Ian Coulter: "In the '60s, the area that was the greatest focus of concern happened to be musculoskeletal problems, and there was a narrowing of our focus ... but the research we're now looking into is coming back to visceral pathology. . . . In terms of practice, there probably has been a retrenchment for a large portion of the profession ... away from those [visceral] areas to a focus on musculoskeletal problems. On the other hand, as the research paradigm is starting to develop, what's interesting is in actual fact a return to that area. . . . We are now starting to re-examine that area. We are keeping the door open. We don't teach any specific therapeutic intervention for treatment of visceral problems; this college tends to focus on musculoskeletal problems. It always has. But in the program here we do introduce the notion that there may be these kinds of responses. At the moment we can't substantiate what they are. At the moment the jury is out."

The Future of Chiropractic

In all likelihood, the jury will be in on some of the answers to the basic questions about manipulation long before there is much knowledge of the relationship of manipulation to human disease. Largely in response to the NINCDS conference, researchers have conducted a number of controlled studies to try to determine if manipulation works and when. Chiropractors have been involved in many of the studies, but none of the controlled trials have been conducted by a chiropractic college. Says Dr. Coulter: "Until very recently this institution had neither the resources nor the expertise to do this kind of study. This is not the University of Toronto. The medical faculty of U. of T. has $50 million per year of external funding. Where do you think we're going to get that money?"

Some people criticize the chiropractic profession for not doing controlled trials. Dr. Coulter does not agree. "... You're laying on us an expectation or standard that the rest of science doesn't have to face," he says, and he is certainly right that few controlled studies on the efficacy of back surgery, for example, have been done. "... I think [chiropractors] waste a lot of time and money trying to convince people.... We are subjected to this criticism about clinical trials, and what I find sad is that our profession is responding and saying yes we ought to do this.... That doesn't mean to say that these trials shouldn't be done, by the way. What I'm saying is that I don't want us to get caught into believing that that is *all* we should do.... We have very limited resources.... My preference at the moment is for us to start investigating [the paradigms] and *then* start focusing on those bigger issues." To some people, this sounds a bit like putting the cart before the horse.

Dr. Cassidy is one of the chiropractors who believes in the importance of controlled trials. Now that his observational study is complete, he and his co-researcher Dr. Kirkaldy-Willis have begun to work on the design for a controlled trial, which they hope to undertake at the University of Saskatchewan. If and when the study does take place, it will deal with chronic back pain patients. But it will be different than the 14 trials that have been conducted to date, because it will use manipulation as a therapeutic technique *daily* for two or three weeks. Some of the past trials have used manipulation every other day, but none has tried an everyday-for-two-weeks approach.

At Hamilton's McMaster University, chiropractor Dr. David Brunarski is also in the process of developing the methodology for a controlled trial. If his study gets off the ground – it has been in the works for several years – it will compare manipulation with medical treatment on a minimum of 300 patients who have been suffering from back pain for more than seven weeks but less than five months.

The great hope of those who are in favour of this kind of research is that projects such as these will clarify the ambiguous results of the 14 controlled studies that have been completed to date.

Many of these studies indicate what Dr. Drum has observed – that manipulation works best on acute rather than chronic back pain. Some of them have found that while manipulation works better than other methods (exercise, education and various other physiotherapy techniques, for example) *initially*, there is no difference in the results after several weeks. Other studies have found that manipulated patients recover more rapidly than those treated with exercise alone.

One recent study was conducted at the Wellesley Hospital in Toronto by physiatrist Dr. Charles Godfrey. His group was comprised of 81 patients who had been suffering from back pain for no more than 14 days. In Dr. Godfrey's study, there was no difference between patients who were manipulated and those who were treated with "detuned" electric massage. The massage *felt* like a TENS machine to the patient, but its current was meaningless as a therapeutic technique.

It is common for researchers around the world to argue about the methods used by others in their experiments, and these 14 controlled studies are no exception. (Chiropractors, for example, have complained bitterly that in some of the studies which were not particularly positive about manipulation's efficacy, poorly skilled medical doctors had performed the manipulations.) But a lot has been learned about methodology from these trials; many people in the field hope that if and when the Cassidy and Brunarski studies are complete, their results will be venerated by both medical doctors and chiropractors around the world.

In the meantime, however, it is probable that the hoopla will continue in much the same vein as it has for a hundred years. Those who find chiropractic useful will continue to pursue it, deciding for themselves when it is helpful and when it is a waste of their time. Those who are skeptical will remain on the fence.

And those who, like NINCDS' Dr. Murray Goldstein, want hard data to define manipulation's scope will continue to push for the types of studies that can shed light on its efficacy. " . . . controlled studies," Dr. Goldstein concluded at the NINCDS conference, "provide the only scientific means presently available for the solution of the clinical research issues identified in this analysis."

19

Hypnosis: The Power of Suggestion

To many people, hypnosis conjures up the image of the Svengali-type character seducing a sweet young thing, or a sitcom plot in which the hypnotized hero runs about in boxer shorts clucking like a chicken. According to modern hypnotists, however, both of these images are just bits of fiction dreamed up by Hollywood writers.

The *Webster's Dictionary* defines *hypnosis* as: "a sleeplike condition psychically induced, usually by another person, in which the subject loses consciousness but responds, with certain limitations, to the suggestions of the hypnotist." But even that definition does little to satisfy those who practise the technique.

Modern hypnotists describe the hypnotic state as one of "altered awareness caused by a subject focusing in on one thing and screening out all the rest." The supposed benefit of this psychological editing is that it allows the person who is in a hypnotized state to communicate with the subconscious. Once in touch with the subconscious, a subject can "harness" it to help work out all sorts of problems. Dealing with chronic back pain, when the source of that pain cannot be eliminated, is one.

Dr. Margarita Gitev is a Toronto psychiatrist who has successfully used hypnosis on many of her back pain patients. She says that there is a physiological, as well as a psychological, explanation for why the technique works. "Recent studies," she says, "have shown that hypnosis can actually inhibit the release of lactic acid, one of the substances that is produced by muscles when they contract." This is relevant because built-up lactic acid is one of the things that can cause muscular pain.

During strenuous exercise, the muscles become contracted, the blood supply to them decreases, and lactic acid is produced. When the muscles are stretched out after exercise, the blood supply to them increases, and the lactic acid that has been produced can be dissipated before it has had a chance to build up. On the other hand, when a muscle is in chronic spasm, it remains contracted. The blood supply to it is restricted, lactic acid continues to be produced and, eventually, it builds up. "Experiments have shown that under hypnosis, patients can learn to prevent this lactic acid build-up," says Dr. Gitev.

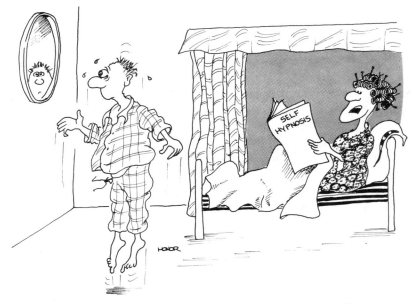

"It might make more sense dear if you lowered the mirror!"

The History of Hypnosis

The first reference to hypnosis was found in an Egyptian papyrus dating to 1000 B.C. In ancient Greece, there were "sleep temples" where patients with various ailments were cured by hypnotic techniques. The history of modern hypnosis, however, is generally thought to have begun in the late 1700s when an Austrian physician, Franz Anton Mesmer, began to practise the technique. It is from Mesmer that the term *mesmerize* was derived.

Mesmer believed that everyone has a magnetic polarity, which he called animal magnetism. He was also of the opinion that certain gifted individuals, such as himself, could exert their magnetism with great force. By passing his hands over a subject's body, he believed he could transmit his "animal magnetic fluid" into the body of the subject, thereby producing a trance.

For almost a century, this explanation prevailed, enjoying more prominence in some decades than in others. Then, around the middle of the nineteenth century, a British physician named James Braid contradicted Mesmer's explanation. Dr. Braid insisted that the passing of hands induction method only worked because subjects believed that it would. Braid's alternative explanation was that "the power of suggestion" was inducing the trance. He tried, successfully, to induce patients by using verbal suggestions and eye contact. It was he who coined the words *hypnotism* and *hypnosis* from the Greek word *hypnos*, which means "sleep."

Sigmund Freud tried hypnosis late in the nineteenth century and then abandoned it, saying that a deep trance was necessary in order for hypnosis to work at all. From that time until after World War II, the use of the technique waned. Then, in the mid-1950s, a British Medical Association committee studied hypnosis and recommended that physicians be given approval to use it. Today, in North America, very few medical schools actually offer courses in the use of hypnosis. But it has been estimated that between 20 and 50 thousand doctors, psychologists and dentists have taken hypnosis workshops and use the technique.

How Hypnosis Works

Heather Strong, a 45-year-old waitress, had been suffering from back pain off and on for 21 years when she tried hypnosis as a last resort. "Physicians couldn't find anything specifically wrong with my back — at least nothing that they seemed to be able to do anything about. There were times when I thought I'd go crazy." By this time, she had developed a dependency on pain-killers and was depressed about the restrictions her back pain was putting on her life. On several occasions, she had had to quit her job, and each time she applied for a new position she was terrified that a prospective employer would find out about her chronic back problem and refuse to hire her.

"I was skeptical about hypnosis at first," she says, "but after eight 90-minute sessions, my life began to change. I have actually learned how to alter the quality and severity of my pain . . . . At first, the pain itself didn't change. It was more a matter of being able to focus on it less. After several months, however, I did begin to get a sense that my back pain was actually diminishing. I believe that my anxiety about my pain had been increasing its intensity, and perhaps causing muscle spasm, for many years . . . . I've been hypnotizing myself for about 18 months now. I can get "under" in less than 20 seconds. I'd say that over the past six months I haven't taken more than a few aspirins for back pain. Hypnosis almost always works as well as pain-killing drugs."

Dr. Rickey Miller, a psychologist, runs a pain management course at the Toronto General Hospital where Heather Strong learned self-hypnosis. According to Dr. Miller, anyone can learn self-hypnosis, which she describes as "a natural state that we all experience at times, but just don't bother to label. We all tend to focus on one thing and screen out the rest when, for example, we drive a car or become totally engrossed in a good book. Almost everyone is capable of not noticing the annoying sounds around them," she says.

"What's different about hypnotherapy is its context. There is a therapist-guide and a subject, or patient. They work together to achieve a specific goal."

For Dr. Miller and her back pain patients, that goal is not to alleviate *all* back pain but rather, as Heather Strong describes it, to change the way in which patients perceive and respond to their pain. Dr. Miller tries to teach people to regard their back pain as "background noise," which they can screen out when they choose to. Once back pain is in the background, rather than in the foreground, they become free to participate in other activities. Participating in other activities will, in turn, take their minds off their back pain even more.

"If you can gain the power to determine what you are going to focus on, you can gain significant control over your life," says Dr. Miller.

A further benefit of hypnosis is that like massage or yoga, it can give people the opportunity to feel what it is like to be totally relaxed. "When they have chronic pain, people become chronically tense," says Dr. Miller. "This frequently leads to what is known as 'pain behaviour'. Unconscious hunching of the shoulders, or grimacing, are two common examples. The problem is that pain behaviour itself can cause chronic muscle contraction which, in turn, leads to more pain. When patients are in the relaxed hypnotic state, they can learn to recognize and give up pain behaviour. They can also learn to recognize what triggers them to begin the vicious circle."

Says Heather Strong: "Under hypnosis, I began to realize that when my lower back was hurting, I'd carry my tray around with my shoulder blades up around my ears. I didn't even realize that I was doing it. Now, I can take a short break and, using hypnosis, 'suggest' to myself that I relax my shoulders. The hunching almost always goes."

Pain behaviour can be verbal as well. Dr. Miller sometimes helps patients to recognize what she calls their cognitive approach to pain. While they are in a hypnotic state, she will ask them to describe their internal dialogue. Often, her patients discover that they have become used to adopting a pattern of negative thinking: "My back hurts; I might as well forget about getting anything done today."

"Instead of dwelling on the fact that your back hurts and your day is therefore ruined," says Dr. Miller, "you can learn to change your internal dialogue to something more positive: 'My back hurts more than usual today, so I think I'll go for a swim a little later on, or make an appointment for a massage. By tomorrow, I'll probably feel fine'."

Back pain can also become exacerbated through what Dr. Miller calls unconscious negative pain imagery. Through hypnosis, she says, patients can become aware of how they visualize their back pain. For example, an engineer in one of her courses kept imagining his back pain as a knife that was stabbing him in the back. Not surprisingly, this image made his back pain feel even worse. Under hypnosis, he was first able to become aware of the image and then change it. By switching to a more positive image – that of a strong massage – his perception of his back pain changed.

People with different personalities have different types of pain imagery. Dr. Alan Banack, a Toronto hypnotherapist, explains that a visually oriented person might "see" back pain as the colour red. Under hypnosis, that person can learn to imagine a calm wave of cool blue washing over the burning red. "Changing the image of pain from red to blue," he says, "can influence a person's perception of that pain. Blue tends to recede into the background while red tends to dominate."

With patients who are scientifically oriented, Dr. Banack has had success with another visual technique. Under hypnosis, he asks these people to imagine the nerves and the spinal cord as a sort of personal telephone switchboard. "Under hypnosis, these people learn to 'disconnect' the switchboard, cord by cord. Metaphorically, they are unplugging their pain."

How to Achieve the Hypnotic State

How is the hypnotic state reached? Most hypnotherapists ask their patients to either lie down, or sit, provided they can find a comfortable sitting position. Usually, the hypnotist will suggest that the patient is feeling very relaxed and drowsy. To get the eyelids to close spontaneously, the subject is asked to focus on an object. Then, the hypnotist will focus on another part of the subject's body, often the hands, and suggest that they feel as if they are floating. Most hypnotists try to find a "setting" that is particularly relaxing to the individual who is being hypnotized. A beach, where the sand is warm and the water can be heard lapping against a rock, might be perfect for one person but impossible for the next. Once she has helped the patient find a relaxing situation to fit his or her unique needs, Dr. Gitev usually makes a tape for the patient to take home and practise with.

A problem that plagues hypnotherapists is patients who have been told that the back pain they feel is not real. Like Heather Strong, many of these people try hypnosis as a last resort but without much hope of success. By the time they reach the hypnotherapist's office, they no longer really believe that any professional can help. "When someone's defences are up, it is usually impossible for them to relax enough for hypnosis to be successful," says Dr. Banack. "The first thing I do is reassure them that their back pain is real. Then I ask them to describe the pain in great detail. Often, people are able to take the first step toward controlling their back pain when a therapist finally takes them seriously."

As part of this process, Dr. Banack's patients are asked to rate their pain on a scale from one to ten. This allows them to mark an improvement, if and when an improvement comes. "Seeing even small amounts of progress can convey the message that they are gaining control," he says.

It is not realistic, however, for someone who suffers from chronic back pain to become dependent upon a hypnotherapist over the long term. For hypnosis to be effective, people must learn to hypnotize themselves. Dr. Jeva Lougheed, a former staff anaesthetist at Women's College Hospital in Toronto, currently practises hypnotherapy full time, focusing on self-hypnosis. "The main task of a hypnotherapist should be to teach patients how to induce themselves," she says.

"Once patients have learned to put themselves into a hypnotic state," says Dr. Lougheed, "they should be able to do it in five or ten seconds." She encourages people to induce themselves three times a day. "While it's true that some people are more suggestible than others, even the most suggestible patients won't benefit from hypnosis if they don't practise. At the same time, with perseverance, even the least suggestible person can learn."

If a patient turns out to be a "bad subject," the most likely reason is that the patient-therapist match isn't right. If you're an anxious person by nature, you may not feel comfortable working with a hypnotherapist whose manner is overly calm. A therapist whose predilection is toward sound imagery might not be the best match for a patient who feels more comfortable with visual imagery.

Many people who consider trying hypnosis are concerned about the guy in his boxer shorts who is clucking like a chicken. Will a person under hypnosis, especially someone who is particularly suggestible, do something weird?

"Definitely not," says Dr. Miller. "People won't do anything under hypnosis that they don't want to do, especially anything that is against their own personal code of ethics. I might also add that it is nonsense to believe that you can get stuck in a hypnotic state." Many hypnotherapists do bring their subjects out of the hypnotic state by counting backward from ten. But people will return to normal by themselves, especially if an emergency arises.

"When I'm at home in a hypnotic state," says Heather Strong, "I won't hear the phone ring when there are other people around to answer it. If, on the other hand, I'm home alone and waiting for an important call, I'll hear the phone on the first ring, come out of my hypnotic state and answer it."

The limits of hypnosis are far from known. But Dr. Victor Raush, a dental surgeon from Waterloo, Ontario, made medical history when he underwent abdominal surgery with hypnosis as the only anaesthetic. He hypnotized himself prior to surgery and joked with the medical personnel during the operation – to lessen *their* tension. He controlled not only the pain, but also his pulse and blood pressure.

Most people, of course, are neither interested nor capable of learning to accomplish such a feat. But the fact that it has been done does tend to make you wonder about the potential of this drugless technique. While it has been used for thousands of years, hypnosis for back pain is a relatively new technique. "As far as I am concerned," says Heather Strong, "it has given me a new lease on life."

Ontario is the only Canadian province that regulates hypnosis; to practise the technique, you must be a physician, a registered psychologist or a dentist. For more information, Ontario residents should contact The Ontario Society of Clinical Hypnosis, 200 St. Clair Avenue West, Toronto, M4V IRI. In British Columbia, contact the Canadian Hypnosis Society, B.C. Division, 100 – 3077 Granville Street, Vancouver, V6H 3J9. In Saskatchewan, contact the Saskatchewan Society of Clinical Hypnosis, 102 Medical Arts Building, Saskatoon, S7K 3H3. In other provinces, the provincial colleges of physicians and surgeons can provide more information on who practises hypnosis and their qualifications.

20

Massage: There's the Rub!

No one considers massage to be a miracle cure for back pain. But because it can alleviate, or at least decrease, back pain for a few hours, a few days and sometimes even longer, thousands of people seek out this centuries-old technique. Just the thought of a good massage can conjure up an image of being pain-free, of taking a holiday from stress.

Massage works to varying degrees for various people. But exactly why is difficult to say. No scientific studies on the treatment have been done. Information is available from two sources only: those who give massages and those who get them.

Christine Sutherland, director of education for the Sutherland-Chan School of Massage and Clinic in Toronto, gives them. Her rudimentary explanation is that massage helps contracted muscles to relax. In turn, relaxed muscles allow blood circulation to increase. Increased blood circulation eliminates toxic wastes, including lactic acid, from body tissues more rapidly. It *is* a scientific fact that contracted muscles produce lactic acid and that a build-up of lactic acid can produce pain.

Most massage therapists maintain that a chronically tight muscle sometimes requires a number of massages in order to relax permanently. The theory is not illogical. A muscle will go into spasm to protect an injured, or strained, area; the spasm acts like a natural splint, if you will. For one reason or another, however, the mechanism that should allow the spastic muscle to relax once the injury has healed does not respond. Sometimes, especially when back muscles are involved, a painful "protective splint" can remain in place for months, or even years, after an injury has healed. In addition, adhesions may have formed. (See page 39.) While one massage may alleviate both spasm and adhesions to some degree, the spasm will return with the slightest increase in stress, simply because being in spasm has become normal. A number of massages over a period of several weeks, however, will often help the spasm to relax completely, and stay relaxed.

Some professionals have a tendency to promote their own discipline to the detriment of all others. Massage therapists are a notable exception; almost all of them agree that their technique is most effective for back pain when it is combined with other treatments.

Kristi Magraw is a massage therapist who has been working in Toronto for more than a decade. She encourages her back pain patients to exercise and improve their posture while they use massage as a therapeutic technique. Her own preferences lean toward swimming, yoga and t'ai chi (an ancient Chinese martial art that is now used by some people as an exercise form) as types of exercise particularly suited for back pain. She also recommends the Alexander Technique for back pain associated with poor posture. "Body awareness is extremely important in the management of back pain," she stresses. "And that's exactly what most of the people I treat lack."

"Until last Christmas, I didn't know I had a back," says Dan Street, a 45-year-old journalist. Working with correspondents in far-flung corners of the world, usually in times of crisis, his job is a virtual inventory of stress. With no on-the-job outlet for his frustrations, Dan Street spends long hours hunched over the phone or typewriter. The fact that he stands over six feet, four inches tall is no bonus; tall people have a propensity toward back pain because they literally don't fit well into their environments. (Office chairs, for example, were not created for the very tall or very short. In addition, many tall people feel uncomfortable towering over their colleagues and acquire a tendency to slouch.)

Dan Street always felt that the way to release tension – and quell the occasional backache – was to exercise, the harder the better. That changed one wintery day when he was frantically shovelling snow and back pain (accompanied by sciatic pain in his right leg) struck with a vengeance. When a week later, the pain had not subsided, Street's doctor prescribed total bed rest. At the end of a three-week purgatory, he felt better, but was certainly not pain-free.

Dan Street credits massage – coupled with physiotherapy – for his improvement, which was gradual. From a physiotherapist, he learned that he had been doing exercises incorrectly, and that his posture, especially while sitting, couldn't have been worse. But exercise and good posture weren't enough. "The fact that I went to a massage therapist meant I needed something more," he says. "I can best describe it as emotional support for me as a person. Sure massage relieves kinks and aches, but just as important is the tremendous sense of physical well-being it imparts. It has taught me – unlike any other type of therapy – to be aware of how unnecessarily hard I am on my body, not only when I shovel snow, but most of the time."

Dan Street had never thought about the concept of relaxation as an honourable goal. "For many people with demanding jobs, nothing is more difficult than learning to relax," he explains. "Learning to recognize and *enjoy* the sensation of being relaxed is even more difficult. I used to feel that relaxing was tantamount to being unproductive, lazy even. I'd feel guilty about taking time off. In the beginning, I begrudged the time it took to have a massage. I'd race back to the office at lightning speed, and by the time I got there I'd feel just as bad as when I'd left. Then I'd feel guilty about having taken off time to go! Eventually, I learned that I had felt good for an hour — imagine, a whole hour! — and after a couple of months, I learned to prolong that feeling and recognize when I was beginning to lose it again. . . . I'm not saying that massage can cure back pain, or prevent it from ever fouling up my life again, but if I had known then what I know now, I would have started having massages a couple of times a month years ago."

The History of Massage

That certainly would have been possible; massage is anything but a modern discipline. As far back as 1200 B.C., Homer was writing about warriors who, upon returning from battle, "were rubbed and kneaded." Eight hundred years later, around 400 B.C., Hippocrates wrote that "the physician must be experienced in many things, but assuredly also in rubbing."

Little is known about massage during the Dark Ages. But by the fifteenth and sixteenth centuries, notable European medical writers were again describing its effects. During that period, the emphasis changed from kneading to heavy pressure. Early in the nineteenth century, Peter Ling, a Swedish gymnast, began to advocate yet another new variation: the combination of light stroking in one direction with deep pressure in another. The concept gained acceptance and Ling is credited as the originator of the Swedish massage, the method the majority of North American massage therapists use.

A smaller percentage of North American massage therapists practise a quite different type of massage. It is called shiatsu, and it originated in the Orient thousands of years ago. Like acupuncture, shiatsu is based on the concept of energy pathways called meridians, and its proponents are more concerned with organs than with muscles.

Ken Saito, director of Toronto's Shiatsu Dohjoh, explains the theory: "Some people wake up in the morning, put their hands on their kidneys and say 'Oh my aching back.' We apply pressure to certain specific points, rather than rubbing the whole area, and by doing so, we find out which meridians are blocked." According to those who practise shiatsu, a block can occur in an organ of the abdomen, for example, and still affect the back.

The Power of Touch

Whichever theory their technique is based upon, massage therapists generally agree on two aspects of massage. The first is that for massage to be successful, there should be some interaction between the client and the massage therapist. The second is that simply being touched by another person has nourishing, or healing, benefits.

Says Susan Lucas, another Toronto massage therapist, "It's a mistake for clients to think of themselves as totally passive. People lose some of the therapeutic benefits of massage if they cut themselves off and don't participate in the healing process."

Adds Kristi Magraw: "It's wonderfully relaxing to 'bliss out' now and then. But by doing so, you miss the chance to learn how stress in one part of your body can act upon another part and what it feels like when tension, or a muscle spasm, lets go. The ideal state to be in during a massage is known as the alpha state. It's a difficult concept to describe. You're both relaxed *and* alert. You observe your body and how it feels – but without trying to dissect or figure things out logically. The problem with being logical is that it distances you from an experience and you lose part of the sensation."

The concept of touch as an instrument of pain relief is becoming more commonly accepted. Studies have shown that cancer patients experience less pain when they are simply being touched by a member of their family or a close friend. According to Susan Lucas, "An exchange of energy is involved in the touching aspect of massage. It can help a person feel less alone and more connected to the world."

"Touch is the most powerful stimulus for relaxation," says Christine Sutherland. "That is why so many people open up to their hairdressers or facialists – people who are more often than not complete strangers. Touch is the unspoken language which can provide crucial emotional support for people who have to deal with chronic pain.

"Not having that kind of emotional support can increase a person's tension, and it is commonly accepted that increased tension can cause pain to feel worse. On the other hand, I have seen chronic pain subside to a significant degree when people fall in love and have physical affection and an outlet for caring."

Approximately one-quarter of the people who take massages at the Sutherland-Chan Clinic are referred by psychotherapists who believe that massage can help the emotional as well as the physiological healing process. Says Dan Street, "I wouldn't have been able to admit this when I first began taking massages, but there is a lot of truth to the aspect of its psychological benefits. Having chronic back pain for months on end is a total emotional drain. I resented that pain, and I believe I also resented the people I am closest to because there was no way they could share it. It was different, however, with my massage therapist. She was able to touch those knots and understand their relevance to my entire life. I realized, through this experience, that part of the debilitation of back pain is the loneliness you experience. Sharing it somehow helps to dissipate that isolation."

Kristi Magraw explains the emotional component of back pain and its application to massage in a logical way: "Back pain is often related to poor posture which, for many people, is connected to self-esteem. Our attitude toward ourselves is expressed through posture. Slouching, for example, is not caused by simple laziness. It's connected to one's self-image and the need to hide feelings such as anger or sadness."

Recently, Kristi Magraw worked with a 47-year-old woman, Anne Baker, who had extreme back pain. A chronic contraction of the iliopsoas muscles – the long muscles which run from the lower lumbar vertebrae to each knee – was thought to be at the root of her problem. "It was a postural habit that created the problem," says Kristi Magraw, explaining that because of the contraction, Anne Baker's lumbar lordotic curve was accentuated which, in turn, was putting strain on the facet joints of the lumbar spine. "Through massage we were able to reduce some of the chronic contraction and that relieved some of her pain. But it was also necessary for Anne to make some major postural changes. To do that, she had to do some stretching exercises, but she also had to change her attitude toward herself. During this difficult period, massage provided her with emotional support."

In Ontario and British Columbia, there are registered schools of massage which will provide names of registered therapists. In other provinces, contact the provincial Massage Therapists' Association for more information.

216

21

The Alexander Technique: Heads Up!

Try describing the colour red to someone who is colour-blind and you'll get an idea of how difficult it is to explain the Alexander Technique.

It's not a drug, or even a set of exercises. Rather, the creation of a turn-of-the-century Australian actor, F. Matthias Alexander, is a method of reorganizing, or *restructuring*, the posture. It is based on the premise that to have an efficient and healthy body – and a back that is pain-free – the head and neck must be properly balanced at the top of the spine.

According to those who support the Alexander Technique, this delicate balance is an easy-to-maintain posture, once you have learned it and integrated it into your life-style. Its benefit is that it allows muscle tension to be reduced to a minimum. When the posture is correct, say Alexander Technique proponents, a person will exert the smallest possible amount of strain on the muscles when standing, sitting or moving around. An analogy is a first class lever which, to move an object, requires less force, or strain, than either a second class lever or a third.

Young people tend to assume a balanced posture naturally say Alexander Technique teachers. But as they get older, especially if they lead sedentary lives, this balance frequently deteriorates. The entire physical system degenerates into a state which F. Matthias Alexander labelled *disorganization*. Had he been a chiropractor, he would probably have used the term *misaligned*.

Once he had coined the word, Alexander saw disorganized bodies everywhere he went. The most prevalent example was the person who stands with the chin jutting forward, the shoulders rounded, the chest caved in, and the stomach stuck out. When you visualize a person in a posture such as this, *disorganized* becomes not a bad choice of words. It is then also easy to accept Alexander's second premise: that maintaining such a posture requires an enormous amount of muscle strain, most of it redundant.

Most of us have somehow become conditioned to think that the human anatomy is more, rather than less, relaxed in a slouched posture. Proving to back pain sufferers that slouching actually puts *more* strain on the muscles became the battle cry of Alexander and his followers. Although it is not a well-known method for dealing with back pain, the Alexander Technique has withstood the test of time. Today, almost 100 years after

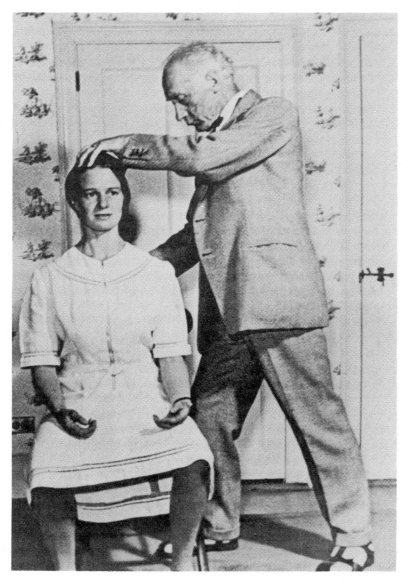

F. Matthias Alexander and patient.

the technique was developed, there is at least one Alexander Technique teacher in almost every major North American city. Almost all of these teachers have graduated from the three-year Alexander Technique diploma course of the London, England, Alexander Trust Fund School.

Describing the Alexander Technique

"So, when you learn the Alexander Technique, you learn to sit up straight?" asked Lorraine Wells, a 33-year-old high school teacher who was trying to decide if the technique could possibly help *her* constant battle with low back pain.

"Not exactly," her Alexander teacher told her. "It's rather more like allowing your back to lengthen."

"So you mean that I'd learn to stretch my back?" she asked.

"Well, not really. There is this principle of 'non-doing'."

"Oh, I see," she said slowly. "Deep breathing and relaxation exercises. . . ."

"Yes and no again," was what had to be explained.

Most people equate relaxing with slouching. If you tell them to relax more, they just slouch more. But when they learn the Alexander Technique, they gradually learn to sit tall, without becoming rigid. In that sense, they've learned to be relaxed. Eventually, sitting or standing in a stretched position becomes natural and relaxed. And at that point, *slouching* causes pain!

Alexander teachers are not proponents of 20-minutes-a-day back exercise programs or of the deep-breathing exercises taught in yoga. What good, they ask, are back exercises done for 20 minutes each day if you go back to slouching for the other 23 hours and 40 minutes? They pose the same question when it comes to breathing exercises. How much good can deep breathing exercises for 20 minutes a day do when a person forgets about good breathing habits the rest of the time?

The only way to "organize" the body, say Alexander Technique teachers, is to learn an almost entirely new way of using it. Once you've mastered this, however, you practise it *unconsciously* all the time. There's no need for an exercise program in the morning or a deep breathing session at night.

This difficult-to-put into-words notion that Alexander Technique teachers try to impart to their students over a period of several months, F. Matthias Alexander perfected slowly, over the course of a decade. He was a Shakespearean actor, working in Australia in the late 1890s, when his vocal cords suddenly seized up. Obviously, he reasoned, if his speechless situation were to remain unresolved, it would put a quick end to his budding career.

Alexander sought traditional treatment but nothing worked. Feeling he had no alternative, he retreated into self-analysis. Eventually, he concluded that the source of his problem was neither his larynx nor his lungs. It was due to the fact that he had been misusing his entire muscular system for years.

For the next nine years Alexander experimented on himself. He spent hours observing his posture in a mirror. In the end, he maintained that he cured himself. Some members of the medical profession argued that the return of Alexander's voice was due to "spontaneous regression." But the fact was that in the process of curing himself, he also worked out a technique that he believed could correct many of the general problems of the "psycho-physical" being. When he died in 1955, at the age of 86, Alexander was still teaching his personal students. Among the faithful were George Bernard Shaw, John Dewey and Aldous Huxley.

When Alexander opened his London school in the 1930s, many of the people who enrolled were actors and musicians. They believed that learning the Alexander Technique would improve their performances. Others were people with long-standing physical symptoms, the most common being back pain. The same types of people with the same sorts of problems consult Alexander Technique teachers today.

Brad Thomas is a composer and musician who divides his time between Montreal and New York. He became interested in the Alexander Technique for both reasons. Thomas chose M. Cohen-Nehemia, Toronto's longest-practising Alexander Technique teacher. Of the Toronto-based Alexander teachers, Nehemia Cohen, as he is known, sees the most people with back pain.

"For me, it was absolutely dramatic," Brad Thomas says. "My back pain was so bad that at times I could barely walk. I would feel better almost immediately after I had an Alexander session. After several weeks, I felt infinitely better."

Several months after he stopped taking Alexander Technique lessons, Brad Thomas found himself overworking once again and letting himself slip back to his former disorganized postural habits. His back pain returned.

"When my back pain is at its worst, I can hardly work. I started taking lessons again and it improved. Say what you want, that it's nothing but learning to relieve tension in the back muscles . . . the point is, I now know a way of relieving my pain, when I put my mind to it."

One of the things Thomas learned from studying the Alexander Technique is that his sedentary life-style was aggravating his back problem. He now frequently composes standing up, with one foot on a footrest. He finds that this posture puts less strain on his back than sitting. He has cut out calisthenics and jogging; instead, he swims and walks for exercise. He has changed his sleeping position (he used to sleep on his stomach) and fights a constant, though not always conscious, battle against slouching. Brad Thomas has become, in a word, *aware*.

Another Toronto Alexander teacher is Robert Rickover. His particular interest is in helping people become aware of *specific* stressful actions that they have picked up – and then helping them develop ways of changing these actions. Typists, for example, tend to sit in a fixed, or locked, position. This puts an enormous amount of strain on the muscles of the neck and upper back. First consciously – and later unconsciously so they're not constantly dwelling on the problem – Rickover has taught typists how to change their position every couple of minutes. "The change needn't be dramatic to be effective," says Rickover. "Even subtle postural changes can relieve tension in the many tiny muscle groups of the back."

How the Alexander Technique Works

But how does all this happen? What actually goes on during an Alexander Technique lesson? Most Alexander teachers begin their lessons by having their students sit in a chair and learn how to stand up properly. And, amazing as it might seem, the second thing most students learn to do is relax when they are lying down!

Most written accounts of the results of these two experiences leave readers frustrated. Of all the attempts to decribe a kinesthetic sensation to people who have never experienced it, only the one by Frank Pierce Jones, in *Body Awareness in Action*, seems to succeed.

Jones's Alexander teacher was, in fact, F. Matthias's brother A.R. Alexander, who was generally referred to by his initials alone. A.R., like most Alexander teachers, would begin each lesson by having Jones sit in a straight-backed chair. From a seated position, A.R. would guide Jones to a standing position. It all sounds ridiculously banal until Jones describes how A.R. made the exercise into an experience. By ensuring that Jones maintained the proper head-neck relationship during the entire motion, A.R. was able to show him how it feels to get up, sit down and remain seated without using more effort than is absolutely necessary.

Wrote Jones, "I [began to become] conscious of being moved by a set of reflexes whose operation I knew nothing about. The most striking aspect of the movement was the sensory effect of lightness it induced."

As he continued with his lessons, Jones began to notice what he couldn't believe he had been missing for years. How, he wondered, could he have been so oblivious to the amount of tension his sitting posture was exerting on the muscles of his back? Since injuring his back in an automobile accident, he had never been able to sit at a desk for very long without a lot of discomfort. He had always thought the problem was unsolvable until, through the Alexander Technique, he discovered that part of his discomfort was due to the fact that his sitting posture was so awkward.

Never having observed his posture before in a mirror he had had no idea that " . . . whenever I leaned forward to read or write, I displaced my head downwards and allowed my chest to collapse." This meant that he was placing the entire weight of his torso – some 80 pounds – on the discs of his lumbar spine.

Like most of us, Jones had always assumed that the only alternative to a collapsed type of posture while sitting is a ramrod straight position, which is the posture most people are taught at school. Whenever he tried this sitting position, however, Jones's discomfort increased. Through the Alexander Technique, Jones learned that there is an alternative – a straight, yet easy-going posture, which involves making small movements, almost constantly, that allow the muscles to alternately relax and contract. Says Robert Rickover, attempting to explain the theory: "The body is like a tree. Its branches, the arms, want to move constantly, want to sway, even when the body is stationary." Eventually, Jones learned how to work at his desk for hours without ever really being completely still and without discomfort.

The second posture which most Alexander teachers concentrate on is the supine position. The student reclines on a table and the teacher gently moves the head and the limbs. This experience releases tension but more importantly, it helps the student feel what it's like when the joints are moving efficiently.

James Laidlaw, who has been teaching the Alexander Technique in Toronto for several years, puts it this way: "*Gently* rotating a student's leg, for example, can give a person the experience of freedom in the hip joint. Most people don't know how to move freely. They throw themselves around. Their movements are uncoordinated and jarring. They use the maximum, rather than the minimum, amount of effort for even the smallest motion."

Most Alexander Technique students experience a feeling of lightness and tallness at first. Then, for some students, there is a period of discomfort, as they become aware of the fact that they have been keeping their muscles needlessly tense for years. Some students realize that they have been feeling discomfort for years but haven't been aware of it.

At first, most students experience a feeling of lightness only during the lesson. But after a few weeks, the light feeling begins to endure. The ultimate aim, as Robert Rickover explains it, is for a teacher to show a student how to recognize when tension is beginning to build up. Eventually, students should progress to the point of not needing a teacher.

Nevertheless, most Alexander Technique students take a couple of refresher lessons every couple of months. Like Brad Thomas, they have become so conditioned to their postural bad habits, that they need occasional guidance. Otherwise, they begin to drift back to their old, disorganized ways.

"The Alexander Technique is not a cure-all," James Laidlaw tries to emphasize. "But it can help people learn to use their bodies beneficially instead of harmfully."

In a pensive moment, Laidlaw tries to explain his version of why there are so many people with back problems in modern North American society. "The proper use of the body has become almost vestigial. It is withering away," he says. "This deterioration has a lot to do with the fact that we sit so much."

F. Matthias Alexander himself often lamented that one of the reasons most people could benefit from his technique was that, from an early age, they were confined at a desk in school without being taught how to sit properly and without many opportunities to take a break to release tension.

"If they had learned in school what it felt like to be relaxed," says Robert Rickover, "people prone to back pain would be able to sense the beginnings of it and connect that to how they were misusing the rest of their body. They could stop and realize, 'Oh, I'm tensing my shoulders; I don't *have* to do that'."

If you would like more information about the Alexander Technique or would like to inquire about teachers in your area, write to: Robert Rickover, Society of Teachers of the Alexander Technique, 190 St. George St., Toronto, Ontario, M5R 2N4.

22

Yoga: Tying It All Together

Mary Bernier of Halifax was advised by her doctor to try yoga for her back pain, which he felt was being exacerbated by stress and a lack of flexibility. As she pondered his suggestion, an image came to her mind. Her vision was of a 1960s-style, esoteric discipline characterized by mysticism, spaced-out passivity and 90-year-old gurus who could hold their breath for days. But when she actually signed up for hatha yoga — by far the most popular form of yoga practised in North America — Mary Bernier found to her surprise a class of quite normal-looking students from a variety of backgrounds; some of them, like her, were even middle-aged! Rather than the grit-your-teeth, military atmosphere of many of the exercise groups she had attended in the past, the ambience was pleasantly serene. Instead of panting and jumping, students were stretching slowly and their breathing was calm. More to the point, the yoga teacher was helping each student to correct a posture, breathe better, or hold a stretch longer at his or her own, individual rate.

Assuming specific postures and marrying them to proper breathing techniques is what hatha yoga, the physical variety, is all about. (Other types of yoga, such as raja, tantra, and jnana yoga, all tend to emphasize meditation, detachment and spiritual growth.) It has been used as a therapy for back pain for hundreds of years.

No one is exactly sure when yoga was first developed, but it is thought to have originated in India about 4,000 years ago. Observing how animals moved and stretched, sages and mystics used them as role models to develop a system of postures which they called *asanas*. When they realized that part of the naturalness of an animal's movement has to do with the fact that, unlike humans, they breathe without constraint, another essential component was added to the system. This is called *pranayama*, which means "breath control." The union of asana and pranayama is yoga.

"The literal meaning of yoga is 'union'," says Esther Myers, who teaches the discipline in Toronto. "It is the union," she goes on to explain, "between the self and the world, the mind and the body, the body and the breath."

According to yoga experts such as Esther Myers, everyone's body has a *natural* sense of unity. Problems begin largely because people slouch constantly and lose their unity. Back problems, they maintain, are often a result of poor postural habits, stress, and structural imbalances. These result from our modern sedentary society, a society in which people have become almost totally unaware of how they use their bodies. "I sometimes wonder if some people realize they have bodies at all," says Esther Myers.

Esther Myers believes that studying yoga can help people become aware, and then change, the way they perceive and use their bodies. Practising the yoga postures, or asanas, she explains, will automatically lead them to become aware of the strong and weak aspects of their bodies, as well as which areas are particularly tight. Learning even the simplest postures can teach people to recognize how they distribute their weight, how they use (or worse do *not* use) their spines, and what weak points they have a tendency to favour or compensate for.

Yoga proponents also believe that there is a direct connection between people's emotions and how they breathe. They maintain that feelings such as anger, hatred, fear and grief can cause *physical* as well as emotional tension. By adding pranayama to the postures, students can learn to assert some control over how their emotions affect their physical well-being. The result is a restoration of the body's natural state, a state yoga enthusiasts describe with words like *harmony* and *balance*.

In yoga, the spine is the central core of the body. "All the postural exercises that we do in yoga classes are focused on the spine," says Esther

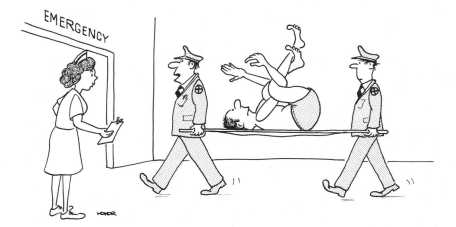

"His back pain has gone. He is in complete harmony with the world. But he's also in a reef knot!"

225

Myers. "We work toward toning the body, rather than making it muscle bound. But the greatest emphasis is on lengthening the spine and gently getting it realigned." Once the spine has become aligned, and they are aware enough to keep it that way, many people find that they can control a good deal of their back pain.

The term *aligned* is used frequently enough to be familiar to most people, but not everyone is able to describe an aligned body. Says Esther Myers, "If the body is aligned, a plumb line dropped from the shoulders will run through the hips and ankles in a straight, vertical line." The physiology is much the same as that which physiotherapists use but for yoga proponents the imagery changes. "The feet will be the base," says Esther Myers. "The pelvis will provide the foundation out of which the body will emerge. The balanced image is of a plant growing out of a pot."

Most people who treat back pain, yoga teachers included, agree that the most common misalignment is a sway-back: normal lumbar lordosis is accentuated, placing an abnormal amount of stress on the facet joints of the lumbar spine.

The second most common misalignment is a head that tilts back; you see people who stand with their chins jutting out. If your head is tilted back, you have a 12- to 15-pound weight to hold up. It has to be counterbalanced by something and that "something" is bound to be muscle tension in the upper back.

"From the way most people with chronic back pain move," says Esther Myers, "you'd think their lower vertebrae were functionally fused to the pelvis. When they move, these people scarcely rotate the pelvis at all. Yoga can help people to free their spines from all these 'burdens'."

To the people who study with Esther Myers, these concepts are crystal clear. To the uninitiated, however, the concept of "unloading burdens" may seem metaphysical. Wendy Cole, who teaches at the Toronto Yoga Centre, uses more literal terms to explain the usefulness of yoga for people who have back problems. "Yoga makes sense for people with back problems," she says, "because of its emphasis on stretching, body awareness and doing it all at your own speed." In yoga classes, students warm up and then begin by stretching out the back and the neck area. Before every posture, there is some preparation in the way of stretching.

The one aspect of yoga that Wendy Cole continually emphasizes is its non-competitive aspect. "You work with your eyes closed," she explains. "You're not concerned with how well the person next to you is doing. You work around your own limitations and your own needs. While you should always tell a yoga teacher, or any other teacher, as much about a specific physical problem as you can, a physical problem such as a back ailment will become apparent almost immediately, simply from the way you move.

An experienced yoga teacher can tell you how to compensate for a particular problem by using a pillow, or altering a posture slightly, until the problem is resolved."

Mary Bernier's experience illustrates what Wendy Cole and Esther Myers have to say. "It was particularly interesting that my doctor had a *general* impression that stress and lack of flexibility were at the root of my back pain. My yoga teacher, however, was able to translate this generalization into specifics by watching how I performed certain postures. For instance, I'd do a pose – at least I'd think I'd be doing it – and my teacher would point out that instead of being balanced above my pelvis, my entire upper torso was twisted to the left. It was as if my pelvis had been inflexible for so long that it had *forgotten* how to rotate."

After a few months of doing gentle exercises that were designed to very slowly increase her range of movement, Mary Bernier began to be able to do the simple postures correctly. At the same time, her back problem began to improve. "I believe," she says, "that this worked far better than if someone had just said to me, 'Look, your pelvis is rigid; do this and that exercise and you'll become more flexible.' Practising with the positive goal of improving an asana rather than focusing on the fact that something is wrong with your back is somehow less intimidating and far less demoralizing. Knowing that all serious yoga students practise for years also gives me the mental and emotional strength to be patient."

When it comes to exercising for back pain, the conventional wisdom has been changing. Just a decade ago, the main goal was to strengthen the abdominal muscles by doing sit-ups. Today, flexibility exercises are considered just as important as those designed to strengthen the back. Ironically, many of the exercises that used to be common only in yoga classes have found their way into traditional exercise programs. In addition, the yoga tenet of doing exercises slowly rather than at neckbreaking speed has also been finding its way into conventional environments.

Says Esther Myers, "Sit-ups work to strengthen the abdominals, and they can certainly help alleviate back pain by allowing a person to compensate for weakness in one area with extra strength in another. But sit-ups do not help a person correct the problem of rigidity, which frequently lies at the root of back pain. Sit-ups also have a compressing, as opposed to a lengthening, action. If they are done in isolation, without corresponding stretching exercises, they can further tighten an already rigid lower back."

Do people who have a tendency to be rigid also tend to develop more back problems? Or do people first develop back pain and *then* acquire the tendency to tense up? Different professionals have different opinions about this issue, but few disagree with Wendy Cole who believes that once they have acquired a chronic back problem, most people commonly inhibit their movements. "Most people with a back problem think they should move as little as possible," she says.

"Restricting your movement makes sense when you are in such an acute phase of a back episode that the slightest motion makes you wince. But otherwise," she says, "not moving only causes your body to stiffen up more.

"If you have a propensity toward back pain," she says, "you should pay particular attention to retaining as much flexibility as possible during the periods when you are pain-free or have only minimal pain. And besides being healthy," she adds, "being able to move easily and freely is such a joy."

Rochelle Brightman, a 36-year-old library sciences professor, learned that lesson five years ago. She had taken yoga classes on and off, until she noticed that it was during her "off" times that back pain would strike. One day, while she was getting out of her car, back pain hit her so hard and so suddenly that, to her companion's amazement, she spent the next ten minutes lying on the sidewalk. The next day, recalling some of the most gentle yoga stretches, she tried lying on her back and moving her pelvis and legs. Breathing slowly, she worked herself up to some mild versions of several simple postures. Since that time, yoga has never been absent from her life for more than three days and totally debilitating back pain has never returned. "I just can't afford not to do it," she says, adding that having a fluid body makes her life richer. "I'm glad now that I *must* remain flexible."

Like the teachers of many of the holistic disciplines, yoga teachers call the lesson that Rochelle Brightman learned so painfully body awareness. Once you learn how to isolate parts of your body and feel how each part moves, you'll be better able to control and protect specific vulnerable parts. Part of this awareness is knowing when to challenge yourself, how much to challenge yourself, and when to let up. "Back pain," says Esther Myers, "is a warning that must be respected, a flashing red light which tells you that something has gone wrong."

Among yoga proponents back pain is considered different, for example, than the pain students often feel in a leg when they first begin a stretch. With a leg stretch, the pain is the first indication that the muscle is starting to lengthen; it is a reflection of how much tension is in that muscle, and if you stay just at the edge of pain, concentrating on your breathing, the tension will ease gradually and your range of movement will increase. You should not, however, attempt to continue stretching a painful back with the goal of easing muscle tension.

One of the side effects of yoga is heightened emotional awareness. To Esther Myers this isn't surprising. "When you withhold your emotions, you tighten your muscles and restrict your breathing. When those muscles relax and your breathing becomes more natural, it will follow that your emotions will be able to flow out."

Esther Myers uses as an example a 50-year-old homemaker with chronic back pain who studied with her for several years. Her striking physical improvement carried with it emotional changes. "She had a new sense of standing tall that was transmitted to her feelings about herself as a person. She went out and got a job, and became more assertive. She still has trouble coping with being a person who asks for things — that she sees as aggressive behaviour. But now there's at least a choice; she doesn't have to be a shrinking violet all the time."

One of the greatest benefits of yoga is that unlike many disciplines, age is no barrier. You can study yoga all your life, and start it at any age with the expectation of improvement. To benefit, a yoga student needn't subscribe to any of the various life-style philosophies that devotees tend to pick up. The challenge is inherent in the *process* of learning asana and pranayama. Whatever suits you is an acceptable goal.

Yoga classes are generally offered at Y's and health clubs, as well as at yoga schools. Some courses are listed in the telephone directory. If they are not listed, look for notices on health food store bulletin boards.

23

Feldenkrais Method: The Israeli Connection

Try this experiment. Look straight ahead, noting the spot where your eyes make contact with the wall in front of you. Turn your head 45 degrees to the right and pick a spot on the part of the wall you are facing now. Good. Now look straight ahead again. Turn your head toward the spot to the right once more, but this time leave your eyes where they were, focused on the wall straight ahead. To most people, moving the head without moving the eyes feels slightly awkward, or at least unusual.

Now try this movement. From a starting point of looking straight ahead, move your eyes to the right but your head to the left. For most people, at least on the first try, this second combination of movements is virtually impossible to perform.

Now try another, much simpler experiment. Clasp your hands together in your lap and notice which thumb is on top. Now clasp your hands again, but this time reverse your thumbs, so that if your right thumb was on top of your left thumb the first time, you are now positioning them the other way around. To almost everyone, clasping the hands the opposite way seems strange. Something about it feels awkward or wrong.

That it feels odd to do something as simple as placing a right thumb on top of a left thumb instead of the other way around is in itself strange. After all, half the world does it one way and half does it the other; why shouldn't we be able to reverse the way we perform this simple motion at will without feeling odd? And the second experiment – moving the eyes one way and the head the other – certainly it's not the way we are used to moving. Nevertheless, at least in theory, performing this eye-head motion seems like it ought to be a fairly simple task to co-ordinate. How could it possibly be so hard?

According to Moshe Feldenkrais, the Russian-born Israeli physicist who developed the Feldenkrais Method of Movement more than 40 years ago, there is an explanation. The awkwardness in doing frequently performed movements a different way, he maintains, stems from the fact that at a young age, humans develop precise patterns of movement that become habits. These habituated patterns, he says, are actually registered in the motor cortex, the area of the brain that controls how we move.

For each pattern of movement – everything from clasping the hands, standing up, sitting down or rolling over in bed – there is a mini-computer program that is kept in a "file" in the brain. Each time you instruct your brain to turn your head to the right, clasp your hands, stand up, sit down, roll over or whatever, a message is transmitted via the nervous system to the brain. The brain goes to its file, calls up the appropriate program and dials it into the computer. The computer sends the message back to the muscles that are responsible for that particular motion, and you make the move, the same way each time. Unless you make an effort to do it differently – and sometimes even when you do – you will always perform a particular movement the same way. Each person, however, is unique. The combination of muscles *you* use when you stand up from your office chair, and particularly the way in which you use them, may not be the same combination of muscles that the person sitting next to you will use to do precisely the same thing.

Performing a movement the same way each and every time would be just fine – if we did it in a way that was good for us. The trouble is, say Moshe Feldenkrais and his proponents, most of us are merciless on our bodies when it comes to moving. Instead of moving gracefully and efficiently, in a way that puts the least amount of strain on our joints and muscles, we tend to throw ourselves around. Rather than being aware that there is more than one way of getting from Point A to Point B and picking the one which takes the design – that is, the physics – of the human body into account, most of us *add* to our burden. When we stand up from our chairs, for example, most of us don't simply move our legs. We arch our backs, putting far more strain than is necessary on the facet joints of the lumbar spine. When we roll over in bed, most of us not only move our torsos, but also crane our necks forward – night after night, year after year. Spend a few hours on a street corner watching people walk by, and you'll quickly realize how many people keep their backs stiff and knees virtually locked. You'll also begin to wonder how our bodies manage to last as long as they do and why most people are not always in pain.

Bruce Holmes, a runner and writer who also teaches the Feldenkrais Method in Illinois, blames our education – or at least the lack of it – for the fact that so few of us are graceful and efficient when we move. "We have all watched the process [of learning to move] in infants," he explains in a 1984 article for *Yoga Journal*. "A child stands, wobbles slightly, finds its balance and then takes a few tentative steps. But just as a smile of triumph erupts, a foot catches on the carpet and the child falls. Then one day the child does not fall, and this is called success. If you think about it for a second, that is just about the only criterion we do have for successful movement. We were not taught to move intelligently. We simply arrived, through a system of trial and error, at a pattern that would keep us from falling on our faces."

The Feldenkrais Movement Sequences

By the time he died in the fall of 1984 at the age of 80, Moshe Feldenkrais had spent 40 years perfecting the Feldenkrais Method of efficient movement. He divided his teachings into two parts. For one part, which is in the form of classes called "Awareness Through Movement," Feldenkrais created thousands of different movement sequences, some of which are similar to the ones already described. The other part, which people who are either permanently disabled or in a phase of acute pain can benefit from more easily, is in the form of private, hands-on sessions called "Functional Integration." During a 45-minute Functional Integration session, the person who is being treated lies on a table and the Feldenkrais practitioner *guides* the body through specific movements in order to teach it new and better habits. In some ways, the technique is not dissimilar to the one Alexander Technique teachers use to illustrate body awareness principles to their students.

To the uninitiated, the Feldenkrais movements – whether performed *by* the patient himself or *on* him by the Feldenkrais practitioner – often appear so simple that it's difficult to believe they could possibly lessen someone's pain. But to those who practise the technique, many of whom suffer from back pain, the Feldenkrais Method makes infinitely good sense. Delicate and inconsequential though the Feldenkrais movement sequences may seem when they are described, actually doing them – or having them done to you – achieves a number of different ends.

Some of the sequences can help you become aware of the inefficient movement "programs" you have on file in your brain. Others, such as moving the eye and head in opposite directions, can help you to break bad habits, to "clear the screen" so that alternative, efficient methods of movement can be programmed in. Still others actually illustrate alternative ways of moving which put less stress on muscles and joints.

Most of the Feldenkrais movements are done while lying on the floor to eliminate the effects of gravity. You don't tell yourself to stop tensing; you simply learn to move in ways that make it impossible for tension to develop. Gently rolling up from the floor into a sitting position, or rocking back and forth on a specific part of the hips, may not seem significant, but when these new *functional* ways of moving become habits, chronic muscle strain will dissipate. The result, say many Feldenkrais students, is an increase in flexibility, a feeling of freedom and joy when moving, and a decrease in pain. As one student marvelled, "I never knew that inside this awkward klutz for whom moving could be such a pain was a graceful person just dying to get out."

Marion Harris is a Toronto Feldenkrais practitioner who learned her craft from Moshe Feldenkrais himself. She agrees with others who say that it is far easier to experience the effects of the Feldenkrais Method than to have them explained. But the way she describes how the Feldenkrais Method affects people's physiology makes sense. "When you move in a balanced and aligned way," she says, "the weight of your body is distributed throughout the entire skeleton." This means that no one part of the body will be over-exerted. The smallest muscles – one thinks of the hundreds of pairs of tiny back muscles – will not be burdened with

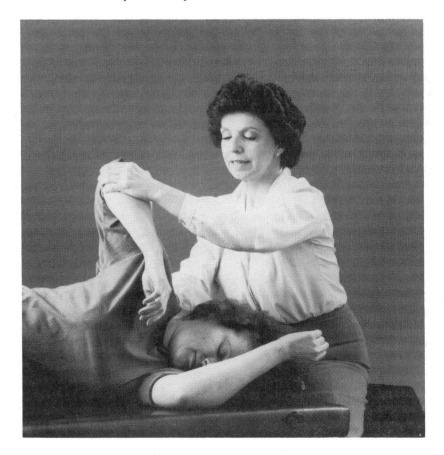

Marion Harris and a patient during a functional integration session

more than they can handle. The larger muscles, on the other hand, will carry more of the body's weight. "The body," she says, "should operate at maximum efficiency."

When she describes the Feldenkrais Method, Marion Harris stresses that each person is unique. According to this discipline, there are no rigid rules, for example, about good posture. Teachers emphasize individual fine-tuning, positions that feel right for you. "Good posture," wrote Moshe Feldenkrais, sounding a lot like F. Matthias Alexander, "is actually dynamic, with the body frame constantly readjusting itself rather than being held in a fixed and rigid way." It is better to sit erect, he used to say, but the main advantage of sitting erect over slouching is simply that it's easier to be dynamic – to make these tiny adjustments – when you are upright than when you are hunched over.

Feldenkrais teachers like Marion Harris believe that even if you've been misusing your body for many years, relearning can still take place. Sometimes changes will occur almost immediately. At other times, they will happen slowly over time. So smart is the brain, wrote Feldenkrais himself, that even after doing something the wrong way a million times, doing it right even one time feels so good that the brain recognizes this immediately as right. "The body has miraculous regenerative powers," says Marion Harris. "When you give it a new alternative that's better than the old one, it takes it."

Don Himes is another Toronto Feldenkrais teacher. "The more you do the movements," he says, "the more you reinforce good habits." Bruce Holmes agrees. In his opinion, changes can occur after doing an exercise once – but they don't always last because partial change just isn't enough. "If you change only a small segment of how you function and leave the rest as it has always been, the remaining pattern will recondition the old behaviour," he explains. "The body," he reminds us, "is an interrelated system."

Sometimes students of the Feldenkrais Method say that while they are aware that changes have taken place, they don't know how, or when, they have happened. Says Don Himes, "The way [the Feldenkrais Method works to produce change] is indirect. People don't always know consciously what their body has learned. But through tiny movements, we re-educate the nervous system." When these movements are done correctly, he says, muscles that have been chronically tight due to over-exertion learn to let go.

For several days before an important business trip, Jane Himmel, a 38-year-old travel agent, spent long hours at her desk, preparing her reports. When it came time to pack, she found that she couldn't walk without pain and when she began to feel that familiar old sciatica shooting down her right thigh, her first reaction was that she'd have to cancel the trip. "I couldn't believe I'd done it again," she said, explaining that she'd had enough years of back pain to know better than to sit hunched over files for 12 hours a day. "I'd been taking Feldenkrais classes for about a month at that point. My teacher had warned me to move around for a minute or two every half hour to prevent my back pain from appearing. 'Walk around the room and think about what your next sentence will be,' she told me. 'It's not a waste of time. You'll find your work will get done faster.' But I didn't listen and once again I was in a mess.

"At first I tried doing some stretching exercises, thinking I could work out the muscle spasm and stress that way. But even the easiest ones just made me feel worse." Then she tried the Feldenkrais approach. "I tried to imagine that my body was in a knot that I'd have to patiently untie," she explained. Lying on the floor on her back with her knees pulled up to her chest, one hand on each knee, she tried some of the gentle circular movements she'd learned in a Feldenkrais class. Noticing the tension in her shoulders, she performed some of the delicate Feldenkrais head and shoulder movements designed to release some of the stress. "I had the sense that everything was connected," she says, "and that by working out one area, the rest of my body would benefit. When I got on the plane the next day, I wouldn't say I was pain-free. But I was at least able to go. Probably the person sitting next to me in the plane thought I was a bit weird when I kept shifting around. But I got through it. During my four days in Montreal, I kept offering to get people coffee. Perhaps they thought I was being polite. In fact, it was an excuse to keep moving around."

The Man Himself

Those who knew Moshe Feldenkrais say that had he been in need of a walk during a meeting, he would have taken one and to hell with anyone who thought he was acting out of place. He has been labelled both feisty and irrascible. Says Marion Harris, "You loved him, you hated him. He was outrageous and compassionate."

Born in Russia, Feldenkrais fled the Revolution, arriving in newly created Palestine on his own at the age of 14. In 1928 he went to Paris where he founded Europe's first judo club. At the same time, he attended the Sorbonne University, earning degrees in mechanical and electrical engineering as well as a doctorate in applied physics. Then, in 1940, Hitler's army arrived in the French capital and Feldenkrais fled to Britain where he worked as a weapons scientist for the British admiralty.

Toward the end of the war, he began to have trouble with his knee, a flare-up from an old injury he had sustained while playing soccer as a youth. Reluctant to undergo knee surgery, which is what his orthopaedic surgeon recommended, he began instead to think about body mechanics.

With a physicist's orientation, he read everything he could find in German, Russian, French, English and Hebrew on the structure and function of the nervous system and anatomy. Combining the practicality of his engineering background with the creative approach of the physicist, he went on to explore the relationship between human development, education and movement. Eventually he developed a set of therapeutic movements, which were designed to teach his brain how to use his "bad" knee painlessly. This was the beginning of the Feldenkrais Method.

In the late 1940s, he published his first book, *Body and Mature Behaviour*. Several years later, he returned to Israel to practise and teach. Some of his early admirers included violinist Yehudi Menuhin, director Peter Brook, anthropologist Margaret Mead and Israel's first prime minister David Ben-Gurion. Feldenkrais treated Ben-Gurion daily for back pain for 17 years.

It took almost 20 years, however, before researchers in North America began to take notice of the Feldenkrais Method. But by the mid-1960s, Feldenkrais was being asked to lecture regularly at California's Esalen Institute, and noted Stanford University neuropsychology researcher Dr. Karl Pribram was studying the Feldenkrais Method's effects. Dr. Pribram concluded that Feldenkrais is not "just moving muscles around. He is actually changing the ways things are organized in the brain, and the results are better movement."

The Medical Establishment's Reaction

The medical establishment, however, has been skeptical about Feldenkrais's theories. To date only one hospital in the world, the Ottawa General, has a Feldenkrais practitioner on staff. (Several American hospitals invite Feldenkrais practitioners to teach part time.)

The Ottawa General's Feldenkrais program was started by physiotherapist Nancy Parker, who took her first weekend workshop with Moshe Feldenkrais in Toronto, in 1979, and was smitten by the technique. "It didn't make much sense to me at first," she says. "Like all physiotherapists I had been taught to encourage people to work a little harder and try a little more, and there was this man Moshe Feldenkrais urging us to do a little less. And yet there I was, wondering how it could be that for the first time in my life I was able to touch my foot to my head!" The next year, Nancy Parker enrolled in the first part of the Feldenkrais program, which is taught over four years, for nine weeks each year.

Several years later, Nancy Parker suggested that the Feldenkrais Method be incorporated into the physiotherapy department at the Ottawa General. At first, the hospital executives were reluctant. Then, the head of the physiotherapy department, a woman who suffers from multiple sclerosis, found that the Functional Integration treatments which Nancy Parker was giving her were providing relief, and Parker was given the opportunity to begin a Feldenkrais trial. "We began in April '84," she says, "and so far, although I get few referrals from doctors, word of mouth recommendations have filled my appointment book."

Nancy Parker admits that explaining the Feldenkrais Method to physicians is difficult. "It's hard for them to understand what it's all about because they don't think in terms of total body function," she explains. As one neurologist told her, "I can't understand what it's all about but it does seem to help."

It may not be long, however, before the medical profession finds a way of explaining the Feldenkrais Method in scientific terms. Only a decade ago, many physicians were calling acupuncture "a load of hokus pokus with no scientific basis." But now, since it was discovered that acupuncture needles stimulate the brain to produce pain-killing chemicals called endorphins and enkephalins, few doctors brush the technique aside. By the same token, many neuroanatomists now believe that damaged nerves can sometimes be reawakened by sensory input. Says Nancy Parker, "Moshe used to say that 90 per cent of the brains of so-called normal people are unused, partly because some parts inhibit others. You can retrain the nervous system and you can see the results."

The theory is not dissimilar to the now accepted belief that if one part of the brain is damaged, another part can sometimes take over a particular task. Nancy Parker translates that notion into functional terms, using disc degeneration as the example: "I've got degenerated discs in my lumbar spine. But that means only that I must be particularly aware of dividing my body's load among all the vertebrae. It doesn't mean the body can't work properly."

In a pensive moment, the English-trained physiotherapist tries to put the Feldenkrais Method – its past and its future – into perspective. "I trained at St. Thomas's Hospital in London, England," she says. "I worked with Dr. James Cyriax, the orthopaedic physician. You know, 35 years ago, when you trained at St. Thomas's, you'd apply for a job and they'd say to you, 'Okay, but you're not going to do any of that Cyriax stuff around here.' Now they line up to learn his techniques; not only physiotherapists, but doctors as well.

"People start using a technique and they expand upon it and it becomes blended into the other things that they do." That happened with Cyriax, she goes on to explain. Many physios now use some of Dr. Cyriax's basic principles, but not everyone labels it orthopaedic medicine. "The same thing," she says, " will likely happen with the Feldenkrais Method of Movement. People will start incorporating Moshe's theories on movement into their work, but not everyone will call themselves Feldenkrais practitioners.

"Our systems are geared toward homeostasis, toward being balanced,"

237

she says. "If you can show someone a better way of moving that is also pleasurable, that they can learn in total comfort, they'll do it. You won't do very well if you want to teach someone who knows nothing about mathematics how to add two and two and you stand there screaming at them to count faster or try harder. But if you put down four little sticks — two here and two there — and gently show them how to add them up, they'll grasp it. And they'll retain it. I just don't see how the Feldenkrais Method can be a passing fad," she adds. "It's just too intelligent."

Okay, one more experiment. Look straight ahead and find a focal point on the wall. Now turn your head to the right as far as it will go with total comfort, noting the focal point on the wall. Look straight ahead again but this time turn your head to the right while moving your eyes to the left. Gently. Now repeat this simple Feldenkrais movement 20 times. Slowly. Good. Now turn your head to the right again as far as it will comfortably go and note the new focal point on the wall. Almost everyone who practises this exercise finds that they have increased the range of their movement by 15 or 20 per cent. Effortlessly and painlessly. It's the mystery of Moshe.

To find out more about the Feldenkrais Method and those who practise in Canada write: Feldenkrais Teachers, 1867 Yonge Street, Suite 600, Toronto, Ontario, M4S 1Y5 or call (416) 626-5465.

To obtain an international directory of Feldenkrais practitioners or the names of books written on the technique write: The Feldenkrais Guild, P.O. Box 11145, Main Office, San Francisco, California, 94101 or call (415) 550-8708.

V

Advice for Special Situations

24

Sports: Good or Bad for Your Back?

If you suffer from chronic back pain, there is always some element of risk associated with participating in sports activities. Obviously, some sports (particularly those that involve body contact or movement at high speeds) are riskier than others. But excluding traumatic injuries, caused by falls or collisions, there are really only three main reasons why people who suffer from chronic back pain get themselves into trouble.

First, and probably foremost, is the fact that most people are unaware of the importance of warming up and stretching before playing, and then stretching again and cooling off after playing.

Secondly, too many people fail to take their level of proficiency and general physical condition into account when competing.

Thirdly, most people simply don't understand how to recognize and compensate for the potential pitfalls of a particular sport vis-à-vis back pain. Unfortunately, many people with chronic back pain avoid sports completely when all three problem areas could be solved.

Warming Up and Cooling Down

The logic behind warming up before playing a sport is simple. When you warm up, you prepare your body for the increased stress it is about to endure. When the heart rate increases, circulation increases proportionately and the muscles can react more quickly without being strained. Slow jogging, easy cycling or easy skipping for five minutes are all excellent warm-up activities, although you can also warm up "passively" by taking a hot shower, a sauna, or whirlpool bath. It is important to remember that a warm-up should be gradual; at the end of it, you should be perspiring slightly.

Once you have warmed up, you are ready to begin stretching. This is logical because only warm muscles are able to lengthen to the limit of their range without strain. It is amazing how many people think that the proper way to prepare for a game of tennis, squash, or a day of skiing is to do stretching exercises *before* warming up. If, in addition, you suffer from chronic back pain, stretching your hamstring and low back muscles while they are cold is probably more harmful than if you didn't bother to stretch them at all.

Which muscles you concentrate on stretching depends upon the sport you are about to do. It would be difficult to compile a comprehensive list of all the muscles it is possible to stretch, but basically the parts of the body being stressed while you play a sport should be stretched beforehand. For example, if you are going to play a racquet sport, the shoulders, arms and legs should be stretched as well as the lower back. If you don't stretch the extremities, you run the risk of straining them, and when they are strained, the most common way of compensating is to put additional stress on the back.

It is as important to cool down when you have finished playing a sport as it is to warm up beforehand. The idea is to return the body gradually to its normal resting state. It may not be as obvious, but changing suddenly from a high rate of activity to a low rate of activity is just as jarring to the circulatory system as serving a tennis ball without warming up is to the musculoskeletal system.

Stretching *after* participating in sports is neglected most of all. When muscles contract during strenuous exercise, the blood supply to them decreases to an abnormal level. As well, there is frequently a build-up of lactic acid, which can cause muscular pain if it is not given a chance to dissipate. When you stretch the muscles that have become contracted by strenuous activity back to normal, the blood supply to them increases and waste products (including lactic acid) can be carried away.

Some tips on stretching. Some people tend to bounce in order to expand their range of movement, but bouncing strains the muscles. Stretching exercises – both before and after a sport – should always be done slowly. You should feel a sensation of pulling but no pain. Most experts advocate that you hold a stretch for 20 to 60 seconds while breathing in order to get the maximum benefit. For specific stretching exercises, see page 162.

Understanding "Murphy's Law of Competition"

The law is very simple. If you are highly competitive, you are much more likely to sustain an injury or exacerbate your chronic back problem than if you play a sport for fun. The moves that probably precipitate the most number of disasters are those made to retrieve an opponent's well-placed ball when it is clearly beyond your normal range of motion. (Most experts also feel that the expenditure of energy through heroic saves is not worthwhile; you would be far better off conceding those points – half of which you lose anyway – and doling out your reserves consistently.) The next most common competitive fault is playing when physically or mentally fatigued. In particular, "weekend" athletes who overdo it to prove an egotistical point probably sustain more injuries and unnecessary exacerbation of chronic back pain than any other type of athlete.

Knowing the Potential Pitfalls of Particular Sports

Understanding the potential pitfalls of each sport and how to compensate for them is not as difficult as it may appear. Basically, there are four types of movements or postures that can exacerbate a back problem. Ironically, they are all performed routinely as we go through our daily activities; they cause problems only when they are performed either in excess of the body's normal range of motion, or repetitively.

These four movements or postures are: flexion or forward bending; extension or arching; rotation or twisting; and lifting, which may or may not include throwing.

FLEXION • Have a look at Dr. Nachemson's chart on page 42. Of the standing postures, standing hunched over is half again as stressful on the discs of the lumbar spine as standing upright. Standing hunched over while holding a weight is more than twice as stressful on these discs. (A comprehensive explanation of *why* these postures are so tough on the discs can be found on page 42.)

It stands to reason that if you have a disc problem, you should try to avoid excessive flexion whenever possible.

For example, if you play tennis, or any other sport that involves a ball, how many times in the course of an hour do you have the choice of either bending your back or bending your knees to pick up the ball? What most people don't realize is that the effects of forward bending are cumulative; it makes sense to most people that bending over 30 times to touch the toes will exacerbate a disc problem, but it frequently doesn't register that doing the same thing sporadically during a set of tennis will accomplish the same negative end. Another example: Take a look at a bench full of players waiting their turn to go up to bat or onto the ice. My estimate is that at least 80 per cent of them will be sitting in a position of sustained flexion. The irony of it is that they are causing more stress to their backs while waiting to play than while playing. References to flexion are also made in the section on specific sports which follows.

EXTENSION • Any activity that involves excessive extension movements will stress the facet joints of the lower back. (For an extensive explanation as to why, see page 45.) As with flexion, the effects of excessive extension can be cumulative. But while it makes sense to most people that standing in a posture of hyperextension for eight hours can exacerbate a worn facet joint problem – for example, the saleswoman who wears high heels – most people don't make the connection that *repetitive* strain can be as deadly as *prolonged* strain. For example, the serve in tennis involves repetitive hyperextension and the higher you throw the ball, the more dramatic that hyperextended posture will be. Gymnastics obviously involves a tremendous amount of hyperextension, both repetitive and prolonged.

ROTATION • The facet joints of the neck were designed to rotate, while the joints of the lower back were not. This is why it is so much less painful to turn the neck 90 degrees than it is to have a pile of 200-pound football players cause the lumbar spine to rotate the same amount! With certain sports, however, it is impossible to eliminate rotational movements to the lower back completely. However, it is frequently possible to alter your technique so that rotational movements can be reduced to a minimum. The section on specific sports gives suggestions on how to accomplish this.

LIFTING (WITH OR WITHOUT THROWING) • The rules for proper lifting techniques are described in greater detail on page 185. Basically there are four:
   1. Keep the object you are lifting as close to the body as possible.
   2. Bend your knees and use the thigh muscles to bear as much of the weight as possible.
   3. Keep the lower back in a pelvic tilt position (see page 167) and lean forward slightly for balance.
   4. If it is necessary to turn, step with the feet rather than twisting at the waist.
   Unfortunately, it is not always possible to follow these rules when participating in a sports activity. Bowling, for example, requires you to support an object away from the body rather than close to the body. Windsurfing frequently requires you to pull up the sail while the lower back is in a position of hyperflexion. The only advice is to try to incorporate as many of the proper lifting techniques as possible. Bend the knees and keep the lower back in a pelvic tilt whenever possible instead of ignoring all the rules when only one or two are impossible to incorporate into your technique.

Aerobics

Three possible pitfalls make aerobics a potentially high risk sport for people who suffer from chronic back pain: an instructor who is poorly educated vis-à-vis spinal anatomy and physiology; peer pressure; and poor footwear.

Basically speaking, an aerobics class should begin with slow warm-up exercises and should then move on to more strenuous strengthening and stretching exercises. At the end, there should be a cool-down period of slow stretching exercises. Excessive extension, or arching, of the back can exacerbate a facet joint problem, central spinal stenosis or a back problem caused by osteoarthritic changes. Excessive bending at the waist can be stressful for people who suffer from a disc problem. If you stay within your own range of movement, however, aerobics should be fine. Many people feel pressured into keeping up with others in the class who do not suffer from chronic back pain. Don't! Most workout books and tapes do not consider the needs of those with chronic back pain and should be avoided. Keep in mind that if your shoes are ill-fitting, or provide inadequate support to both the sides and soles of the feet, your lumbar spine will absorb the additional shock.

Aquabics

Aquabics is an excellent, low risk activity for the chronic back pain sufferer, mainly because it is difficult to exacerbate a spinal condition when you are weightless. The only exercise you may want to avoid, or alter, is the hamstring and low back stretch, which is sometimes done with both feet flat against the side of the pool, and both hands grasping the edges. You can limit the range of your stretch by stretching one leg at a time (while holding on with one hand instead of two) or keeping your feet a minimum of 12 inches apart.

Badminton

If you play consistently and avoid heavy competition, badminton can be a low to medium risk sport. The chronic back pain sufferer who plays badminton once every few months is more likely to strain muscles, ligaments and joints than the person who plays two or three times a week. The main pitfalls for those who suffer from chronic back pain (and these, in fact, apply to all racquet sports to varying degrees) are: failure to warm up and stretch before playing, especially when playing on a cool indoor court; hyperextending and rotating the back on backhand shots; and changing direction with rapid and jerky movements to chase down an opponent's well-placed shot. If you are over 40 and suffer from intermittent back pain due to the normal degenerative changes that accompany the aging process, you may find that your pain is exacerbated by badminton. If you play indoors on a cool court, wear a sweater that covers the hips for the first 20 minutes. Make sure that you allow enough time for a cool-down period of gentle stretching exercises.

Ballet

Faulty technique is cited as the most common cause of back injuries among professional ballet dancers. However, even dancers with impeccable technique frequently suffer from back pain; the human body was simply not designed to withstand the strain of ballet's many convoluted positions, and for this reason it is rated as a high risk activity.

The Russian method of training emphasizes more arching of the back and dramatic movements than the western school. Many experts feel that, while it may produce more world-class dancers whose bodies are more sleek, the Russian method is harder on the back. Injured professional dancers also tend to return to their training programs too quickly because of intense competition. If you are a ballet hobbyist, however, your risk is far less. Be on guard for neck injuries from spinning – the body revolves first and the head snaps to catch up. And watch out for facet or hip joint pain from hyperextension and rotary movements, such as those required by the *arabesque*. (Keeping the hips level as much as possible as one leg is raised will help prevent using your back to increase speed.)

If your child is interested in ballet, ensure that he or she is not suffering from spondylolysis or spondylolisthesis (see page 55), which can be exacerbated by ballet. If your child has enrolled in a serious ballet program and suffers frequently from severe muscle cramps, consider the possibility that these may be caused by an electrolyte imbalance due to a stringent diet designed to keep the weight below normal levels. If your youngster has a short Achilles tendon, or a lumbar spine that is stiffer than normal due to the structure of the bones (have these checked by a physician or physiotherapist), ballet is probably the wrong pursuit; these two conditions rarely improve, even with practice.

Ballroom Dancing

Ballroom dancing is considered to be a low risk activity for people who suffer from chronic back pain. Simply avoid "dipping" if you suffer from a facet joint problem and, perhaps, the tango, which also involves hyper-extended posture.

Baseball

If you are pitching, your risk of exacerbating a chronic back problem is far higher than if you are playing any other position. Pitchers frequently hyperextend their backs, particularly if they are trying to compensate for a strained shoulder muscle. Other positions are only moderately risky for the person who suffers from chronic back pain. Obviously, avoid crashing into the bases and home plate, and don't lunge beyond your normal range to make the save of the day. Another potential pitfall of baseball is that it is difficult to stay warmed up while waiting for your turn at bat. Concentrate on keeping your swing smooth and try to absorb some of the twisting motion while at bat with your hips and knees rather than your lumbar spine. If you are a weekend player, take extra care to do warm-up and stretching exercises before you play.

Basketball

Basketball is considered a low risk sport vis-à-vis back injuries, even among those who play competitively. Most professionals suffer injuries to their knees and ankles (and to a lesser degree, their hands and feet) rather than to their backs. In fact, in one American study, low back strain accounted for only one per cent of all injuries. Basketball hobbyists who suffer from chronic back pain, however, often find that their pain is exacerbated when they play. Most experts, however, do not blame the sport, pointing out that many hobbyists fail to understand the importance of warming up and often play competitively when they are not in good physical shape. Trunk rotation exercises before the game are essential as are cool-down stretches after the game. Avoid unnecessary hyperextension of the lumbar spine when jumping for the ball.

Bowling

Ten pin bowling can be a high risk sport if you suffer from chronic back pain; it depends mostly upon technique. Bowlers begin their throw with their backs in a flexed position, and the weight of the ball on one side of the body only. This posture can strain both the discs of the lumbar spine and the hip joint on the opposite side of the throwing arm. They end up in a rotated position with the weight of the ball at arm's length, a posture that can put strain on both the discs and the facet joints of the lumbar spine. Additional specific pitfalls for the chronic back pain sufferer are: releasing the ball too late (which means that the arm is extended more than necessary); and using a ball that is too heavy, or one that does not fit the fingers well. Many players find that wearing a corset for a short period of time *after* an acute exacerbation of a chronic back problem prevents excessive rotation of the facet joints and the hip joints. Do not play until a painful episode has subsided completely. Five pin bowling is less stressful, mainly because of the lighter ball. With either ball, good technique is the best way to avoid back injuries.

Boxing

Potential brain damage far outweighs the possibility of injuries to the spine. Boxers can suffer neck injuries when their heads repeatedly snap back as a result of being punched. Injuries to the lower back are infrequent and occur mostly due to falls.

Break Dancing

If you suffer from chronic back pain, you are likely too old to be interested in break dancing, which is a high risk activity. Its main pitfall is that it demands violent moves and rapid changes from postures of full flexion to full extension. Spinning on the head is not great for the neck. If your child is interested in break dancing, ensure that he or she is not suffering from spondylolysis or spondylolisthesis (see page 55).

Curling

Curling is considered to be a high risk sport for people who suffer from chronic back pain. The main potential pitfall of curling is that hobbyist participants are frequently in poor shape. A cool curling rink is not conducive to a pre-game warm-up and keeping warm during the game can be difficult since so much time is spent standing around in the cold. If you have a chronic disc problem, sweeping in the flexed posture can exacerbate your condition. If you have a facet joint problem, try to avoid releasing the rock too late, which involves a hyperextended posture. If you suffer no back pain at all and follow the simple guidelines for sports, it is doubtful that curling will cause you to develop back pain.

Cycling

Cycling, whether indoors or on the open road, is generally rated as a low risk sport for those who suffer from chronic back pain. The only pitfalls are: a high seat, which will cause you to hyperextend your lumbar spine if you are riding upright, and curved handlebars, which make it necessary to hunch forward, causing excess stress on the discs of the lumbar spine. Adjust your seat height so that when your foot rests on the lower pedal, your knee is still slightly bent. If you suffer from intermittent sciatic pain, you should avoid sitting for long periods without a break (this applies to sitting on a bicycle as well as sitting at a desk). Otherwise, cycling is an excellent sport, which will take care of your aerobic requirements as well as your back. Five or ten minutes of easy cycling is also an excellent way to warm up before doing stretching exercises.

Diving

Diving is a high risk activity for the chronic back pain sufferer and is definitely not recommended. For those who do not suffer from back pain, the main pitfall of this sport is poor technique, particularly when entering the water. For example, the jackknife hyperextends the lower back to an abnormal degree, and this can cause injury if entry into the water is too early or too late. Diving can also cause spondylolysis, which can lead to spondylolisthesis (see page 55). It goes without saying that diving into shallow water has been the cause of many severe neck injuries; always check water depth before you dive.

Exercise Machines

For people who suffer from chronic back pain (and even for people who don't), exercise machines are a high risk activity unless you use them properly. Regardless of the type of equipment you use (Nautilus, Universal, Hydra-gym, etc.), if you are not properly trained, or you are unaware of the specific exercises that must be performed in a posture of hyper-extension, you can exacerbate your back problem or cause one; if you suffer from back pain, avoid hip flexor and abductor/adductor exercises. Always maintain a pelvic tilt (see page 167) while using this type of equipment. As well, be sure to warm up (five or ten minutes on an exercise bicycle is excellent) before you begin your repetitions, and be sure to do adequate stretching exercises afterward. Some instructors advocate quick repetitions to build sleek muscles rather than slow repetitions to build bulk. This is fine, but be sure that you are capable of maintaining an excellent pelvic tilt if you are going to proceed rapidly. Don't be tempted to do full sit-ups quickly on the tilted exercise board; they look like good value for your time, but half sit-ups are better for your abdominal muscles as well as your back.

Football

Whether you have the world's strongest back or a severe back problem, *don't do it*. There is absolutely nothing good to say about football; merely pointing out that it is a high risk sport falls far short of describing the potential for disaster when playing this sport. It causes more low back and neck injuries (not to mention knee and ankle injuries) than any other sport. It is hard on the discs of the spine, the facet joints, the muscles and the ligaments. It involves excessive twisting, weight-bearing and hyperextension. Most tackling is done with the back flexed more than 45 degrees; most players who get tackled land with their spines hyperextended or rotated. Studies have also shown that football causes four times as many spondylolysis injuries than any other sport.

Touch football is obviously less stressful, but when played by weekend players who are out of shape, it is frequently the cause of strains and sprains. Many physicians who specialize in sports medicine feel that football should be outlawed completely.

If you (or your child) must play tackle football, it is essential to warm up properly, stretch thoroughly, be in superb physical shape, and learn proper tackling and blocking techniques. Head tackling and blocking should always be avoided. Stretching exercises after a game are also essential.

Golf

If you suffer from chronic back pain, especially a facet joint problem, the rotational movements of the golf swing can be extremely stressful. For this reason, golf is considered to be a moderate to high risk sport. According to pro golfer George Knudsen, however, you can compensate for a back problem by warming up and doing stretching exercises before you play and by altering your swing. Knudsen, who himself suffers from back pain, advises chronic back pain sufferers to adapt the swing so that the legs, hips and feet absorb some of the stress that the back normally takes, and to ensure that the weight transfer from one foot to the other is performed evenly. Since this is difficult to describe, the best advice is to ask a professional to help you learn how to adjust your swing. Too much time on the driving range will likely exacerbate a facet joint problem regardless of the cautionary rules you follow. If you use a golf cart, it is more difficult to keep your muscles and joints warm between holes; on cool days dress appropriately.

Gymnastics

Gymnastics is considered to be a high risk sport even for those who do not suffer from chronic back pain. The main pitfalls are: wear and tear to the facet joints from severe hyperextension of the spine; strained spinal ligaments – particularly the supraspinous ligament – from dramatic flexion postures; and spondylolysis leading to spondylolisthesis (see page 55) from falling off equipment. (According to some studies, ankle sprains are even more common than back injuries!) If you already suffer from chronic back pain avoid this sport completely.

If your child is interested in pursuing gymnastics seriously, keep in mind that a study of Bulgarian gymnasts has shown that 50 per cent developed spinal problems. Basically, the human body was not designed to extend to the degree that it must for many gymnastic postures, nor was it designed to change quickly from a position of full flexion to one of full extension. When you watch the force with which professional gymnasts leap off equipment to end their programs (landing without so much as a ripple), it's obvious that the spine is absorbing a great amount of shock. Youngsters frequently train to the point of exhaustion, and those who are competing sometimes try to perform difficult maneuvers before their musculature has developed sufficiently to support the stress they put on the bones of the spine. Ensure that your child's instructor is fastidious in the use of spotters and is not inclined to push your child too quickly.

Hockey

Hockey is considered to be a low risk sport for those who suffer from chronic back pain. Interestingly enough, only two players associated with the Toronto Maple Leafs during the past 15 years have had to abandon hockey because of persistent back pain. Hockey is a sport that tends to be tough on the knees and ankles, rather than the back.

If your child is interested in pursuing hockey, the main potential pitfall is spondylolysis, which can lead to spondylolisthesis (see page 55). If the team is not highly competitive, however, and there is a minimal amount of body checking, this is rarely a problem. Warming up and doing stretching exercises before the game is essential. Goalies, who spend long periods in a position of hyperflexion, should stretch whenever they get the chance. Former Montreal Canadien goalie Ken Dryden was one of the first hockey players to take stretching exercises seriously and should be applauded for giving stretching a good name! In general, the body movements made by hockey players are more fluid than those made by other team sports players, and this likely accounts for the fact that hockey rarely damages the back or exacerbates a chronic back problem.

The "morning after" stiffness associated with hockey can generally be attributed to the fact that weekend hockey hobbyists rarely spend enough time warming up before the game and cooling down after the game, and are frequently out of shape. If this stiffness lingers longer than a day, try doing a back exercise program (see Chapter 16) three times a week, concentrating on abdominal strengthening exercises. This should adequately prepare you for the strain of your once-a-week hockey game.

Horseback Riding

Most injuries from riding are due to falls and occur to the head and/or face rather than to the spine. For this reason, horseback riding is considered a low to medium risk sport for those who suffer from chronic back pain. The best advice is to proceed with caution while you are recovering from a painful episode; obviously a lot of bouncing around on the lumbar spine can exacerbate an already existing back problem. But if your technique is good, and you don't spend hours on end sitting atop your mount, you should be fine. Poor technique when jumping tends to put the lower back into a position of hyperextension.

Ice Skating and Figure Skating

Ice skating is a low risk sport for those who suffer from chronic back pain as long as stunts and long strides, which require a hyperextended posture, are avoided. The ice makes for fluid movements. (See also Hockey.) In the past, figure skating was also considered a low risk sport. However, in recent years, the competition level has been changing.

If your child is interested in pursuing a figure skating career, you should be aware of the potential pitfalls. Many studies say that youngsters now perform maneuvers beyond the capability of their undeveloped musculoskeletal systems. For example, triple jumps are now commonly performed at the novice level and sometimes even at the juvenile level. When a child whose muscles are not yet strong enough to attain sufficient height attempts to complete three revolutions in mid-air, the lower back must absorb severe rotational forces. On the other hand, children sometimes train so hard that they develop muscles that are stronger than their bones can support. As a result, the area where the muscle is attached to the bone becomes a weak link and damage sometimes results. Most teachers who coach figure skating at the recreational level, however, are fastidious about warming up and stretching exercises. If your child is pursuing this sport at this level, the chances of he or she developing a back problem are not overly high.

Jogging

Jogging, which is considered a medium risk sport for those who do *not* suffer from chronic back pain, is more apt to cause knee, ankle, foot and shin splint injuries than back injuries. However, if you do suffer from chronic back pain, jogging is considered to be a moderate to high risk sport. If you are determined to jog nevertheless, you can decrease your chances of exacerbating your back problem if you follow some rules. If your shoes are poor, your back will absorb far more stress than it would if you invest in jogging shoes that provide excellent support. If you run on pavement, your back will be stressed regardless. Warming up and stretching before running is essential, as is cooling down when your run is over; you should be walking, not running, the last half mile. Running uphill puts the lower spine into excessive flexion; when running downhill, it is extremely difficult to avoid a posture of hyperextension. In fact, if you are practising the pelvic tilt (see page 167), you'll know how much more difficult it is to maintain this posture when walking than when standing still, and maintaining the pelvic tilt when running takes a great deal of concentration and tenacity.

If you have been diagnosed as having central spinal stenosis, jogging may provoke sciatic pain because a position of hyperextension will strain your narrower-than-normal spinal canal even more. Fast walking with attention to the pelvic tilt is probably a better idea. If you have injured your ankle or knee, be careful that you do not put additional strain on your back to compensate. If jogging provokes knee or leg pain, seek medical advice from a physician who specializes in sports medicine; you may be experiencing referred pain from the back.

Martial Arts (Karate, Tae kwon do, Judo, Aikido)

Curiously enough, the martial arts are considered a low risk sport even for those who suffer from *mild* chronic back pain. Most of the various martial arts do not provoke back injuries and, in fact, many people who suffer from mild chronic back pain find that participation in these activities alleviates their back pain as opposed to increasing it. This is probably due to the fact that most martial arts teachers emphasize proper warm-up and stretching exercises, as well as proper technique and falling methods. If you find that aikido or karate do exacerbate your back pain, try taking it easy on the high kicks. Keep in mind that your foot technique is extremely important as are flexible hamstring and hip flexor muscles (see hamstring and hip flexor exercises on page 165). Studies have shown that if you fall badly you are more likely to strain your neck than your lower back.

Rowing (Includes Rowing Machines, Canoeing and Kayaking)

Rowing is a high risk sport for people who do not suffer from chronic back pain and will almost always exacerbate an already chronic back problem. The main pitfall with sweep rowing (where the rower uses one oar only) is that it combines a strong rotational motion with hyperextension and, adding insult to injury, requires that one do this while sitting for long periods of time. When sculling, the rower uses two oars, and this at least avoids most of the rotation. Often it is difficult to distinguish between pain that is due to muscle strain and pain that is due either to the wear and tear of a facet joint or a disc problem. Many physicians suggest that if you are experiencing leg or hip pain rather than back pain, you should take it easy for a few weeks to see if the pain subsides. If it returns again when you resume rowing, you may have to face the fact that this sport is irritating your sciatic nerve and consider whether the potential damage is worth it. If you are using a rowing machine, don't row to your full range of movement, which will cause you to hyperextend your back; stay within comfortable limits.

Kayaking is almost always less problematic for people who suffer from chronic back pain because the posture is balanced.

Sailing

Sailing is considered to be a moderate to high risk sport for people who suffer from chronic back pain. The main problem is that sailors are not always in good physical shape and are often called upon to undertake arduous lifting maneuvers. Concentrate on lifting with your knees. In large boats you may do nothing for an hour or two and then suddenly have to pull up sails when the course or wind changes. Obviously it is difficult to stay warmed up, or to do stretching exercises, on a boat. If you sail a small boat, try to avoid hiking, which puts you in a position of extreme hyperextension.

Skiing (Downhill, Cross-Country and Water-skiing)

Except for the fact that you can suffer a traumatic injury from a fall, downhill skiing is considered to be a low risk sport for people who suffer from chronic back pain. If you do proper warm-up and stretching exercises at the beginning of the day, the gentle motions used while skiing will actually help you to develop pelvic flexibility and will promote the pelvic tilt. If your technique is poor, however, you run the risk of twisting while in an unbalanced posture. If you suffer from chronic back pain, it is more important than ever to do leg strengthening exercises before the season starts. Keep in mind that most injuries occur at the end of the day when skiers are too tired to concentrate on technique.

Cross-country skiing is generally low risk as well. If you suffer from a chronic facet joint problem or central spinal stenosis, try to avoid long strides which hyperextend the back. If you have a chronic disc problem, try to avoid double-poling up a hill, which will put excessive stress on your lumbar discs.

Water-skiing is also considered a low risk sport for those who suffer from chronic back pain as long as you warm up and stretch before you go, and avoid trying to impress the audience with the tricks you haven't performed for 30 years.

Soccer

As long as you warm up and do stretching exercises before you play, soccer is considered to be a low risk sport for people who suffer from chronic back pain. Professional soccer players rarely injure their backs and when they do, the injuries are mostly strains of short duration. I often wonder if soccer players who "head" the ball repeatedly might eventually suffer from joint degeneration in the neck.

Soccer is the fastest-growing sport among American teenagers, and if your child prefers soccer to football consider yourself lucky. The only complication might be if he or she plays on artificial turf. Although I have not seen any formal studies, a number of physicians who specialize in sports medicine have noticed that more soccer players who play on artificial turf suffer injuries, including back injuries, than those who play on natural surfaces.

Squash and Racquet Ball

More stressful on the back than tennis, squash and racquetball are considered to be moderately risky sports for people who suffer from chronic back pain. Several studies have shown that squash players over the age of 40 tend to suffer more leg than back injuries while those under 40 tend to incur more back injuries, perhaps because they are less likely to adapt their competition level to their physical shape. The main potential pitfalls of squash are: the backhand, which involves stressful rotational movements, especially if the shot is a difficult one to reach; the rapid changes from positions of hyperextension to hyperflexion; failure to warm up and stretch properly before the game; and courts which are maintained at cool temperatures.

Generally speaking, the same rules apply to squash and racquetball as to other racquet sports. Lunging to make a save will get you into more trouble than anything else. Try to use your arms and legs more and your trunk less when hitting backhand shots. Adjust your competitive attitude to fit your ability and general physical shape. If you switch to squash when the tennis season is over, keep in mind that squash demands more jarring motions than tennis and is therefore considered to be rougher on the individual who suffers from chronic back pain. The added variable of playing in a constricted area where you have to avoid walls, racquets and opponents also makes squash a more stressful sport than tennis. Warming up and stretching before every game is therefore essential as is cooling down with stretching exercises when you are finished. If the court is cool, wear a sweater for the first 10 or 15 minutes of play.

Swimming

For people who suffer from chronic back pain, swimming can be a low to moderately high risk activity; it all depends upon the stroke and your degree of proficiency. Strokes done on the stomach require a hyperextended posture, particularly the butterfly, but also the breast stroke. The butterfly should be avoided completely, because it forces you to flex and extend at the same time. If you are able to do the breast stroke with your head in the water rather than out of the water, the stress on your back will be reduced. If your technique is good, the crawl is less likely to exacerbate a chronic back problem. Some instructors recommend alternating the breathing side; I myself find that while alternating sides is easier on my back, it is tough on my lungs owing to the fact that I end up drinking half the pool. The back and side strokes are almost always beneficial to those who suffer from chronic back pain. (If you do all your sidestroke lengths facing the same side of the pool, you'll be stretching both sides of your body equally.) Some people have the erroneous idea that swimming is an all-purpose type of exercise. If you have a back problem, it is still necessary to do pelvic tilt and abdominal strengthening exercises as well as stretching exercises. Swimming is great for muscle *tone* and aerobics, and while it will help *maintain* muscle strength, it will not provide the kind of full contraction necessary to *strengthen* your muscles.

T'ai Chi

Technically speaking, t'ai chi is a martial art, but most North Americans practise this Chinese discipline at a more leisurely level. In fact, some people pursue the sport specifically to alleviate back pain. At this level, t'ai chi is considered to be a low risk sport for those who suffer from chronic back pain. The "set" (an approximately 20-minute sequence of slow, fluid movements) develops co-ordination and is excellent for developing pelvic flexibility and improving the ability to maintain a pelvic tilt. It is almost impossible to over-exert the spine while performing the set, and many t'ai chi enthusiasts insist that they have learned how to correct poor postural habits by doing it. T'ai chi devotees believe that their sport is an all-round exercise, and that if you practise it, no other form of exercise is necessary. Those who adhere to a more western concept of body mechanics would probably disagree, saying that people who suffer from chronic back pain should be doing specific back strengthening and stretching exercises in addition to t'ai chi.

Tennis

A low to medium risk sport for people who suffer from chronic back pain, tennis' main pitfalls are more or less the same as those for squash and racquetball but to a lesser degree. If you suffer from central spinal stenosis, or a facet joint problem, serving may exacerbate your back problem. Avoid a hard serve with a twist at the end and practise throwing the serving ball no higher than necessary in order to reduce hyperextension as much as possible. Doubles is easier on the back simply because you are less likely to have to move beyond your normal range of motion to return a tough shot. Footwear with good support is essential. Clay courts are easier on the back than harder surfaces because the game is slower and you can slide into a shot which is less jarring on the back. Some players find that a back brace is helpful when they are getting over a painful episode, but be careful that a back brace is not used to mask symptoms that are a warning sign to quit for the day.

Track and Field

Hurdling, javelin-throwing and pole-vaulting are all high risk sports for people who suffer from chronic back pain and, in fact, can provoke back problems in those who are problem-free. All three involve movements in hyperextended postures. To pole-vaulting add the potential risk of a bad fall. Javelin-throwing involves holding a weight with the arm extended while in a hyperextended position. Warming up and stretching exercises are essential. Technique is as important as it is for gymnastics. Proper footwear will save wear and tear on the back as well as the legs and feet.

Volleyball

A medium risk sport for people who suffer from chronic back pain, volleyball is unlikely to *cause* back pain in someone who is problem-free. The main pitfalls are: playing without doing proper warm-up and stretching exercises; playing seasonally when in poor shape; and spiking the ball which can involve stressful rotational movements. Other than that, if you avoid heroics and play within your range of motion, you should be fine.

Weight Training

Most injuries from weight training are related to the lumbar spine, and it is considered a high risk sport, both for those who suffer from chronic back pain and those who are pain-free. Proper technique is essential; many weightlifters who suffer back injuries lift while in a hyperextended posture, thereby putting hundreds of pounds of stress on the facet joints of the lumbar spine. If your child is interested in weight-training, be aware that overtraining can lead to serious injuries both immediately and down the road.

Windsurfing

Windsurfing is considered to be a high risk sport for people who suffer from chronic back pain. Pulling up the sail is often awkward as well as stressful on the back; moreover, the windsurfer is obliged to hoist this weight while in a flexed posture. Once underway, most people who wind-surf spend long periods of time in a position of hyperextension to achieve maximum speed. If you are not in excellent physical shape, don't do it.

Wrestling

Oddly enough, wrestling is not considered a high risk sport for those who do not suffer from chronic back pain, and those who do have back problems generally don't participate. When injuries occur, it is usually when one wrestler is applying a hold to the other who is struggling to escape, and opposing forces happen to be exerting stress at a weak point – most often, a joint. However, most holds, if not illegal, will not produce an injury and wrestling referees tend to be fastidious in their officiating duties, at least at the amateur level.

Yoga

A low risk sport for those who suffer from chronic back pain, yoga can, in fact, help alleviate back pain. When done properly, it increases flexibility and helps to improve posture. In addition, the breathing exercises of yoga help relieve tension which frequently exacerbates back pain. The non-competitive ambience is also excellent for back pain sufferers. The only potential pitfall is the exercises which demand a posture of hyperextension; people who suffer from a facet joint problem should follow the general rule of thumb "don't do it if it hurts." (See also Chapter 22.)

25

Scoliosis: Don't Let It Throw Your Kid a Curve

When Mark Lewis was 13 years old, his mother noticed what looked like a lump to one side of the middle of his back. At the doctor's office, she and Mark were told that Mark had scoliosis – a sideways curvature of the spine – that in his case was so severe, that unless he had surgery, Mark couldn't be expected to live past middle age. There had been no pain, no symptoms whatsoever. "In fact, the only pain I ever had was *after* the operation," Mark says. "But when they tell you you'll probably only live to age 40, it's not hard to decide to have surgery."

Mark Lewis underwent surgery to correct his scoliosis in 1979. During the operation, two steel rods were inserted into his back to reduce the curve and the vertebrae of the spine in the area of the scoliosis were fused to prevent further deterioration. For two weeks he suffered from post-operative pain, but other than that, it was all uphill. For four months he wore a back brace. For two months he weaned himself from it. Today, at age 20, he goes to college in Toronto and plays hockey in his spare time.

Most of us have heard the word *scoliosis*. Few of us know exactly what it is, why it occurs and how often, and what should be done about it.

Scoliosis is the medical term for a spine that curves sideways. The name *skoliosis* was chosen by Hippocrates, who was the first physician to attempt to treat patients with crude braces. Unfortunately, his efforts failed and it was not until 1911, when the first spinal fusion was performed, that scoliosis could be successfully treated.

In 1946, the Milwaukee Brace was designed by Dr. Walter Blount and Dr. John Moe, who also designed the Twin Cities program in Minneapolis, and, for the first time, conservative treatment for scoliosis became possible.

About 12 per cent of the population has some amount of scoliosis, but often it is so slight that it has remained undiagnosed. Says Chris MacHattie, a physiotherapist at Toronto Western Hospital, "Only two per cent of people with scoliosis require any treatment at all," and cases as dramatic as Mark Lewis's are extremely rare.

Scoliosis can be divided into three categories, according to the severity of the problem. A curve of 30 degrees or less is considered mild and may remain undetected until the person is examined for unrelated backache later in life. With moderate curves of 30 degrees to 60 degrees, there is a noticeable deformity and, in most cases, pain eventually develops. In the severe category are curves of 60 degrees and more. If they go un-treated, they can cause heart failure, severe arthritis, or early death from heart and lung problems due to constriction in the chest cavity. Mark's 70-degree curve put him in this severe category.

Scoliosis is treatable. If treatment is begun early enough, deformity and discomfort are usually preventable. In the 1970s, a number of school boards instituted scoliosis screening programs for 12-and 13-year-old stu-dents, the age at which scoliosis is most likely to appear. Because of budget cuts in the 1980s, however, many of these screening programs were dropped. If there isn't a program in your child's school, you should screen your child yourself.

To check for scoliosis, sit behind your child. He or she should be standing and be naked from the waist up. Make sure that the feet are parallel and that the weight is distributed evenly on both feet. Instruct the child to bend forward slowly, bringing both hands toward the knees. "If you see an asymmetry, or bump, on one side of the spine, take the child to a physician for a thorough checkup," says Chris MacHattie.

Sometimes there is no visible asymmetry from this position. You should therefore also check to see if your child's posture is balanced. Have the child stand, facing you, while wearing as few clothes as possible. The feet must be parallel and the weight evenly distributed. Starting at the top and working down, look for differences in the levels of the shoulders, shoulder blades, collarbones, nipples and hips.

If you do find an imbalance, don't panic. Chances are good that dramatic treatment will be unnecessary. In fact, conservative treatment is now begun so early that, for example, at the Toronto Western Hospital Scoliosis Clinic, surgery for scoliosis has only been performed several times since 1982.

Types of Scoliosis

There are four types of scoliosis: congenital, neuromuscular, traumatic, and idiopathic.

Congenital scoliosis is present at birth. Usually the spinal vertebrae and ribs are poorly formed.

Neuromuscular scoliosis is the umbrella term for a wide variety of conditions. There is always some damage to nerves and muscles and it is caused by such diseases as polio or cerebral palsy.

Traumatic scoliosis is caused by an injury which damages a previously

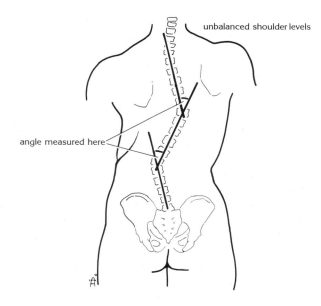

unbalanced shoulder levels

angle measured here

Diagram 32　Scoliosis

normal spine. A spinal fracture, unrelated surgery, radiation treatment, or an injury to muscles and tissues at the side of the spine can all cause traumatic scoliosis.

Idiopathic scoliosis accounts for between 70 and 80 per cent of all cases. Despite extensive research, the precise cause is unknown. Recent studies have been pointing to genetic factors, but further investigation must be done before this can be confirmed.

In children with idiopathic scoliosis, the spine is normal at birth and starts to curve just before or during the adolescent growth spurt. It affects both boys and girls, but almost all of the *severe* cases occur in girls.

Doctors used to believe that once a child with idiopathic scoliosis reached maturity, the curve stopped increasing. Recent studies have shown that this is not always the case. A significant number of adults with idiopathic scoliosis continue to have a gradual worsening of their curves and experience pain and disability as they get older. If you were diagnosed as having mild scoliosis as a teenager, it is a good idea to have your back examined annually.

The Treatment of Scoliosis

There are three main treatments for scoliosis: serial observation, conservative treatment (usually a brace and exercise program combination but sometimes electro-spinal stimulation) and surgery.

For mild scoliosis, which does not appear to be progressing, serial observation will usually suffice. There is no active treatment; the doctor simply examines the patient at regular intervals to ensure that the condition is not getting worse.

Conservative treatment is generally chosen for children whose curves are between 25 and 45 degrees. In most cases, a brace will be prescribed and a special exercise program will be designed. The brace can only be taken off for an hour or two each day. During that time, the child must do the exercise routine which is designed to enhance the effectiveness of the brace as well as preserve normal muscle strength and flexibility. This combination works well for children who still have several years of growth left.

In a few North American centres, electro-spinal stimulation, a new experimental treatment, is being used as an alternative to the brace and exercise program. There are two types of stimulation, but both involve the use of electrodes to stimulate specific back muscles. When these muscles contract, they work *against* the abnormal curve in the spine. The stimulation itself is painless. One type is attached only at night. The second type is surgically implanted in the back muscles and works 24 hours a day.

The only other type of treatment for scoliosis is surgery. During surgery, the curve is reduced and the spine is stabilized. To pull the spine straighter, metal rods are implanted on either side of the spine. Then the spine is fused in the area of the scoliosis.

Whether manipulation is a viable treatment for scoliosis is a difficult question to answer. Chiropractors, for whom manipulation is the treatment mainstay, maintain that manipulation sometimes helps. The medical profession, which generally believes that manipulation is a viable treatment for some back ailments but not others, does not. Chris MacHattie explains the reasoning behind medicine's rejection of manipulation when it comes to scoliosis: "The cause of idiopathic scoliosis is unknown. But studies have shown that in a patient with scoliosis, the muscles and other soft tissue – the ligaments and tendons – are abnormal in their chemical composition. They do not respond to manipulation in the same way as normal tissue, and this is the reason why we do not recommend it for scoliosis patients."

Even severe cases of scoliosis sometimes go unnoticed and never cause serious back problems. Gloria Chan, a 34-year-old homemaker with severe scoliosis, has never experienced much pain. Her father noticed the irregularity of her spine when Gloria was a young child living in Canton. Being a yoga teacher, he designed an exercise program with the idea of strengthening her muscles to counteract the curve. She has followed this exercise program religiously.

Had she grown up in North America, Gloria Chan would probably have been a candidate for surgery, but for her, a diligently adhered to exercise program has allowed her to live a relatively pain-free life. "But if I miss my exercises for even a day," she says, "I feel it."

If you think your back pain may be caused by a slight scoliosis, there are some exercises you can do. First, have your scoliosis checked by a medical doctor in case more than exercise is required. Swimming, which promotes flexibility and strengthens the trunk muscles without stressing the body, is thought by many experts to be one of the best forms of exercise for back problems, including mild scoliosis. In addition, you may be referred to a physiotherapist who can design an exercise program to improve your posture and flexibility.

Where scoliosis is concerned, the best advice is to keep active and maintain a positive attitude. As both Gloria Chan and Mark Lewis well know, even a serious case of scoliosis need not slow you down.

26

The Cervical Spine: That Pain in the Neck

"I've never had a back problem in my life," said Alison Davis, a legal secretary who spends most of her working day pecking at the keys of a word processor. "It's my neck that drives me crazy. Some days I think I'll never be able to turn my head again."

Like many people who suffer from neck pain, Alison Davis is mistaken. A neck problem is a back problem. It's just that it's the upper back – the cervical spine – that hurts.

In most ways, the anatomy of the neck and the pathology, or cause, of pain in it is the same as for the lower back. Figuring out what to do about neck pain can be slightly different than figuring out what to do about a back problem in the lumbar spine. But as with the lower back, poor posture and degenerative changes are most frequently to blame when it comes to a pain in the neck.

Because the head is lighter than the torso, the neck is subjected to a lighter load than the lumbar spine. What it lacks in load, however, is made up for by the demands associated with the fact that the neck must be so much more flexible than the lumbar spine.

The neck suffers from the same types of degenerative changes as the lumbar spine: disc degeneration; disc herniations (although they are far more common in the lumbar spine); facet joint degeneration; osteoarthritic changes; and spinal stenosis. If you haven't read Chapters 1 and 2, it would be a good idea to do so now.

All mammals, even the giraffe, have seven cervical vertebrae. In man, these vertebrae are smaller than those of the other regions of the spine. They are also the only ones that possess an opening in the transverse process through which blood vessels and nerves pass.

The first two vertebrae are called the atlas (C1) and the axis (C2). In addition to having an opening in the transverse process, they are shaped somewhat differently than the other five cervical vertebrae which, in terms of basic structure, more or less resemble the rest of the spinal vertebrae. As well, there is no disc between them.

The atlas is named for the giant in Greek mythology who supports the world on his shoulders. In the case of your atlas, the world is your head! The atlas has virtually no vertebral body at all. Its most striking feature is the hole in its centre, on either side of which are two flat surfaces that support the skull. When you nod your head – the motion you make when you are indicating yes – the skull rocks back and forth on the atlas.

The axis just below is unique in that it has a large post which projects upward on the side that is nearest to the front of the body. This post fits into the ringlike opening in the atlas. When you shake your head – the motion you make when indicating no – the atlas swivels around the axis' post.

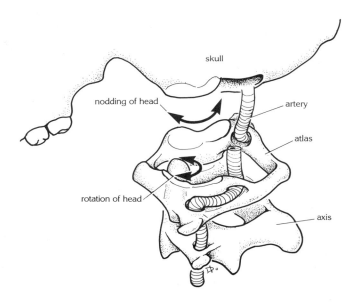

skull

nodding of head

artery

atlas

rotation of head

axis

Diagram 33   The Cervical Vertebrae

The lowest cervical vertebra (C7) has an unusually long spinous process, the end of which you can feel if you run your fingers along the base – or nape – of your neck.

Eight pairs of nerves emerge from the spinal cord at this area. The lower four merge to form the major nerve branches that pass below the shoulders and run into the arms. In the same way as pain from the lumbar spine can be "referred" to a leg, pain from the cervical spine can be felt in an arm. However, pain that radiates into an arm can also be caused by a wrist problem or a shoulder problem, and is sometimes very difficult to diagnose. On occasion, a physician will use a nerve conduction test, which can indicate whether the nerve roots are conducting impulses and, as well, how fast these impulses are travelling. To perform a nerve conduction test, the physician inserts fine needles (similar to the ones used for acupuncture treatments) into the muscles of the arm where nerve impulses ought to be running. Wires attached to the needles measure electrical activity. The procedure, which usually takes approximately 30 minutes, is generally uncomfortable but not painful.

There are several layers of muscle in the neck. The one that tenses up most frequently is the broad, triangular-shaped muscle called the trapezius, which forms the outermost muscle layer. When you see people inadvertently massaging their shoulders, it is the trapezius muscle that they are trying to loosen. The other two muscles of the neck region that have a tendency to tighten are the sternocleidomastoid (often referred to as the sternomastoid) and the scalene muscles. When you see people who spend long hours sitting at their desks trying to loosen the back of their necks by probing the neck muscles with the end of a finger, it is the spasm in these two muscles that they are trying to undo.

The neck is the most flexible part of the spine. It can flex 90 degrees

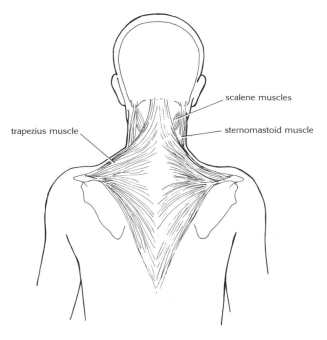

Diagram 34   The Muscles of the Neck

forward, extend or arch 90 degrees back, rotate a full 180 degrees from side to side and tilt about 120 degrees. Because it is curved (it has a lordosis similar to the one in the lumbar spine), it can absorb stress. But because of its amazing degree of flexibility, it has less stability than the lumbar spine and for this reason it can become strained.

Margaret Duffy, a senior physiotherapist at Toronto Western Hospital, estimates that between 30 and 35 per cent of the Western's back pain patients are people who have a pain in the neck.

"Most of the younger patients," she says, "come in with acute 'wry' neck pain. Some have turned awkwardly during the night, perhaps nipping a joint capsule or irritating a cervical facet joint. Others have strained the trapezius muscle due to improper lifting techniques, generally on the job. Still others have injured themselves by twisting suddenly while playing a sport such as squash."

People who are middle-aged are more likely to come in with neck problems that are a result of degenerative changes of the discs and facet joints of the cervical spine. Like the structures of the lumbar spine, those of the cervical spine also go through changes as a result of the natural aging process.

About a third of all the neck problems that Margaret Duffy sees are caused by whiplash – sprained, or torn, ligaments and/or muscles – usually the result of a car accident during which the neck has been forced to move beyond its normal range of motion. If you are in a car that is hit from behind, your head will be snapped backward as your body is thrown forward. In some cases, the head will snap forward again in a recoil motion. Some of these patients go to a physiotherapist while they are in an acute phase of whiplash. Others come in years after the accident complaining of pain that is a result of degenerative changes secondary to the whiplash. "A severe whiplash can speed up the normal degenerative process," Margaret Duffy says.

Many things about the treatment of neck pain have changed in recent years. Says Margaret Duffy, "As few as ten years ago, heat treatments and traction were the mainstays of neck therapy. Nowadays, we use quite a lot of mobilization and some manipulation, which can produce good results much faster than heat and traction on their own."

Manipulation, the technique that is the mainstay of chiropractic treatment, involves forcefully stretching a joint beyond its normal physiological range of movement for an instant. Manipulation can break down adhesions (see page 39) and can also free up a joint that is locked, or fixated, because of protective muscle spasm in the immediate area. The theory in this second case is that once the muscle spasm has decreased, the joint will be free to relocate itself in the correct plane.

"Those of us who are medically oriented look upon manipulation as one form of treatment that is sometimes indicated and sometimes not," says Margaret Duffy explaining some of the differences in philosophy between physiotherapists and chiropractors when it comes to using manipulation to treat a sore neck. Physiotherapists do not believe in *repeated* manipulation. They will generally try the technique once or twice, but if this produces no results, they will move on to another type of treatment. Regular monthly manipulations as "tune-ups" are not prescribed by physiotherapists, who prefer to educate patients to rely on home exercise programs and improved posture for dealing with their neck problems over the long term. "Physiotherapists use a wide range of techniques of which only one is manipulation," says Margaret Duffy.

Mobilization, on the other hand, is less traumatic than manipulation and can be repeated. Physiotherapists also believe that it is a much safer technique than manipulation in certain situations. "With mobilization, you don't go past a joint's physiological range of movement," Margaret Duffy explains. "You stay within the range, moving the joint rhythmically anywhere from the beginning of the range to the end. Its advantage over traction, for example, is that it is a far more specific type of treatment." By gently moving a joint at the mid-point of its range of motion, a physiotherapist can loosen up protective muscle spasm and reduce pain. This is what techniques such as massage, the application of heat, short wave diathermy (deep heat) and ultrasound can also accomplish, but with mobilization, the treatment can be applied to one particular joint. (See also Chapter 14.)

The use of TENS machines in the treatment of neck pain has also been gaining popularity in recent years (see page 148). TENS is generally used for pain relief rather than to correct the source of the problem. But pain itself can produce protective muscle spasm which, in turn, produces more pain and more spasm. "TENS therapy can also break up that pain/spasm cycle," she says.

Sometimes a cervical collar will be prescribed for someone who is going through an acute phase of neck pain. A patient who is suffering from strained paraspinal muscles, which are the muscles at the back of the neck, can sometimes benefit from a collar; the collar can take some of the strain off these muscles, transfering the weight of the head to the collarbones. However, a cervical collar is not recommended over the long-term. If it is worn *full time* for more than two or three weeks, a patient can actually become "addicted" to it. "Full time use of a collar for more than three weeks *at the outside* will cause the neck muscles to become weak," says Margaret Duffy. "At that point removing the collar may cause increased pain."

The best way of avoiding "collar addiction" is to wear a collar for two or three hours and then take a one-hour break. When it comes time to wean yourself from a collar, try wearing it only while performing activities involving neck flexion combined with arm activity: dishwashing, typing or other desk work.

The majority of neck pain, however, is muscular, due to poor posture while sitting, standing and sleeping, and does not require professional intervention. If you spend a substantial amount of time sitting at a desk and you find that you frequently suffer from neck pain by the end of the day, reread Chapter 17 on Posture. If you frequently wake up with a sore neck, have a look at the section on sleeping in that chapter; your pillow, mattress, or sleeping position may be to blame. If you think you may be interested in one of the holistic alternatives, the Alexander Technique, which is based on neck alignment, may also be of interest.

You will also likely find that a few simple exercises, which take no more than a minute each, will relieve a great deal of your muscular neck pain. Most of them are isometric and can even be done while sitting at a desk.

Neck Exercises

1. CHIN TUCK STRETCH (ISOMETRIC CONTRACT-RELAX TECHNIQUE FOR RELIEF OF A TIGHT TRAPEZIUS MUSCLE) • This exercise can be done while sitting or standing. Place the left hand on the left side of your forehead. Let your head drop forward to the end of its range of motion. Tilt the head slightly to the left, turning the chin a little to the right. While resisting with your hand, push the head down into the hand and hold this contraction for five seconds. Relax and let your head fall forward again. Repeat the isometric push. Relax and let your head fall forward. Repeat isometric push a third time. By the time you have repeated this exercise three or four times, you will find that your range of motion has increased and your right trapezius muscle will feel looser.

Repeat the exercise, this time with your head tilted slightly to the left.

This exercise is an excellent adjunct for those who are wearing a cervical collar, particularly if muscle spasm or tension are complicating the problem. Just remember to do the exercise gently.

2. EXTENSION STRETCH (ISOMETRIC HOLD-RELAX TECHNIQUE FOR TIGHT SUB-OCCIPITAL MUSCLES, WHICH ARE THE ERECTOR SPINAE MUSCLES OF THE NECK) • This exercise is similar to the Chin Tuck Stretch. Place one hand behind the head. Push the head against the hand while the hand resists. Relax, letting the head fall forward and keeping the chin tucked in. Repeat three times. Some physiotherapists believe that the Chin Tuck works better; if you find that this version does not provide relief, don't bother with it.

This exercise is also excellent if you are weaning yourself from a cervical collar and are concerned about tight neck muscles.

3. SIDE BEND STRETCH (ISOMETRIC CONTRACT-RELAX TECHNIQUE FOR RELIEF OF TIGHT SCALENE MUSCLES) • This exercise can be done while sitting or standing. To stretch the right scalene muscles, position your head so that your face is vertical and your eyes are focused straight ahead. Then tilt the head to the left side as far as possible without strain. Place the heel of your left hand on the left side of your head just above the ear. Push the head sideways into your left hand while resisting movement with your hand. Relax and repeat three times. Then repeat in the opposite direction using the right hand to resist movement in the opposite direction.

Note: Always start this exercise with the head bent as far as possible without discomfort; the appropriate muscle should be stretched fully.

4. SIDE BEND STRETCH (ISOMETRIC HOLD-RELAX TECHNIQUE FOR TIGHT SCALENE MUSCLES) • As in exercise 3, tilt the head to the left until the right scalene muscles are stretched to their maximum without discomfort. Placing the left hand just above and slightly behind the right ear, push your head sideways against your left hand, using the left hand to resist any movement. Relax and let the head stretch further. Repeat three times. This exercise is similar to exercise 3. Try both and then pick the one that works better for you.

5. NECK AND SHOULDER RELAXERS • Stand or sit with arms hanging loosely at your sides. Shrug the shoulders up as high as you can. Count slowly to ten and relax. Repeat a minimum of ten times.

In the same position as above, pull the shoulder blades back together, as if you were trying to create a furrow in the middle of your back. Hold for a count of ten and relax. Repeat a minimum of ten times.

In the same position as above, bring the shoulders forward into a hunched position. Hold for a count of ten and relax. Repeat a minimum of ten times.

27

Osteoporosis: Prevention Is the Key

The meaning of *osteoporosis* is simple – "porous bone." But the exact causes of this disease, which like diabetes, for example, takes many different forms, are complex and far from completely understood. What is known is that unlike most back ailments which tend to affect middle-aged people, osteoporosis typically affects those who are over the age of 65. It also strikes four times as many women as men.

When osteoporosis occurs, bone density decreases. The bones become more porous, as the name of the condition would suggest. They also become more brittle, resulting in an increased susceptibility to fractures. In fact, if the disease has progressed to a severe stage, a bone fracture can occur spontaneously. The vertebrae of the spine are at greatest risk; in extreme cases, the weight of the upper body can literally crush the vertebrae of the lumbar spine.

Mildred Holmes, a 72-year-old retired book-keeper, was told that she had osteoporosis four years ago when she began to suffer from low back pain for the first time in her life. "I was shocked," she says. "I hadn't fallen or done anything that seemed serious enough to cause something to break but there, on the X-ray, was the line of a fracture at the front of a vertebra. I could see it plain as day the moment my doctor pointed it out."

Most fractures caused by osteoporosis eventually heal in the sense that the two lines of fracture "knit" together, but if the vertebra has been crushed into a wedge shape it remains that way. If several fractures have occurred, the person can lose up to several inches in height as a result of being hunched forward.

There are few national statistics on the prevalence of osteoporosis in Canada, but the American numbers, divided by ten, provide a fairly accurate picture of its incidence, which many physicians believe is becoming epidemic.

• Osteoporosis currently affects an estimated 4 million Americans (400,000 Canadians), and this number is likely to increase as the proportion of the elderly in our population goes up.

271

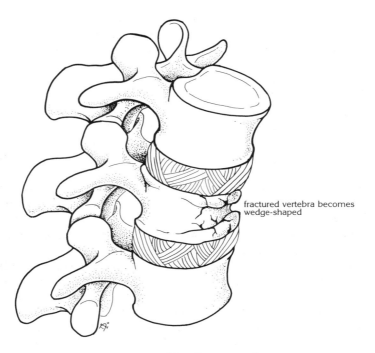

fractured vertebra becomes wedge-shaped

Diagram 35   Osteoporosis

• In the United States, approximately 700,00 fractures (70,000 in Canada) are attributed each year to osteoporosis, the majority being fractures of the vertebrae of the spine. Between 12 and 20 per cent of women who sustain hip fractures due to osteoporosis die within six months due to complications.

• Few studies on the incidence of osteoporosis in men have been conducted, but according to some researchers, the disease may affect only one-quarter as many men as women. Studies have shown that 25 per cent of women over the age of 50 will suffer a bone fracture due to osteoporosis. By age 75, the American statistics indicate, half of all Caucasian females will have already suffered a vertebral compression fracture due to osteoporosis. (Unfortunately, by the time the disease has progressed far enough to show up on a normal X-ray, between 30 and 50 per cent of bone density has already been lost. By this point, the disease is considered to be serious and fractures are likely to occur.)

How Osteoporosis Affects the Bones

The only way to understand how osteoporosis affects the bones of the spine is to acquire a basic understanding of how bone forms, or ossifies.

Most of us tend to think of bone as inert. It is, on the contrary, very active. Our bones produce blood cells and store minerals – mostly calcium which gives it its strength. As well, bone is constantly dissolving and being generated. If you could monitor over a seven-year period the composition of a bone in the body of an active person, you would see that all of its cells and all of the bone minerals have been replaced.

Cells in bone called osteoblasts are responsible for production. Other cells called osteoclasts reabsorb bone cells that have either died or are no longer functioning. Osteoclasts are also thought to be responsible for maintaining normal calcium levels in the blood which are required by nerves and organs. If this level becomes too low, the body will signal the osteoclasts to reabsorb enough calcium from the bones to make up for the deficiency.

Normally, a balance exists between the activity of the osteoblasts and that of the osteoclasts. Enough new bone is produced to make up for the amount that is reabsorbed. When the osteoclasts reabsorb more bone than the osteoblasts can produce, however, the net amount of bone decreases. The result is called osteoporosis. An easy way of visualizing what is going on is to think of the bone tissue as a slice of Swiss cheese. As osteoporosis develops, the holes in the cheese become bigger and bigger. The result is less cheese, or in the case of the body, less bone.

Why Osteoporosis So Frequently Affects the Bones of the Spine

Exactly why osteoporosis develops, doctors do not know. They are not even certain why osteoporosis tends to affect the bones of the spine more frequently than the other bones of the body, an exception being the bones of the hips. But there are theories.

The basis for the most widely accepted theory is not difficult to understand. It has to do with the fact that all bones are composed of two basic substances: cancellous bone and cortical bone.

Cancellous bone is often found in the interior of the bone and has a meshlike structure. Cortical tissue, which is hard, forms the exterior portion of the bone. Cancellous tissue is responsible for the production of the blood cells; it is also where the many items which move in and out of the marrow are stored. Because it is more active, the cancellous portion of any bone is thought to be more sensitive to metabolic changes in general, some of which have been linked to osteoporosis. Most doctors explain the high susceptibility of the vertebrae and hip bones to osteoporosis by the fact that these bones contain more cancellous tissue than most other bones.

The Causes of Osteoporosis — Who Is at Risk?

Osteoporosis has been attributed to the aging process. It is logical in the sense that as our bodies get older, their mechanisms wear out and less tissue is generated. But the specifics are not quite as simple. Osteoporosis, say most of the researchers, is a condition with multiple causes.

It has been linked to inactivity, diet, the decrease of estrogen production in women, and a host of other factors, including certain drugs and high alcohol consumption. Most of these tend to pertain more to the elderly than the young.

INACTIVITY • Amazing as it may seem, activity contributes to the production of bone mass. When they are under strain, the osteoblasts increase their production of bone tissue. The greater the amount of strain that is placed on a bone and the heavier the load it has to carry, the more bone it produces.

The bones of athletes, for example, are significantly heavier than those of people who do not engage in sports. When a person with a broken leg bone that is immobilized in a cast continues to walk on the opposite leg, the bone of the unused leg becomes thin as its calcium content declines; the bone in the other leg remains normal. Activity, for reasons which are not well understood, provokes the osteoblasts to produce bone. Inactivity causes a slow down in the production process and, eventually, as old bone wears out, the net amount of bone decreases.

DIET — CALCIUM DEFICIENCY • In some cases, osteoporosis is thought to be caused by a calcium deficiency. Either an insufficient amount of the mineral is being consumed; or, in some instances, the body is not able to absorb the calcium it takes in.

Recent studies have shown that North Americans, particularly women, tend to consume an insufficient amount of calcium. Many researchers blame our society's preoccupation with slenderness for the fact that our diets tend to be so low in calcium-rich foods. Many women diet constantly. As well, during pregnancy and while a woman is breast-feeding, the calcium intake should increase substantially. Unfortunately, many women are unaware of their calcium needs. Says Dr. Charles Gold, a gynaecologist at Toronto General Hospital, "I advise pre-menopausal women to take at least 1,000 milligrams of calcium daily. Many women find it difficult to get this amount from dairy products and other calcium-rich foods and take calcium supplements. If you take calcium supplements, it should be elemental calcium. I also advise women to ensure that the supplements they buy contain no lead." If you are taking calcium supplements, it's a good idea to ask your general practitioner to check the calcium levels in your blood and urine to ensure that they are normal.

There are a number of reasons why some people's bodies are not able to utilize the calcium they consume.

First of all, various nutrients, including vitamin D and phosphorus, are essential in the absorption process of calcium. In order for calcium and phosphorus to be absorbed, vitamin D must be present. Once absorbed and transferred to the bones, the two minerals combine chemically. If either calcium or phosphorus is lacking, they cannot combine and for this reason, both are essential. The proper calcium/phosphorus ratio is 2.5:1 and approximately 400 milligrams of vitamin D is required daily. Generally speaking, North Americans do not suffer from a deficiency of either vitamin D or phosphorus. In fact, North Americans tend to consume more phosphorus than calcium rather than the other way around.

DIET – AN EXCESS OF PHOSPHATE AND PROTEIN • In studies on animals, an excessive amount of phosphate was found to increase the risk of osteoporosis. This evidence has never been substantiated in humans, however. On the other hand, diets extremely high in protein have been linked to osteoporosis in humans. One study has shown that people who increase their daily protein intake from 70 grams to 100 grams increase their annual bone loss by one per cent.

DIET – COFFEE AND ALCOHOL • Some studies have shown that people who drink large amounts of coffee tend to lose more calcium than those who do not. The mechanism, however, is not well understood. Severe alcohol use causes an increase in the amount of calcium that is excreted by the body. But in these studies, too, the mechanisms are vague and researchers point out that calcium deficiency among alcoholics may be due to the fact that their diets are also poor.

THE DECLINE OF ESTROGEN PRODUCTION IN WOMEN • The ovaries of post-menopausal women produce far less estrogen than the ovaries of women who are still menstruating and, eventually, they stop producing estrogen completely. A study conducted in the United States showed that shortly before menopause, the average woman lost approximately .3 per cent of bone mass per year. For five to eight years after menopause begins, the average yearly loss was nine times that amount (2.7 per cent) and then there was a levelling off.

Researchers have known for many years that the incidence of osteoporosis is much higher among post-menopausal than pre-menopausal women. Most of them believe that estrogen plays an important role in the development of the disease, but the exact nature of this role has yet to be determined.

Some studies have indicated that a high level of estrogen decreases the amount of calcium that is excreted by the kidneys; from this, researchers have concluded that post-menopausal women may excrete more calcium than women who are still menstruating.

The presence of estrogen is also thought by some researchers to keep the amount of calcitonin produced by the thyroid glands at a high rate. A high level of calcitonin is thought to stop the osteoclasts from reabsorbing calcium. When estrogen levels are low, little calcitonin is produced and, so the theory goes, the osteoclasts reabsorb greater amounts of calcium from the bones.

For reasons which are not well understood, overweight women produce more estrogen than slender women and develop osteoporosis less frequently. Some studies indicate that after menopause, fat cells may produce estrogen.

DRUGS • Osteoporosis has been cited as a side effect of corticosteroids, drugs which have a tendency to inhibit calcium absorption and which promote the excretion of calcium in the urine. Other drugs which have been linked to osteoporosis are: Heparin and aluminum-containing antacids. If you are taking either of these drugs, and especially if you are also female and over the age of 40, you should discuss the increased risks of osteoporosis with your doctor.

The Treatment of Osteoporosis

The loss of bone caused by osteoporosis can seldom be replaced. The challenge is early detection. The sooner the condition is discovered, the sooner steps can be taken to arrest its progression.

Unfortunately, osteoporosis is difficult to diagnose. X-ray changes become visible only after 30 to 50 per cent of bone mass has been lost, and by this time the patient will have already reached the stage at which fractures occur.

It is hoped that in the near future, more cases of osteoporosis will be diagnosed long before so much bone mass has been lost. In one research project, which is being conductd by Dr. Joseph Houpt's team at the Mount Sinai Hospital in Toronto, patients' bone mass is measured with a machine called a Dual Photon Absorptiometer. The amount of bone mass is then compared to what is considered normal for a person of that age. At the moment, the stickler is trying to determine exactly what is normal since the research in this area is relatively new. In Dr. Houpt's project, women who are approaching the age of menopause as well as certain high risk patients are being studied. In the future, it is hoped that all high risk women will be able to be screened. Says Dr. Houpt, "As investigators prove the clinical usefulness of methods such as these, hopefully larger numbers of women will have their bone masses measured so that earlier detection of osteoporosis will be possible for more people."

The main treatment – whose aim really is to prevent the disease from progressing – is a combination of calcium supplements and exercise. In some instances, estrogen supplements are prescribed to women who are post-menopausal. Research into the use of sodium fluoride, which in some cases can actually bring bone mass up to normal levels, is also being conducted in several North American centres.

CALCIUM SUPPLEMENTS AND EXERCISE • For both men and women who are suffering from osteoporosis, a dose of 1,500 milligrams of elemental calcium per day is generally prescribed along with as much exercise as possible. On rare occasions, when the metabolization of calcium is of concern, approximately 400 units of vitamin D per day will be prescribed in addition to the calcium supplements. (In the past, much larger doses of vitamin D were prescribed for patients with osteoporosis, but its use has become less common in recent years.)

Calcium supplements, however, do not increase bone formation. They can only act to suppress the mechanisms by which bone is reabsorbed. Furthermore, calcium and vitamin D in extremely high doses can sometimes cause adverse side effects. Megadoses of calcium have been linked to kidney stones and constipation; overdoses of vitamin D can also lead to kidney stones, as well as abnormally high levels of the vitamin in the blood. (Generally speaking, however, a person who is taking calcium supplements need not worry about overdosing; moderately excessive amounts of calcium are merely excreted by the body, or stored in the long bones for future use. Most doctors believe that painful calcium deposits such as those of bursitis and scleroderma are not caused by an excess of dietary calcium.)

Exercise, on the other hand, can increase bone formation, although it cannot reverse the toll taken by bone mass which has already been lost. The difficulty is, of course, that osteoporosis patients who have suffered a painful bone fracture are hardly in the mood to exercise. Nevertheless, once a fracture has healed, and the pain has subsided to some degree, most doctors recommend that their osteoporosis patients try, at least, to walk as much as possible. Dr. Gold recommends a minimum of 20 minutes of brisk walking at least three times a week.

ESTROGEN REPLACEMENT THERAPY • Like calcium supplements, estrogen supplements can suppress bone reabsorption, at least in some women. The still unanswered question is for whom. For a number of years, in the late 1960s and early 1970s, estrogen was frequently prescribed to women in their fifties who were suffering from hot flashes and other symptoms that frequently accompany the onset of menopause. The drug worked in that it decreased these symptoms and, although it was not realized until some years later, it also prevented osteoporosis in many cases. But estrogen also increased the incidence of cancer of the endometrium, the lining of the uterus. Since then, the use of estrogen for both the symptoms of menopause and osteoporosis has been controversial.

Some researchers believe that if progesterone — which brings on a "period" during which the endometrium is shed — is added for the last 10 to 14 days of the cycle, the risk of endometrial cancer becomes significantly reduced. Others disagree, saying that unless a woman has had a hysterectomy (in which case there is no uterus in which cancer can develop) estrogen therapy can be risky. One thing is certain; if you are taking estrogen supplements, it is advisable to take progesterone as well. In addition, your doctor should be monitoring you frequently for pre-cancerous changes in the cells of the endometrium.

FLUORIDE AS A TREATMENT FOR OSTEOPOROSIS • The early results of studies being conducted at the Bone and Mineral Metabolism Unit of the University of Toronto on the use of sodium fluoride are showing it to be promising as an agent that can increase bone mass. Says Dr. Timothy Murray, Director of the Metabolic Bone Clinic at St. Michael's Hospital, "The current status of sodium fluoride is that it is still in the research stage. . . . I think it is going to turn out to be a useful treatment in the future. But the really exciting thing about this fluoride research is that it has shown that it is possible to take an osteoporitic skeleton and get it to form new bone. Until now, there was nothing that could do this. . . . We may find that fluoride is not the ultimate, but the fact that it's possible really turns around your way of thinking, and when you start changing your thinking, all kinds of things can happen." Other studies are being conducted at the Mayo Clinic and at the Henry Ford Hospital in Detroit.

At the moment, several aspects of sodium fluoride remain to be resolved. Some studies on animals have shown that the bone produced when sodium fluoride is used differs from normal bone in that it is more brittle. This is not to say, however, that the results on humans will be the same. Says Dr. Murray, "The data on humans is difficult to gather for many reasons, one simple one being that you can't put human bones in a vice and hit them with a hammer. You have to wait and count the number of fractures to tell if the bone that is produced is strong, and that takes an incredible amount of time and work."

Some people absorb sodium fluoride more efficiently than others, making it difficult to determine correct dosages. There are also side effects:

approximately ten per cent of the patients in the St. Michael's Hospital study suffer from such side effects as joint pain and irritation of the gastro-intestinal tract. "These side effects are probably largely dose-related and most can be handled one way or another," says Dr. Murray. "But when you talk about the side effects these patients face, the risks of fluoride treatment are not all that significant compared to what else may result from the osteoporosis itself. About a third of patients seem not to respond at all."

The Prevention of Osteoporosis

It's not difficult to see that the key to osteoporosis is prevention: a proper diet, exercise and education. Says Dr. Houpt, "The people we have to talk to are young women and women who have just had a first baby because the time to achieve your peak bone mass is before the age of 35."

American studies show that the average daily calcium intake is as low as 500 milligrams per day. Children need 400 to 700 milligrams of elemental calcium daily. Adolescents require 1,300 milligrams; pre-menopausal women and adult men require approximately 1,000 milligrams. Post-menopausal women who are not on estrogen replacement therapy should be consuming the same amount of calcium as a woman who is pregnant – 1,500 milligrams per day. For post-menopausal women who are taking estrogen supplements, 1,000 milligrams of calcium are recommended. While a woman is breast-feeding, some physicians advise up to 2,000 milligrams of calcium per day.

But there is no substitute for exercise for preventing osteoporosis. The minimum amount that is recommended is one hour, three times a week. If you're not getting this much, you are likely increasing your risk of developing osteoporosis in the future.

Just about any type of exercise – jogging or fast walking, cycling, aerobics, hiking – where there is stress on the long bones of the body should be beneficial in the prevention of osteoporosis. (Swimming is not considered to be as beneficial in the prevention of osteoporosis since you are weightless when you swim; it is, however, considered a good exercise for people since it will not further stress a weakened skeleton.)

An American study compared a group of women who exercised for an hour, three times weekly, to women who did no exercise. The comparison went on for a year. At the end of the year, the women in the active group had increased their total body calcium by 2.6 per cent; those in the inactive group found that their total body calcium had *decreased* by 2.4 per cent. That's a five per cent difference in only a year! While more long-term studies are required in this area, there is no doubt that exercise should be a part of your life.

EXAMPLES OF FOODS THAT ARE RICH IN CALCIUM •

• milk and milk products such as cheese and yogurt — a 228 millilitre glass of milk contains 300 milligrams of calcium.

• green leafy vegetables such as spinach and broccoli — a cup of cooked broccoli spears contains 132 milligrams of calcium and a cup of steamed dandelion greens (if you're so inclined) contains 252 milligrams of calcium!

• seafood — a pound of shrimps contains 325 milligrams of calcium, a pound of clams, 248 milligrams

• canned salmon — a pound with the bones contains 1,168 milligrams of calcium compared to tuna which is only 36

• canned sardines — a pound has 1,234 milligrams of calcium

If you are interested in acquiring more information about osteoporosis, you can contact the Osteoporosis Society of Canada, 76 St. Clair Avenue West, Toronto, Ontario, M4V 1N2, (416) 922-1358.

28

Pregnancy: Is Back Pain Inevitable?

"Back pain during my pregnancy? My doctor told me it was inevitable. I just tried to grin and bear it, hoping that in time it would go away."

Margaret Rice
Architect

"The back pain came on so suddenly and with such intensity that one morning I just couldn't get out of bed. I felt as if I'd been run over by a truck in my sleep."

Bev Randall
Teacher

"By the time I was in my fifth month my back was hurting so much that I couldn't stand for more than ten or fifteen minutes."

Alice Turner
Sales Clerk

"I finally figured out how to use a lot of pillows to prop myself up in bed at night and I'd try not to move around very much."

Sandra Belford
Homemaker

"I'd heard about postural changes and back pain during pregnancy, but I was confident I wouldn't have any problems. I was in good shape. I'd always exercised regularly and was rather arrogant about my physical condition. For my arrogance I had back pain for five months. I couldn't believe it."

Terry Anne English
Journalist

These five women, all pregnant for the first time, experienced one of the more common side effects of pregnancy: back pain. According to some obstetricians, the phenomenon (due mostly to postural and hormonal changes) is inevitable. "Of course you'll have back pain when you're pregnant," says one Toronto obstetrician who doesn't feel that there is very much you can do about it.

Kim Swigger, a Scarborough, Ontario public health nurse and prenatal instructor, disagrees. In her experience, 60 per cent of women suffer from back pain during pregnancy. "Some of them describe their back pain as a mild, quite bearable ache," she says. "Others describe it as all-consuming." But she firmly believes that most women could beat back pain during pregnancy if they understood the basic changes that the body goes through and how to counterbalance them with good posture, proper body mechanics, exercise and rest.

The Changes that Take Place During Pregnancy

In the middle of the menstrual cycle, ovulation takes place. While the egg is travelling from the ovary to the uterus, a small gland in the ovary called the corpus luteum begins to produce the hormone progesterone. The function of progesterone is to build a lining in the uterus, or womb, where the fertilized egg can develop. If the egg is not fertilized, however, this lining becomes unnecessary and the production of progesterone stops. The egg is expelled from the body, and a menstrual period follows, during which the built-up uteral lining is shed.

If, on the other hand, fertilization does occur, the lining of the uterus continues to build up and more, rather than less, progesterone is needed. Around the fourteenth week of pregnancy, the body also starts to change shape in order to accommodate the growing fetus. Progesterone is involved in these changes as well. Massive amounts of it are required and the placenta starts to produce it.

The increase of progesterone causes several changes to take place which, in turn, cause other changes. The broad ligaments that support the uterus and hold it in place relax so that the uterus can expand. The connective tissue linking the right and left sections of the abdominal muscles softens so that the abdomen too can expand. As the abdomen expands, the body's centre of gravity begins to change. As the centre of gravity changes, many women develop an excessively lordotic, or hyper-extended, posture which frequently causes muscle spasm in the lower back. As the fetus continues to grow and develop, pressure on the large blood vessels of the abdomen increases. This pressure can cause circulation to the legs to decrease. In addition, the developing fetus requires more and more calcium which, if not available from dietary sources, will be taken from the mother's calcium reserves. Many physicians believe that an inadequate supply of calcium during pregnancy — less than 1,500 milligrams per day — can result in cramping and muscle spasm in the legs.

How the Uterus Expands

Have a good look at Diagram 36. The uterus is located within the pelvic girdle in the space created by the round shape of the hip bones. There are three joints within the pelvic girdle: the right and left sacroiliac joints, which attach the hip bones to the sacrum by means of taut and powerful ligaments; and the pubic symphysis, the fibrous cartilage which joins the pubic bones at the pelvis' front. Chris MacHattie, a physiotherapist at Toronto Western Hospital, explains the changes that take place. "By the twelfth week of pregnancy, the uterus will have expanded to the point where it takes up all the space in the pelvic girdle. In order for further expansion to take place, progesterone acts on these ligaments, causing them to relax."

Normally, the sacroiliac joints are rigidly fixed by their ligaments, but when these ligaments relax, movement can take place. Nature is not always precise in matters such as these, however, and many women's sacroiliac joints move more than necessary, straining the ligaments. Rotational movements in particular (vacuuming or rolling over in bed are two good examples) put excessive strain on the sacroiliac joint ligaments. "If, around the fourth or fifth month of pregnancy, you begin to experience pain in the posterior hip areas directly over the sacroiliac joints, strained ligaments are most likely the cause," she says.

Much of the pain from strained sacroiliac ligaments can be avoided, or

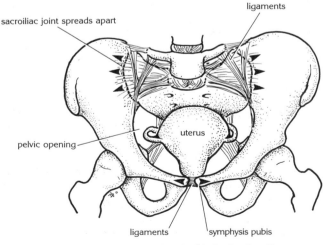

Diagram 36   The Pelvic Girdle During Pregnancy

at least reduced, if you avoid rotational movements as much as possible. For example, when you get out of bed, first roll to one side, and use your arms to push your body into a sitting position. Then sit for a moment before standing. When doing household chores, move your feet to face your task rather than twisting the upper body. Try to carry two light bags of groceries, one on either side, rather than one heavy bag. Avoid bending over with the legs straight and pay particular attention to lifting techniques (see page 185), especially if you have a young child. "It may take a little longer to go through your normal routine," says Chris MacHattie, "but it will also save you a whole lot of pain."

How the Abdomen Expands

The three sets of abdominal muscles act like a strong girdle to hold the upper body erect: the internal and external oblique muscles, the left and right transversus abdominis muscle, and the left and right rectus abdominis muscles (see Diagram 36).

Normally, the rectus abdominis muscles are attached in the centre by strong, taut connective tissue. As progesterone production increases, this

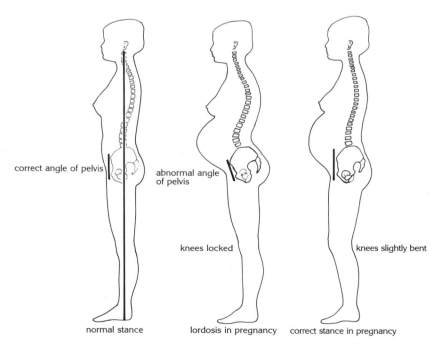

correct angle of pelvis

abnormal angle of pelvis

knees locked

knees slightly bent

normal stance   lordosis in pregnancy   correct stance in pregnancy

Diagram 37   Lordosis in Pregnancy

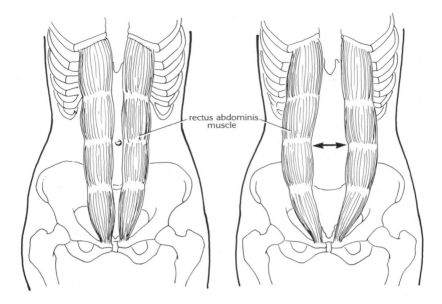

rectus abdominis muscle

Diagram 38   Diastasis Recti

connective tissue begins to relax so that the rectus abdominis muscle can stretch and the abdomen can expand. As the abdomen expands, the rectus abdominis muscle loses some of its ability to keep the spine erect. This, as well as the change in the centre of gravity (see Diagram 37), frequently cause pregnant women to assume a hyperextended posture. Women who have a tendency to stand with their knees locked seem to develop this excessive lordosis most often.

As explained in more detail in Chapter 2, excessive lordosis puts strain on the anterior longitudinal ligament of the spine and the anterior fibres of the discs' annuli, causing the facet joints to become weight-bearing. Either of these conditions can lead to back pain.

But in addition, a vicious circle sometimes results. The problem of excessive lordosis also causes additional strain on the two halves of the rectus abdominis muscle which, in turn, causes even more lordosis.

Most serious of all is a condition called diastasis recti. Diastasis recti sometimes develops when so much strain is placed on the two halves of the rectus abdominis muscle that they not only stretch but also separate. To understand what actually happens, have a look at Diagram 38. "A good analogy of diastasis recti is a zipped-up zipper that has separated in the middle while remaining done up at both ends," says Chris MacHattie.

Neither excessive lordosis nor diastasis recti are inevitable conditions of pregnancy. If you pay attention to your posture and practise pelvic tilt exercises regularly, excessive lordosis and diastasis recti can almost always be prevented. When the pelvis is tilted, lordosis decreases, the baby can be held properly within the pelvic girdle and the abdominal muscles will have to endure less strain. Read Chapter 17 on posture and practise the exercise program (emphasizing pelvic tilt exercises) described in Chapter 16. Eliminate those exercises which require you to lie on your stomach as well as any which you personally find uncomfortable. You may also want to add the exercises described at the end of this chapter, which are especially helpful during pregnancy.

Even if you exercise faithfully, it is a good idea to make sure that you are checked for diastasis recti after you have given birth to your baby. Normally, you will want to get back to a general exercise program as soon as possible after delivery. "If you have had some separation of the rectus abdominis muscles," says Chris MacHattie, who herself experienced this condition when her son was born, "you should avoid sit-ups and any other exercises which will cause the abdominal muscles to contract *isotonically* [see page 158]." Diastasis recti can take anywhere from six weeks to a year to heal although an average is about three months. *Isometric* abdominal strengthening exercises, such as the one described at the end of this chapter, are recommended.

Muscle Spasm

Another condition associated with pregnancy is muscle spasm in the legs as well as in the lower back. Most of the time, muscle spasm can be attributed to poor posture, although inadequate calcium in the diet and poor circulation can also play a role.

A calcium deficiency is simple to correct. Adult females require 700 milligrams to 1,000 milligrams of calcium per day; if you are pregnant, however, this amount should be increased to 1,500 milligrams per day. (While breast-feeding, you require 2,000 milligrams per day.) For foods that are rich in calcium see page 280. To avoid gaining excessive amounts of weight, stick to skim milk, rather than whole milk products.

Finding a way to get relief from the muscle spasm caused by poor circulation is more difficult. Some women find it helpful to sit on the floor with one leg bent and grasp the foot of the straight leg with both hands, bending the toes forcefully upward toward the knee. Others find that placing a hot water bottle, or heating pad, under the cramped muscles for no more than 20 minutes at a time will provide relief. Fiona Rattray, a Toronto massage therapist, suggests that massages during pregnancy can also provide immediate short-term relief from muscle spasm. "It's soothing to have rhythmic pressure applied and released, and massage also helps to remove toxins and built-up lactic acid," she says.

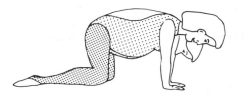

I. CAT STRETCH • The Cat Stretch will gently strengthen your back and neck muscles as well as stretch them out.

Kneel on the floor on your hands and knees keeping your arms straight and your back parallel to the floor. Do not lock the elbow joints. While exhaling, round the back toward the ceiling, pulling the buttocks in and bringing the chin close to the chest. Hold this position for three seconds without inhaling. Now inhale, letting the lumbar spine sink to the horizontal position once again. Exhale and relax. Repeat this exercise a minimum of five times.

A variation of the Cat Stretch is the Spinal Stretch. Assume the Cat Stretch starting position. Inhale. Keeping the back parallel to the floor, exhale and stretch the right leg straight behind, the toes pointed toward the floor and the leg parallel to the floor. Raise the head and look straight ahead. Inhale and return the knee to the floor. Relax and repeat five times. Start again, this time stretching the left leg.

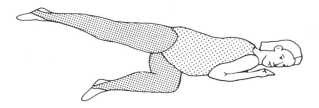

2. SINGLE LEG RAISE • The single leg raise will help to strengthen the abdominal, buttock and thigh muscles while stretching the spine.

Lie on the floor on your left side with the body stretched straight and the right leg on top of the left. Bend the left elbow and rest your head on your left hand. Bend the bottom leg so that the knee is in front of the body thus flexing and protecting the lumbar spine. Assume the pelvic tilt position. Inhale and lift the right leg about three feet off the floor, pulling the toes of the right foot back. Hold for three seconds. Exhale and return the leg to the starting position. Repeat this exercise a minimum of ten times. Turn to lie on your right side and repeat lifting the left leg.

3. INNER THIGH STRETCH • The inner thigh stretch will stretch the thigh muscles and help to align the spine.

Sit on the floor with the legs bent at the knees, the soles of the feet together and the heels as close to the body as possible. Hold on to the toes with your fingers. Inhale and straighten the spine while tilting the pelvis and tightening the buttock muscles. Hold this position to a count of three. Exhale while gently pushing the knees to the floor, keeping the back straight and the pelvis tilted. (It is normal to feel a good stretch along both sides of the spine, as well as the inside of the thigh.) Hold this position for 10 to 30 seconds and then relax. Move the legs and knees up and down for several seconds to relax the muscles and then repeat the exercise a minimum of three times.

Acknowledgements

The back pain sufferers who have shared their experiences have made this book unique. Too numerous to mention, they are the members of the Back Association of Canada, and I am grateful for their support. Their stories appear throughout *Your Guide to Coping with Back Pain*; while the names have been altered to protect their anonymity, the facts are unchanged.

The medical illustrations in this book bring to reality concepts that words alone cannot adequately describe. They are the work of Dorothy Irwin, B.Sc., A.A.M. and her associate Jan Pèrez Vela, A.A.M.

The cartoons of Peter Honor and Susan Goobie first appeared in the Back Association's journal *BACK TO BACK*. They add a touch of humour to *Your Guide to Coping with Back Pain*. The illustrations for specific exercises and proper posture also appeared in *BACK TO BACK*. They are the work of Gill Cameron.

Some of the information in this book appeared in a different form in articles that were prepared for *BACK TO BACK*. I would like to thank the people who contributed to that journal: Dawn Davis, a mystery novelist and recent mother, with Toronto Western Hospital physiotherapist Chris MacHattie: "Pregnancy"; Chris MacHattie with Sandra Svatos, teacher and educational editor: "Scoliosis"; Linda Rosenbaum, Health Promotion Consultant, Toronto Department of Public Health: "Some Practical Advice for Dealing with Health Care Professionals"; Maxine Sidran, a producer for CBC's "Venture": "Microsurgery"; "Addiction"; and much of the research for "The CT Scanner"; "Acupuncture"; and "Chymopapain"; Stan Solomon, a Toronto writer, with Toronto Western Hospital sports medicine physiotherapist Joanne Piccinin: "Sports"; Jacqueline Swartz, a Toronto journalist who writes about health topics for medical journals and the popular press: "Psychiatry"; "Hypnosis"; "Massage"; "Yoga"; "The Alexander Technique"; and much of the research for "Feldenkrais Method"; Hal Tennant, a Toronto journalist who collaborated with Dr. Hamilton Hall on *The Back Doctor*: "Surgery"; and "Myelograms and Discograms", Peter de Vries, a Canadian medical journalist who currently lives in New York City where he writes for *Emergency Medicine*: "Orthopaedic Physicians."

While any errors that may exist in the text are solely my responsibility, I am particularly indebted to four physiotherapists who each reviewed large sections of the manuscript: Margaret Duffy, Judy Flaschner, Chris MacHattie and Joanne

Piccinin. Judy Flaschner is in private practice in Toronto. The others are staff physiotherapists at Toronto Western Hospital.

I am also grateful to the dozens of professionals who agreed to be interviewed in the interest of conquering back pain:

Carl von Baeyer, Ph.D., Clinical Psychologist, Pain Management Service, University Hospital, University of Saskatchewan; Associate Professor of Psychology, University of Saskatchewan; Alan Banack, M.D., Courtesy Staff, Department of Family Medicine, North York General Hospital; Consultant, Department of Plastic Surgery and Burn Unit, Hospital for Sick Children; Teaching Faculty (workshops), Ontario Society for Clinical Hypnosis and American Society for Clinical Hypnosis; David Brunarski, B.Sc., D.C., F.C.C.S.(C), Lecturer, Applied Chiropractic Studies, Canadian Memorial Chiropractic College; J. David Cassidy, D.C., B.Sc., Research Fellow, Department of Orthopedics, University Hospital, University of Saskatchewan; Paul Caulford, B.Sc., M.Sc. (Physiology), M.D., Staff Physician, Toronto East General and Orthopaedic Hospital; M. Cohen-Nehemia, S.T.A.T., Teaching Member, Society of Teachers of the Alexander Technique; Director, The Canadian Centre for the Alexander Technique Ltd.; Founder and Director, The Mitzvah Technique Centre Ltd.; Faculty Member, The Royal Conservatory of Music of Toronto; Wendy Cole, a Toronto yoga instructor; Ian Coulter, Ph.D., President, Canadian Memorial Chiropractic College; Elvio DelZotto, Q.C., President, Tridel Corporation, Toronto; David Drum, D.C., Toronto; Ken Dryden, Youth Commissioner, Province of Ontario; former goalie, Montreal Canadiens; Margaret Duffy, Dip. P.T. (Irl.), Senior Physiotherapist, Department of Rehabilitation Medicine, Toronto Western Hospital; Leonard Faye, D.C., Ottawa; Judy Flaschner, P.T., Toronto; Donald M. Fraser, M.D., F.C.F.P, C.C.F.P., Clinical Assistant Professor of Orthopedics, Faculty of Medicine and Dentistry, University of Rochester, Rochester, N.Y.; President, North American Academy of Manipulative Medicine; Vice President, International Society of Orthopaedic Medicine; Jerry A. Friedman, M.D., F.R.C.P (C), Staff Psychiatrist, Toronto General Hospital; Lecturer, Department of Psychiatry, Faculty of Medicine, University of Toronto; Margarita Gitev, M.D., C.C.F.P, F.R.C.P. (C), Dip., Child Psychiatry; Psychiatric Consultant, Scarborough Board of Education, Ontario; member, Canadian Psychiatric Association; member, American Academy of Child Psychiatry; member, American Society of Clinical Hypnosis; Charles Godfrey, M.A., M.D., F.R.C.P. (C), Director, Department of Rehabilitation Medicine, The Wellesley and Princess Margaret Hospitals; Professor Emeritus, Department of Rehabilitation Medicine, Faculty of Medicine, University of Toronto; Consultant, Department of Rehabilitation Medicine, Sunnybrook Medical Centre; Charles Gold, M.D., F.A.C.O.G., F.R.C.S. (C), Staff Obstetrician/Gynaecologist, Toronto General Hospital; Assistant Professor, Department of Obstetrics and Gynaecology, Faculty of Medicine, University of Toronto; Director, Genesis Research Foundation; Stanley Greben, M.D., F.R.C.P. (C), F.R.C. Psychiatry, F.A.C.P.; Psychiatrist-in-Chief, Mount Sinai Hospital; Professor of Psychiatry and Professor of Psychotherapy, University of Toronto; Diplomat, American Board of Psychiatry and Neurology; Adrian Grice, D.C., F.C.C.S. (C), Professor, Applied Chiropractic Studies, Canadian Memorial Chiropractic College; Hamilton Hall, M.D., F.R.C.S. (C), Associate Professor of Surgery, Faculty of Medicine, University of Toronto; Staff Surgeon, The Orthopedic and Arthritic Hospital; Staff Surgeon, Women's College Hospital; member, International Society for the Study of the Lumbar Spine; Marion Harris, relaxation movement educator, certified teacher of the Feldenkrais Method, Toronto; Don Himes, certified teacher of the Feldenkrais Method, Toronto; Richard C. Holgate, M.D., F.R.C.P. (C), Associate Professor of Radiology and Director of Neuroradiology, Medical University of South Carolina, Charleston, South Carolina; Joseph B. Houpt, M.D., F.R.C.P. (C), Director, Rheumatic Disease Unit and Bone Disease Group, Mount Sinai Hospital; Associate Professor of Medicine, Faculty of Medicine, University of Toronto; Past President, Canadian Rheumatism Association; Brian Howard, D.C., M.B.Ch.B., Resident in Radiology, University of Toronto; J. David Imrie, M.D., Director, Back Care Centre, Toronto; Peter Kogon, D.C., F.C.C.R. (C), D.A.C.B.R., Associate Clinical Professor, Clinical Training, Canadian Memorial Chiropractic College; James Laidlaw, S.T.A.T., member, Canadian Society of Teachers of the F.M. Alexander Technique, Toronto; John Lama, President, Lama Orthopedic Chairs, Toronto; Geoffrey J. Lloyd, M.B., Ch.B., F.R.C.S. (Eng.), F.R.C.S. (C); Staff Surgeon, Toronto Western Hospital; Associate Professor of Surgery, Faculty of Medicine, University of Toronto; Orthopedic Consultant, Hugh McMillan Centre; Director, B.A.R.C. Clinic, Workers' Compensation Board of Ontario; Jeva Lougheed, M.D., F.R.C.P. (C), member, International Society of Hypnosis; member, American Society of Clinical Hypnosis; member, the Society for Clinical & Experimental Hypnosis; member, Canadian Anaesthetists Society; Susan Lucas, R.M.T., Toronto; Kristi Magraw, R.M.T., Toronto; John McCulloch, Associate Professor, Northeastern Ohio Universities College of Medicine; Staff Orthopedic Surgeon, Akron City Hospital, Rootstown, Ohio; member, International Society for the Study of the Lumbar Spine; Angela Hamodraka Mailis, M.D., F.R.C.P. (C), Staff Physician, Department of Rehabilitation Medicine, Toronto Western Hospital; Director, Pain Investigation Unit, Toronto Western Hospital; Lecturer, Department of Rehabilitation Medicine, Faculty of Medicine, University of Toronto; Chris MacHattie, P.T., Staff Physiotherapist, Department of Rehabilitation Medicine, Toronto Western Hospital; Marion McIntosh, M.D., C.C.F.P. Head, Family and Community Medicine, Addiction Research Foundation, Toronto; Rickey Miller, PH.D., Staff Psychologist, Toronto General Hospital; Klaus Minde, M.D., F.R.C.P. (C), Professor of Psychiatry and Pediatrics, Faculty of Medicine, University of Toronto, and Director of Psychiatric Research, The Hospital for Sick Children, Toronto; Timothy Murray, M.D., F.R.C.P. (C), Director, Metabolic Bone Clinic, St. Michael's Hospital; Co-ordinator, Endocrinology and Metabolism, University of Toronto; Professor, Faculty of Medicine, University of Toronto; Chairman, Medical Advisory Board, Osteoporosis Society of Canada; Esther Myers, yoga teacher, Toronto; James Nethercott, M.D., F.R.C.P. (C), Professor and Director, Occupational and Environmental Health, Faculty of Medicine, University of Toronto; Director, Occupational Health Unit, St. Michael's Hospital Toronto; Glenn O'Reilly, Business Development Manager, Travenol Canada Inc., Toronto; Nancy Parker, M.C.S.P., Staff Physiotherapist, Department of Physiotherapy, Ottawa General Hospital; Joanne Piccinin, P.T., Senior Physiotherapist, (sports medicine specialist), Department of Rehabilitation Medicine, Toronto Western Hospital; Carolyn Posen, B.Sc., Phm., Toronto; Linda Rapson, M.D., Director of Education, Acupuncture Foundation of Canada; Marcel Reux, P.T., student, Canadian Memorial Chiropractic College; Robert Rickover, S.T.A.T., teaching member, Society of Teachers of the Alexander Technique; member, American Association for the Alexander Technique; Frank Roberts, President, Obus Forme Ltd., Toronto; Gail Robinson,

291

M.D., F.R.C.P. (C), Staff Psychiatrist, Toronto General Hospital; Associate Professor of Psychiatry, Faculty of Medicine, University of Toronto; Ken Saito, Shiatsu Dohjoh, Toronto; Ahmed Sakoor, M.D., L.R.C.P. & S. I., L.M.C.C., Family Physician, Raxlen Clinic, Toronto; Hart Schutz, M.D., F.R.C.S. (C), Assistant Professor of Neurosurgery, Faculty of Medicine, University of Toronto; Staff Surgeon, Toronto Western Hospital and Mississauga Hospital; Michael L. Schwartz, M.Sc, M.D., F.R.C.S. (C), Staff Neurosurgeon, Sunnybrook Medical Centre; Assistant Professor of Neurosurgery, Faculty of Medicine, University of Toronto; member, Canadian Neurosurgical Society and American Association of Neurological Surgeons; founding member, Trauma Association of Canada; Geoffrey Squires, B.Sc., Phm., Product Manager, Ayerst Laboratories, Montreal; J. David Stewart, B.Sc., M.D., D.E.C.H, C.C.F.P., Medical Director, Department of Occupational Health and Safety, Sunnybrook Medical Centre; Director, Occupational Health and Safety, CBC; Christine Sutherland, R.M.T., Director of Education, Sutherland-Chan School and Teaching Clinic, Toronto; J.C. (Carl) Sutton, Jr., M.D., F.R.C.S. (C), Director of Orthopedic Surgery, St. Mary's Hospital, Montreal; Associate Professor of Surgery, McGill University, Montreal; Allan G. Swayze, M.D., D.Psych., F.R.C.P. (C), Associate Psychiatrist-in-Chief, Women's College Hospital; Co-ordinator, Psychosocial Support Team, High Risk Obstetrical Service, Women's College Hospital; Associate Professor of Psychiatry, Faculty of Medicine, University of Toronto; Associate Staff Psychiatrist, Toronto General Hospital; Ronald R. Tasker, M.D., F.R.C.S. (C), Head, Division of Neurosurgery, Toronto General Hospital; Professor of Surgery, Faculty of Medicine, University of Toronto; council member, American Society for Stereotactic and Functional Neurosurgery; council member, International Association for the Study of Pain; Marvin Tile, M.D., B.Sc. (Med), F.R.C.S. (C), Deputy Surgeon-in-Chief, Sunnybrook Medical Centre; Professor of Surgery, Faculty of Medicine, University of Toronto; President-Elect, International Society for the Study of the Lumbar Spine; member, Canadian and American Orthopedic Associations; Paul Waitzer, President, The T. Milburn Company Limited, Toronto; George Wortzman, M.D., F.R.C.P. (C), Radiologist-in-Chief, Mount Sinai Hospital; Professor of Radiology, Faculty of Medicine, University of Toronto.

I would also like to thank the following people and institutions for their permission to use the following illustrations and photographs: Prof. Dr. Med. Hanns Schoberth, staff physician, Ostseeklinic, Damp, West Germany, for the illustration on page 180 from *Correct Sitting at the Workplace*; The Canadian Society of Teachers of the F.M. Alexander Technique for the use of their photograph, page 218; *Spine Magazine*, Harper & Row Publishers Inc. and Dr. Alf Nachemson, professor of orthopaedic surgery, Göteborgs Universited, Göteborg, Sweden, for the use of the illustration on page 42, which has been reproduced from the March 1976 issue of *Spine*; J. David Cassidy and the *Journal of Manipulative and Physiological Therapeutics* for permission to reprint the photographs on page 198, which appeared in *J.M.P.T.*, Vol. 2, 1979, in the article "Motion Examination of the Lumbar Spine" by Dr. Cassidy.

I would also like to express my gratitude to my literary agent Beverley Slopen and the Back Association of Canada's secretary Sharlene Samuel, who provided encouragement and support during the years it took to complete this book.

Bibliography

BOOKS

Altman, Nathaniel. *The Chiropractic Alternative*. Los Angeles: J.P. Tarcher, 1981.
American Medical Association. *The American Medical Association Book of Back Care*. New York: Random House, 1982.

Berkeley Holistic Health Center. *The Holistic Health Handbook*. Berkeley: AND/OR PRESS, 1978.
Bonica, John J., ed. *Pain*. New York: Raven Press, 1973.
Brecher, E.M. et al., eds. *Licit & Illicit Drugs*. Boston: Little, Brown, 1972.

Cheng, Richard Shing Sou. *Mechanisms of Electroacupuncture Analgesia as Related to Endorphins and Monoamines; An Intricate System Is Proposed*. Toronto: University of Toronto, 1980.
Cyriax, James. *Manipulation: past and present*. London: Heinemann, 1975.
————. *The Slipped Disc*. Epping: Gower, 1980.

Delvin, David. *You and Your Back*. London: Pan Books, 1977.
Duke, Marc. *Acupuncture*. New York: Pyramid House, 1972.

Feldenkrais, Moshe. *Awareness Through Movement*. New York: Harper & Row, 1972.
————. *The Potent Self*. New York: Harper & Row, 1985.
Fine, Judylaine. *Afraid to Ask: A Book About Cancer*. Toronto: Kids Can Press, 1984.
Francis, Carl C. *Introduction to Human Anatomy*. Saint Louis: C.V. Mosby, 1973.
Friedmann, Lawrence W., and Galton, Lawrence. *Freedom from Backaches*. New York: Simon and Schuster, 1973.

Genant, Harry K., ed. *Spine Update 1984: Perspectives in Radiology, Orthopaedic Surgery, and Neurosurgery*. San Francisco: Radiology Research and Education Foundation, 1984.
Graedon, Joe. *The People's Pharmacy*. New York: Avon, 1976.
Guyton, Arthur C. *Basic Human Physiology: Normal Function and Mechanisms of Disease*. Philadelphia: W.B. Saunders, 1971.
————. *Function of the Human Body*. Philadelphia: W.B. Saunders, 1969.

293

Hafen, Brent Q., and Frandsen, Kathryn, J. *From Acupuncture to Yoga*. Englewood Cliffs, N.J.: Prentice-Hall, 1983.

Haldeman, Scott, ed. *Modern Developments in the Principles and Practice of Chiropractic*. New York: Appleton-Century-Crofts, 1980.

Hall, Hamilton. *The Back Doctor*. Toronto: Macmillan, 1980.

Imrie, David. *Goodbye Backache*. Toronto: Prentice-Hall/Newcastle, 1983.

Inglis, Brian. *The Book of the Back*. New York: Hearst Books, 1978.

Jones, Frank Pierce. *Body Awareness in Action: A Study of the Alexander Technique*. New York: Schocken, 1976.

Keim, Hugo, A. *How to Care for Your Back*. Englewood Cliffs, N.J.: Prentice-Hall, 1981.

Kelner, Merrijoy; Hall, Oswald; and Coulter, Ian. *Chiropractors: Do They Help?*. Toronto: Fitzhenry & Whiteside, 1980.

Klein, Arthur C., and Sobel, Dava. *Backache Relief*. New York: Times Books, 1985.

Kogun, Gerald, ed. *Your Body Works*. Berkeley: Transformations Press, 1980.

Kurland, Howard D. *Back Pains: Quick Relief Without Drugs*. New York: Simon and Schuster, 1981.

Leach, Robert A. *The Chiropractic Theories: A Synopsis of Scientific Research*. Mississippi: Mid-South Scientific Publishers, 1980.

LeCron, Leslie M. *The Complete Guide to Hypnosis*. New York: Harper & Row, 1971.

Levin, Arthur, ed. *Health Services: The Local Perspective*. New York: The Academy of Political Science, 1977.

Levine, David B. *The Painful Low Back*. New York: P W Communications, 1979.

Long, James. *The Essential Guide to Prescription Drugs*. New York: Harper & Row, 1982.

Macnab, Ian. *Bachache*. Baltimore: Williams & Wilkins, 1977.

Melzack, Ronald, and Wall, Patrick. *The Challenge of Pain*. Harmondsworth: Penguin, 1982.

Notelovitz, Morris, and Ware, Marsha. *Stand Tall!: Every Woman's Guide to Preventing Osteoporosis*. Toronto: Bantam, 1985.

Pribram, Karl H., ed. *Mood, States and Mind*. Harmondsworth: Penguin, 1969.

Root, Leon, and Kiernan, Thomas. *Oh, My Aching Back*. New York: Signet, 1975.

Rothenberg, Robert E. *The Complete Surgical Guide*. New York: Signet, 1974.

Silverman, Harold, and Simon, Gilbert. *The Pill Book*. New York: Bantam, 1979.

Smith, Adam. *Powers of Mind*. New York: Summit Books, 1982.

Stoddard, Alan. *The Back: Relief from Pain*. Toronto: Prentice-Hall, 1979.

Taylor, Malcolm G. *Health Insurance and Canadian Public Policy*. Montreal: Queen's University Press, 1978.

Thomas, Lewis. *The Lives of a Cell*. New York: Viking, 1974.

———— *The Youngest Science: Notes of a Medicine-Watcher*. New York: Bantam, 1984.

Weil, Andrew. *Health and Healing*. Boston: Houghton Mifflin, 1983.

Weisenberg, Matisyohu, ed. *Pain: Clinical and Experimental Perspectives*. Saint Louis: C.V. Mosby, 1975.

White, Augustus A. III. *Your Aching Back*. Toronto: Bantam, 1983.

Wilcox, L. DeWitt. *Where Is My Doctor?*. Toronto: Fitzhenry & Whiteside, 1977.

Wong, Joseph, and Cheng, Richard. *The Science of Acupuncture Therapy*. Toronto: Acupuncture Foundation of Canada, n.d.

Zauner, Renate. *Speaking of: Backaches*. New York: Consolidated, 1978.

Zebroff, Kareen. *Back Fitness the Yoga Way*. Vancouver: Fforbez Publications, 1982.

PERIODICALS

Agre, Karl et al. "Chymodiactin Postmarketing Surveillance." *Spine*, Vol. 9, No. 5:485 (September, 1984).

Arato, Rona. "Smoothed Out: Why Ergonomics Makes the Living Easy." *The Financial Post Magazine:* 32-34 (January 1, 1985).

Ayerst Laboratories. "Treating Your Disc Problem: The Chemonucleolysis Decision." *Ayerst Laboratories* (1984).

Barbor, Ronald. "Sclerosant Therapy." From the proceedings of *Reunion Sobre Patologia de la Columina Vertebral*, Murcia, Spain (March 30, 1977).

Barnes, Colin G. "The differential diagnosis of backache." *British Journal of Hospital Medicine:* 219-231 (February, 1971).

Bell, Gordon R. et al. "A Study of Computer-Assisted Tomography," *Spine*, Vol. 9, No. 6:552-556 (June, 1984).

Bernhang, Arthur M. "Equestrian Injuries." *The Physician and Sports Medicine*, Vol. 11, No. 1:90-97 (January, 1983).

Berson, Burton L. "An epidemiological study of squash injuries." *American Journal of Sports Medicine*, Vol. 9, No. 2:103-106 (1981).

Birrer, Richard et al. "Injuries in Tae Kwon Do." *The Physician and Sportsmedicine*, Vol. 9, No. 2:97-103 (February, 1981).

————. "Martial Arts Injuries." *The Physician and Sportsmedicine*, Vol. 10, No. 6:102-108 (June, 1982).

Boeckh, Sherry. "Paying Pain's Price." *The Financial Post Magazine:* 25-30 (June, 1979).

Botta, Joseph R. "Chiropractors: Healers or Quacks?" *Consumer Reports* (2 Parts):542-547 and 606-610 (September and October, 1975).

Brady, Thomas A. et al. "Weight training-related injuries in the high school athlete." *The American Journal of Sports Medicine*, Vol. 10, No. 1:1-5 (1982).

Bromley, John W. et al. "Double-Blind Evaluation of Collagenase Injections for Herniated Lumbar Discs." *Spine*, Vol. 9, No. 5:486-487 (September, 1984).

Brower, Brock. "Oh, My Aching Back: You don't die from back problems – it isn't that easy." *Esquire:*101-102, 134, 136 (November, 1980).

Brown, John R. "Low Back Pain Syndrome: Its Etiology and Prevention." *Ontario Ministry of Labour, Labour Safety Council* (1977).

Bullock, Carole. "From the Pain Clinics' Pain Clinic, the Word: Get Them Functioning." *Medical Tribune:* 1, 16-17 (March 28, 1984).

Cassidy, J. David et al. "Manipulative management of back pain in patients with spondylolisthesis." *The Journal of the Canadian Chiropractic Association:*15-20 (March, 1978).

————. "Motion Examination of the Lumbar Spine." *Journal of Manipulative and Physiological Therapeutics,* Vol. 2, No. 3:151-158 (September, 1979).

Clarke, Kenneth S. et al. "Women's injuries in collegiate sports." *The American Journal of Sports Medicine,* Vol. 8, No. 3:187-191 (March, 1980).

Day, Nancy Raines. "Neck Owner's Manual." *Patient Information Library,* Daly City, California (1981).

Deburge, A. et al. "The Diagnosis of Disc Sequestration." *Spine,* Vol. 9, No. 5:496-499 (September, 1984).

Deyo, Richard A. "Chymopapain for Herniated Intervertebral Disc." *Spine,* Vol. 9, No. 5:474-478 (September, 1984).

Dowling, Patrick. "Prospective study of injuries in United States Ski Association freestyle skiing – 1976-77 to 1979-80." *The American Journal of Sports Medicine,* Vol. 10, No. 5:268-275 (1982).

Dupuis, Pierre R. "Radiologic Diagnosis of Degenerative Lumbar Spinal Instability." *Spine,* Vol. 10, No. 3:262-276 (March, 1985).

Dvorine, William. "Kendo: A Safer Martial Art." *The Physician and Sportsmedicine,* Vol. 7, No. 12:87-89 (December, 1979).

Eagle, Robert. "A pain in the back." *New Scientist:*170-173 (October 18, 1979).

Ende, Leigh S. et al. "Ballet Injuries." *The Physician and Sportsmedicine,* Vol. 10, No. 7:101-118 (July, 1982).

Feldenkrais, Moshe. "Self-Fulfillment Through Organic Learning." *Journal of Holistic Health,* Vol. 7:27-34 (1982).

Feriencik, Kazimir. "Trends in Ice Hockey Injuries: 1965 to 1977." *The Physician and Sportsmedicine,* Vol. 7, No. 2:81-83 (February, 1979).

Ferkel, Richard D. et al. "An analysis of roller skating injuries." *The American Journal of Sports Medicine,* Vol. 10, No. 1 (1982).

Ferstle, Jim. "Figure Skating: In Search of the Winning Edge." *The Physician and Sportsmedicine,* Vol. 7, No. 2:129-133 (February, 1979).

Gainor, Barry J. et al. "The throw: biomechanics and acute injury." *The American Journal of Sports Medicine,* Vol. 8, No. 2:114-118 (1980).

Garrick, James G. "Epidemiology of women's gymnastics injuries." *The American Journal of Sports Medicine,* Vol. 8, No. 4:261-264 (1980).

Gelabert, Raoul. "Preventing Dancers' Injuries." *The Physician and Sportsmedicine,* Vol. 8, No. 4:69-76 (April, 1980).

Godfrey, Charles M. et al. "A Randomized Trial of Manipulation for Low-Back Pain in a Medical Setting." *Spine,* Vol. 9, No. 3:301-304 (September, 1984).

Goldstein, Murray, ed. "The Research Status of Spinal Manipulative Therapy." NINCDS Monograph no. 15, *National Institutes of Health, Department of Health, Education and Welfare,* Bethesda, Maryland (1975).

Graham, Mrs. Duncan. "Canadian Physiotherapy Association: An Historical Sketch." *Canadian Physiotherapy Journal:*9-13 (November, 1939).

Gray, Charlotte. "New Ways to Win the War on Chronic Pain." *Chatelaine:* 52, 92-108 (June, 1981).

Gunby, Phil. "Chymopapain: Tropical tree to surgical suite." *Journal of the American Medical Association,* Vol. 249, No. 9:1115, 1119-1123 (March 4, 1983).

Henry, Jack H. et al. "The injury rate in professional basketball." *The American Journal of Sports Medicine,* Vol. 10, No. 1:16-18 (1982).
Holmes, Bruce. "Moving Well with Feldenkrais." *Yoga Journal:* 30-32 (January/February, 1984).
Howell, Damien W. "Musculoskeletal profile and incidence of musculoskeletal injuries in lightweight women rowers." *The American Journal of Sports Medicine,* Vol. 12, No. 4:278-282 (1984).

The Industrial Accident Prevention Association of Ontario. "Industrial Ergonomics." *The Industrial Accident Prevention Association of Ontario* (1982).

Jessell, Thomas M. "Pain." *The Lancet:*1084-1087 (November 13, 1982).

Kirkaldy-Willis, W.H., and Cassidy, J. David. "Spinal Manipulation in the Treatment of Low-Back Pain." *Canadian Family Physician,* Vol. 31:535-540 (March, 1985).
Korr, Irwin M. "The spinal cord as organizer of disease processes: II. The peripheral autonomic nervous system." *Journal of the American Osteopathic Association,* Vol. 79, No. 2:82-90 (October, 1979).
Kruse, Diana L. et al. "Bicycle accidents and injuries." *The American Journal of Sports Medicine,* Vol. 8, No. 5:342-344 (1980).
Kulund, Daniel N. et al. "Tennis injuries: prevention and treatment." *The American Journal of Sports Medicine,* Vol. 7, No. 4:249-253 (1979).
Kurland, Harvey L. "A Comparison of Judo and Aikido Injuries." *The Physician and Sportsmedicine,* Vol. 8, No. 6:71-74 (June, 1980).
————. "Injuries in Karate." *The Physician and Sportsmedicine,* Vol. 8, No. 10:80-85 (October, 1980).
Kvidera, Dennis J. et al. "Trauma on eight wheels: A study of roller skating injuries in Seattle." *The American Journal of Sports Medicine,* Vol. 11, No. 1:38-41 (1983).

Lowry, Cathy Benton et al. "A retrospective study of gymnastics injuries to competitors and noncompetitors in private clubs." *The American Journal of Sports Medicine,* Vol. 10, No. 4:237-239 (1982).
Lyons, John W. "Cross-Country Ski Injuries." *The Physician and Sportsmedicine,* Vol. 8, No. 1:65-71 (January, 1980).

Maitland, G.D. "The Treatment of Joints by Passive Movement." *Australian Journal of Physiotherapy,* Vol. XVIV, No. 2: 65-72 (June, 1973).
McCall, Iain et al. "Induced Pain Referral from Posterior Lumbar Elements in Normal Subjects." *Spine,* Vol. 4, No. 5: 441-446 (September/October, 1979).

Maravilla, Kenneth R. et al. "Magnetic Resonance Imaging of the Lumbar Spine with CT Correlation." *American Journal of Neuroradiology:*237-345 (March/April, 1985).
McKay, D.H. "Downhill Skiing Injuries." *The Physician and Sportsmedicine,* Vol. 9, No. 1:105-116 (January, 1981).
Micheli, Lyle J. "Low back pain in the adolescent: differential diagnosis." *The American Journal of Sports Medicine,* Vol. 7, No. 6:362-366 (1979).

297

Mior, Silvano A. et al. "Lateral nerve root entrapment: pathological, clinical and manipulative considerations." *Journal of the Canadian Chiropractic Association,* Vol. 26, No. 1:13-20 (March, 1982).

Mostardi, Richard A. "Musculoskeletal and Cardiopulmonary Characteristics of the Professional Ballet Dancer." *The Physician and Sportsmedicine,* Vol. 11, No. 12:53-60 (December, 1983).

Mueller, Frederick O. et al. "Football Injury Update – 1979 Season." *The Physician and Sportsmedicine,* Vol. 8, No. 10:53-55 (October, 1980).

Nathan, P.W. "The Gate Control Theory of Pain: A Critical Review." *Brain:*123-158 (1976).

Olson, O. Charles. "The Spokane Study: High School Football Injuries." *The Physician and Sportsmedicine,* Vol. 7, No. 12:75-82 (December, 1979).

Paris, Stanley V. "Mobilization of the Spine." *Physical Therapy,* Vol. 59, No. 8:988-995 (August, 1979).

Pedegana, Larry R. "Waterskiing Injuries." *The Physician and Sportsmedicine,* Vol. 7, No. 6:109-114 (June, 1979).

Rapson, Linda M. "Acupuncture: a Useful Treatment Modality." *Canadian Family Physician,* Vol. 30: 109-115 (January, 1984).

Requa, Ralph. "Injuries in interscholastic wrestling." *The Physician and Sportsmedicine,* Vol. 9, No. 4:44-91 (April, 1981).

Rosenfeld, Albert. "Teaching the body how to program the brain is Moshe's 'miracle'." *Smithsonian,* Vol. 22, No. 10 (January, 1981).

Rothman, Richard H. "Introduction: A Study of Computer-Assisted Tomography." *Spine,* Vol. 9, No. 6:548 (June, 1984).

Simmons, James W. "Chemonucleolysis: An Alternative to Back Surgery." *Spinal Column,* Vol. 1, No. 1:7, 13 (Fall, 1983).

Sinclair, G.B. "Nature's Opiates." *Saturday Night:* 15-16 (March, 1981).

Smith, Angela D. et al. "Injuries in Competitive Figure Skaters." *The Physician and Sportsmedicine,* Vol. 10, No. 1:36-47 (January, 1982).

Snook, George A. "Injuries in women's gymnastics: A 5-year study." *The American Journal of Sports Medicine,* Vol. 7, No. 4:242-244 (1979).

———. "A survey of wrestling injuries." *The American Journal of Sports Medicine,* Vol. 8, No. 6:450-453 (1980).

Standish, William. "Low back pain in middle-aged athletes." *The American Journal of Sports Medicine,* Vol. 7, No. 6:367-369 (1979).

Stanitski, Carl L. "Low Back Pain in Young Athletes." *The Physician and Sportsmedicine,* Vol. 10, No. 10:77-91 (October, 1982).

Stark, Elizabeth. "Breaking the Pain Habit." *Psychology Today:*31-36 (May, 1985).

Sullivan, J. Andy et al. "Evaluation of injuries in youth soccer." *The American Journal of Sports Medicine,* Vol. 8, No. 5:325-327 (1980).

Szajman, Rena. "Exercise and Pregnancy." *Great Expectations:*54-58 (January, 1983).

Talmi, Alon. "Notes on Functional Integration." *Somatics:*19-20 (Fall/Winter, 1982).

Terrett, Allen C.J. et al. "A Controlled Study of the Effect of Spinal Manipulation on Paraspinal Cutaneous Pain Tolerance Levels." *American Journal of Physical Medicine:* 217-225 (October, 1984).

Touflexis, Anastasia. "That Aching Back." *Time:*24-30 (July 14, 1980).

Waddell, Gordon et al. "Assessment of Severity in Low-Back Disorders." *Spine,* Vol. 9, No. 2:204-208 (September, 1984).

Wallis, Claudia et al. "Unlocking Pain's Secrets." *Time:* 60-70 (June 11, 1984).

Wiesel, Sam W. et al. "A Study of Computer-Assisted Tomography." *Spine,* Vol. 9, No. 6:549-551 (June, 1984).

Zelisko, John A. "A comparison of men's and women's professional basketball injuries." *The American Journal of Sports Medicine,* Vol. 10, No. 5:297-299 (1982).

Index

Numbers of pages on which illustrations occur are in italic.

Abdominal muscles, *26*, 26-27, 170-71, 284
  strengthening of, 157, 161, 167-71, 182, 227
Acetaminophen, 82-83
Acupuncture, 69, 71, 78, 138-44, 148-49
  electroacupuncture, 142
Acupuncture Foundation of Canada, 139-40, 144
Adaptive shortening, 35, 147, 161
Addiction to drugs, 79-85
Adhesion, 39-40, 42, 124, 212
ADL (Activities of Daily Living), 146
Aerobics, 244-45
Aging process, 31-33, 274
Alexander, A.R., 221
Alexander, F. Matthias, 217, *218*, 219-20, 223
Alexander Technique, 11-12, 217-23
Alexander Trust Fund School, 219, 220
Alignment of spine, 12, 35, *44*, 226
Anaphylactic reaction, 126
Anatomy of back, 17-30
Ankylosing spondylitis (Marie-Strumpell Disease), *52*, 52-53, 94
Annulus fibrosus, *22*, 32, 37-43, *37*, 125, 133, 147, 185-86
Anxiety. *See* Stress
Apophyseal joint. *See* Facet joint
Apothecary, 200
Aquabics, 245
Arthritis (arthritic changes), 10, 33-34, *33*, 48-50, 53
  osteo———, 10, 33-34, *33*, 48-49, 53, 92
  osteophyte, 32-34, *33*, 37, 43, 45, 48-50, 90, 92, 114, 120
  rheumatoid, 34, 53
Articular process, *19*, *20*, 21
Asana, 224, 225
Aspirin, 82-83
Atlas, 19, 264, 265, *265*
Axis, 19, 264, 265, *265*
Ayerst Laboratories, 129

Babinski Sign test, 96
Back Association of Canada, 11
Back Doctor, The, 117, 122
Back. *See also* Spinal canal; Spinal cord; Spine
  ache. *See* Diagnosis of back pain; Pain; *see also specific treatments for*

anatomy of, 17-30
muscles, strengthening of, 161, 171-72, 173-74
Backrests, 185
  Obus Forme, 175, *176*
Back Store, The, 176
Back support (brace), 136, 259, 262
BACK TO BACK, 11
Badminton, 245-46
von Baeyer, Dr. Carl, 70
Ballet, 246
Ballroom dancing, 246
Bamboo spine. *See* Ankylosing spondylitis
Banack, Dr. Alan, 209
Barometric pressure, 47-48, 72
Baseball, 246-47
Basketball, 247
Baxter-Travenol Laboratories (Travenol Canada), 128
Bed rest, 13, 91, 93, 111
Beds, 183-84
  water———, 184
Blood tests, 76, 91
Blood vessels, 150
Blount, Dr. Walter, 259
Body awareness, 12. *See also* Alexander Technique; Feldenkrais Method; Massage; Yoga
Bone, 273
  cancellous, 273
  cortical, 273
  mass, 271, 274, 276-77, 278
  osteoblasts, 273, 274
  osteoclasts, 273
Bone scan, 93
Bone-setters, 200
Bone spur. *See* Osteophyte
Bonica, Dr. John, 61, 68-69, 149
Bowling, 244, 247
Boxing, 248
Brace, back, 136, 259, 262
Braid, Dr. James, 207
Brain, 46-47, 62-66, 68, 72, 108, 143
  cerebral cortex of, 62-66, 72
  thalamus of, 62-63, 66
Brandykinon, 65-66, 68
Break dancing, 248
British Medical Association, 207
Brunarski, Dr. David, 203
Bulging disc. *See* Disc

CADUCEUS, 129
Calcium, 273, 274-75, 276, 277, 279, 282-83

Canadian Hypnosis Society
  B.C. Division, 211
  Ontario Society of Clinical Hypnosis, 211
  Saskatchewan Society of Clinical
    Hypnosis, 211
Canadian Medical Association, 79
Canadian Memorial Chiropractic College,
  192, 195, 203
Cancellous bone. *See* Bone
Cancer, 56
  of the spine, 56
Canoeing, 253
Cassidy, Dr. David, 193, 196, 198, 200,
  203
Cauda equina, *29*, 30
Caudal epidural block, 131, 134-35
Caulford, Dr. Paul, 195
Cavitation, 193
Cerebral cortex, 62-66, 72
Cervical collar, 268-69, 270
Cervical spine, 17, 28, 264, 265, 266
Chairs, 178-80
  dimensions for, 179, 180, *180*
  Lama Orthopedic, 175, *178*
  proper posture in, 178, 180
Chemonucleolysis, 128
Cheng, Dr. Richard, 143
Chiropractic (chiropractors), 36, 70, 134,
  191-204
Chiropractors: Do They Help?, 192, 194
Chymodiactin, 129
Chymopapain, 39, 124-30, 136
Clinical examination. *See* Diagnosis
Coccyx, 17-19, *18*
Cohen, Nehemia, 220
Cold packs, 149, 171
Cole, Wendy, 226, 227-28
Communication, importance of, 154
  with children, 154-55
  with health care professionals, 12-13,
    73-78
Conus medularis, 28
Cool-down, after exercising, 158, 242
Correct Sitting at the Workplace, 179
Cortical bone. *See* Bone
Coulter, Dr. Ian, 192, 202, 203
Crelin, E.S., 201
CT (CAT) Scan. *See* Diagnostic tests
Curling, 248
Curvature of spine. *See* Kyphosis;
  Lordosis; Scoliosis
Cycling, 160, 248
Cyriax, Dr. James, 132, 134, 237

Darvon, 84
Degeneration of spine, 31-34, 36-37,
  40-48, 51, 267
Depression, 69, 82, 152-53
Desks, 179

Diagnosis of back pain, 9-10, 42-43, 53,
  75-76, 89-98, 99-110, 137, 145, 194
  clinical, 10, 43, 70, 91, 93-97, 107, 124,
    132-33
Diagnostic test(s), 14, 55
  blood tests, 76, 91
  bone scan, 93
  CT (CAT) Scan, 39, 49, 76, 90, 94, 97,
    99-104, *100*, 112-13, 124, 126
  caudal epidural block as a, 134
  discogram, 39, 43, 55, 99, 101, 104-10,
    125
  myelogram, 39, 43, 55, 90, 99-110,
    105, 124-26
  nerve conduction, 266
  SLR (Straight Leg Raising), 96, 124
  urine sample, 91
  X-rays, 10, 42-43, 70, 76, 90-91, 94, 97,
    132, 192, 197, 198, *198*
Diet
  as a cause of osteoporosis, 274-75
  during pregnancy, 282-83
Disc(s), intervertebral, 9-10, 17, *19*, *20*,
  22, *37*, *41*, *44*
  annulus fibrosis of, *22*, 32, 37-43, *37*,
    125, 133, 147, 185-86
  bulging (protruding), 40-43, *41*, 109,
    131, 134, 147, 150
  degeneration of, 10, 31-34, 36, *44*
  hard disc problem, 133
  herniation of, 36-40, *39*, 42-43, 90,
    92-97, 104-06, 111-15, *113*, 119-20,
    124-30, 134, 147
  narrowing of, 37
  nerve to, 28, *39*
  nucleus pulposus of, *22*, 30, 36-43,
    113, 114, 125, 133
  numbering system for, 21
  sequestration of, 38-39, *39*, *113*, 114,
    119, 147
  "slipped," 38 (*see also* Disc(s),
    herniation of)
  soft disc problem, 133
Discase, 128
Discogram. *See* Diagnostic tests
Discotomy. *See* Surgery
Diving, 249
Dorsal horn, 63-65, *64*
Drugless Practitioners Act, 202
Drugs, 68, 71, 79-85
  addiction to, 79-85
  analgesic (pain-killer), 61, 67, 79, 82, 83,
    139-40
  anti-inflammatory, 53, 67, 82-83
  list of, 83-85
  muscle relaxant, 80, 84
  non-prescription, 82
  prescription, 61. *See also specific*
    names

Drum, Dr. David, 194, 196, 197, 199
Dryden, Ken, 251
Duffy, Margaret, 11, 158, 159, 160, 170, 175, 267, 268
Dura mater, 28, 30, 133, 135, 172

Emotional component of back pain, 61-64, 66, 70-72, 153-55
Endorphins, 12, 67-69, 143, 149, 155
Enkephalins, 67-68, 143, 149, 155
Essential Guide to Prescription Drugs, The, 82
Estrogen, 275-76
  use of for osteoporosis, 277-78
Exercise machines, 249
Exercise(s), 76, 157-74, 213, 263. *See also* Sports
  cooling down, importance of, 158, 242
  hamstring stretch, 162-65
  hip flexor stretch, 165-67
  importance of, 36, 97, 157-61, 274, 277, 279
  isometric, 158
  isotonic, 158
  lactic acid build-up during, 157-58, 205
  low back extension stretch, 173
  low back stretch, 171-72
  pain and, 158, 159-60, 171
  pelvic tilt, 45, 158, 165, 167-70, 182
  sit-up, 157, 170-71, 227
  small muscle group strengthener, 173-74
  strengthening, 157-58, 160-71, 171-74, 227
  stretching, 157-58, 160-73, 227, 241-42
  warming up, importance of, 157, 160, 241-42
Extension. *See also* Lordosis
  hyper——— (hyperlordosis), 35-36, 45-48, 93, 147, 158, 161, 173, 181-82, 183, 226, 244, *284*, 285

Facet, *19*
Facet joint, *19*, *21*, 24, 32-36, 43-48, *44*, 50, 76, 93-95, 134
  alignment of, 35-36, 43-48, *44*
  capsule of, *21*, 36, 47-48, 147
  ligaments as support for, 23, 36
  manipulation of, 150, 193-94, 196, 199, 200, 267
  mobilization of, 150-51, 268
  nerve to, 28
  stiff (hypomobile), 193, 197, 199
  strained, 35-36, 45-48, 160
  synovial fluid of, 47, 193
  unstable (hypermobile), 32, 134, 147, 196, 197
Feldenkrais Method, 11-12, 230-38, *233*
Feldenkrais, Moshe, 11, 230, 231, 232, 234, 235-36, 237

Figure skating, 252
Flaschner, Judy, 145, 146, 147, 148, 151
Flexibility, importance of, 161, 227
Flexion, 243
  hyper———, 42, 243
Football, 249-50
Footstools, 175, *177*, 179, 182
Foramen, intervertebral, *19*, 21, 28, *44*, 105, 114
Fracture, 271-72
  hip, 272
Fraser, Dr. Donald, 131-37
Freud, Dr. Sigmund, 207
Friedman, Dr. Jerry, 153-54, 156
Fusion. *See* Surgery

Gate Control Theory of Pain, 62-63, 65, 67-68, 143
General practitioners, 73-77, 91
Genetic propensity toward back pain, 38
Gitev, Dr. Margarita, 205, 206
Goald, Dr. Harold, 123
Godfrey, Dr. Charles, 204
Gold, Dr. Charles, 274, 277
Goldstein, Dr. Murray, 191, 204
Golf, 250
Gravity, 22
Greben, Dr. Stanley, 12, 152-53
Grice, Dr. Adrian, 12
Gymnastics, 244, 250-51

Hall, Dr. Hamilton, 117, 122
Harris, Marion, 233-34
Hatha yoga, 224
Healthcare professionals, how to deal with, 13, 73-78
Heat, treatment with, 67, 149
Herniated disc. *See* Disc
Himes, Don, 234
Hip, 272, 273
  flexor muscles, 165
Hockey, 251
Holgate, Dr. Richard, 105-09
Holistic approach to treatment of back pain. *See* Alexander Technique; Chiropractic; Feldenkrais Method; Hypnosis; Massage; Yoga
Holmes, Bruce, 231, 234
Horseback riding, 251-52
Hot packs, 67, 149
Hounsfield, Dr. Geoffery, 101
Houpt, Dr. Joseph, 276
Hughes, Dr. John, 68
Hyperlordosis. *See* Lordosis
Hypermobility, 32, 134, 147, 196, 197
Hypnosis, 11-12, 72, 78, 205-11
Hypomobility, 193, 197, 199

Ice, treatment with, 149, 171
Ice skating, 252

Innate Intelligence, 201
Instability of facet joint. See Facet joint
Interferential current, 149-50
International Society of Orthopaedic
  Medicine, 136-37
Intervertebral disc. See Disc
Intervertebral foramen. See Foramen

Jogging, 69, 252-53
Joint. See Facet joint; Sacroiliac joint
Jones, Frank Pierce, 221

Kayaking, 254
Kirkaldy-Willis, Dr. W.H., 200, 203
Knudsen, George, 250
Kosterlitz, Dr. Hans, 68
Kyphosis, 17, 18, 93

Laidlaw, James, 222
Lama, John, 175
Lama Orthopedic Chair, 175, 178
Lamina, 20, 119
Laughter, 69
Lifting. See Posture
Ligaments, 17, 23, 35-36, 51
  adaptive shortening of, 35, 147, 161
  anterior longitudinal, 23, 35, 46
  laxity of, 32, 35-36, 97, 135, 161
  interspinous, 23, 35
  ligamentum flavum (yellow ligament),
    23, 35
  posterior longitudinal, 23, 30, 35, 38
  of sacroiliac joint, 36, 283
  strained, 32-35, 132
  supraspinous, 23, 23, 35
  torn, 35, 161
Ling, Peter, 214
Lipping. See Osteophyte
Lordosis, 17, 18
  hyper——— (sway-back), 35-36, 45-48,
    93, 147, 158, 161, 167, 173, 181-82,
    183, 226, 244, 284, 285
  normal, 173
  "poker" spine, 173
Lougheed, Dr. Jeva, 210
Lucas, Susan, 215
Lumbago, 56

MacHattie, Chris, 259, 260, 283, 285
McIntosh, Dr. Marion, 79-81
McKenzie, Robin, 146-47
  derangement group, 147
  dysfunctional group, 147
  postural group, 146
Magraw, Kristi, 11-12, 213, 215, 216
Mailis, Dr. Angela, 61, 71
Malingerer, 61, 71
Manipulation, 9, 12, 36, 67, 150-51, 191-
  92, 193-94, 196, 199-200, 203-04
  for acute pain, 67, 194, 199, 203

for chronic pain, 194, 195, 199, 200
  of neck, 267
  medical and chiropractic, difference
    between, 133-34, 150-51, 268
  scoliosis, indications as a treatment for,
    262
Marie-Strumpell Disease. See Ankylosing
  spondylitis
Martial arts, 253. See also T'ai Chi
Massage, 11, 51, 70, 143, 148, 150,
  212-16, 286
  shiatsu, 214
  Sutherland-Chan School of, 212
  Swedish, 214
  micro———, 148
Mattresses, 183-84
Mayo Clinic, 103
Melzack, Dr. Ronald, 62-63, 65-67, 143
Meridians, 139, 142, 214
  natural energy flows, 12
Merskey, Dr. Harold, 62
Mesmer, Dr. Franz Anton, 206
Micromassage, 148
Microsurgery. See Surgery
Milburn's Backeaser footrest, 175, 177
Miller, Dr. Rickey, 11, 207, 208, 210
Milwaukee Brace, 259
Minde, Dr. Klaus, 154, 155, 156
Mobilization, 76, 150-51
  how different from manipulation,
    150-51, 268
  of neck, 268
Moe, Dr. John, 259
Morphine, 67-68, 144
Motion (stress) X-rays. See X-rays
Mount Sinai Hospital, 99-103, 105
Murray, Dr. Timothy, 278
Muscle(s), 17, 24, 26, 47-48, 50-51,
  160-61, 212.
  adaptive shortening of, 161
  back, small, 24, 24, 173-74, 179
  erector spinae, 25-26, 25, 171, 179
  gluteus maximus, 28, 97
  hamstring, 162-63
  iliacus, 165
  obliquus externis, 171, 284
  obliquus internis, 26, 170-71, 284
  nerves to, 28, 30
  psoas, 26, 165
  rectus abdominis, 26, 27, 170, 284
  rectus femoris, 165
  relaxants, 80, 84
  scalene, 25, 266, 266
  spasm in, 32-33, 34, 47-48, 50-51, 171,
    179, 205-06, 212, 268, 286
  sternomastoid, 266, 266
  strain, 34, 50-51, 60, 217-18
  transversus abdominis, 26-27, 26, 171,
    284

trapezius, 266, *266*
  weakness of, 34
Myelogram. *See* Diagnostic tests
Myers, Esther, 11, 224-25, 225-26, 227, 228

Nachemson, Dr. Alf, 9, 41, *42*, 175
Naprosyn, 82, 85
Neck, *19*, 43, 180, 264-70, *265*
  exercises for pain in, 269-70
  manipulation of, 267
  mobilization of, 268
  treatment for pain in, 43, 268
Nerve(s), *27*
  brachial plexus, *29*
  branch, *27*, 28, 46-47
  conduction test, 266
  fibre, 62-67
  irritation of root, *41*, 46-48
  L3, 28, 97
  L4, 95-97
  L5, 90, 96-97
  lumbosacral plexus, *29*
  pinched, 38-40, *39*, 41, 46
  root, *27*, 28-29, *29*, 38-43, 46-47, 92-96, 109, 111-12, 114, 135, 143
  sciatic, 28, *29*, 38-43, 46, 120, 124
  S1, 28-29, 92, 95-96
Nerve root. *See* Nerve
Neurological deficit, 92-93, 97, 133
Neurosurgeon, 91, 122-23
Neurotransmitter, 64-65
NINCDS Conference, 191, 204
Nociceptors, 35, 45, 65
Nucleus pulposus, *22*, 30, 36-43, *113*, 114, 125, 133
Numbness, 38, 40

Obus Forme Backrest, 175, *176*
O'Callaghan, Dr. William, 123
Ontario Medical Association, 139
Opiate(s), 67-68, 82, 143
  receptors, 67-68
Organic pain, 60, 70-72
Orthopaedic medicine, 131-37
  Cyriax, Dr. James, 132, 134, 237
  International Society of, 136-37
Orthopaedic physician, 36, 131-37
Orthopaedic surgeon, 51, 77, 91-97, 113-18, 122-23, 136
Osteoarthritis, 33-34, *33*, 48-49, 53, 92
Osteomyelitis, 55
Osteopathy (osteopaths), 201, 202
Osteophyte, 33-34, *33*, 37, 43, 48-50, 90, 92, 114, 120
Osteoporosis, 271-80, *272*
  causes of, 274-76
  prevention of, 279-80
  treatment of, 277-79
Osteoporosis Society of Canada, 280

Ottawa General Hospital, 236-37
Ottewell, Dr. David, 50

Paget, Dr. James, 201
Pain, 30, 38, 59-72, *64. See also*
  Diagnosis of back pain; Posture, contribution to back pain
  acute, 59-60, 149, 159, 199
  back, cost of, 11, 61
  behaviour, 11, 72, 208
  in buttock, 40
  chronic, 60-61, 63, 68-72, 79, 139-40, 146, 152-54, 159, 194, 199, 208, 210, 212, 215, 226, 227-28
  clinics, 61, 69-72
  definition of, 61-62
  from diagnostic tests, 99, 103, 105-10
  discs, role in, 30-34
  drugs for (*see* Drugs)
  exercise when in, 158, 159-60, 171
  facet joints, role in, 30-34, *33*, 45-47, 93
  functional (psychogenic), 60, 70-72, 209
  Gate Control Theory of, 62, 65, 67-68
  in leg (*see* Pain, sciatic)
  ligaments, role in, 30, 35
  muscles, role in, 33, 34
  due to nerve compression, 38-43
  organic, 60, 70-72
  referred, 40, 46-47, 93, 133, 265
  sciatic (sciatica), 38-43, 46, 93-94, 120, 124-27, 138, 142, 160, 162-63, 200
  statistics on, 10, 31, 38, 61, 124-25, 139-41
  from surgery, 111-20
  threshold, 89
  tolerance, 66, 68-72
Pain gate, 63, 65-67
Pain-killers. *See* Drugs, analgesic
Pain receptors, 30, 35, 38, 51, 65
  nociceptors, 35, 45, 65
  mechanoreceptors, 65
  thermoreceptors, 65
Palmer, Daniel David, 201
Papain, 127-28
Papaya fruit, 128-30
Parker, Nancy, 236-37
Pelvic tilt, 45, 158, 165, 167-70, 182
People's Pharmacy, The, 82
Percodan, 79-80, 84
Physicians
  how to deal with, 12-13
  importance of, 13, 145, 194-96
Physiotherapy, 10-12, 51, 70, 76, 91-92, 133-34, 145-51, 157-72
Pia mater, 27-28
Pillows, 185
Pill Book, The, 82
Pills. *See* Drugs
Pinched nerve. *See* Nerve(s)